Pediatric Allergy

Editors

CORINNE A. KEET
PAMELA A. FRISCHMEYER-GUERRERIO
ROBERT A. WOOD

IMMUNOLOGY AND ALLERGY CLINICS OF NORTH AMERICA

www.immunology.theclinics.com

February 2015 • Volume 35 • Number 1

ELSEVIER

1600 John F. Kennedy Boulevard • Suite 1800 • Philadelphia, Pennsylvania, 19103-2899
http://www.theclinics.com

IMMUNOLOGY AND ALLERGY CLINICS OF NORTH AMERICA Volume 35, Number 1
February 2015 ISSN 0889-8561, ISBN-13: 978-0-323-35442-4

Editor: Jessica McCool
Developmental Editor: Stephanie Carter

Immunology and Allergy Clinics of North America (ISSN 0889–8561) is published quarterly by Elsevier Inc., 360 Park Avenue South, New York, NY 10010-1710. Months of issue are February, May, August, and November. Periodicals postage paid at New York, NY and additional mailing offices. Subscription prices are $320.00 per year for US individuals, $454.00 per year for US institutions, $150.00 per year for US students and residents, $395.00 per year for Canadian individuals, $220.00 per year for Canadian students, $577.00 per year for Canadian institutions, $445.00 per year for international individuals, $577.00 per year for international institutions, $220.00 per year for international students. To receive student/resident rate, orders must be accompanied by name of affiliated institution, date of term, and the *signature* of program/residency coordinator on institution letterhead. Orders will be billed at individual rate until proof of status is received. Foreign air speed delivery is included in all *Clinics* subscription prices. All prices are subject to change without notice. **POSTMASTER**: Send address changes to *Immunology and Allergy Clinics of North America*, Elsevier Health Sciences Division, Subscription Customer Service, 3251 Riverport Lane, Maryland Heights, MO 63043. **Customer Service: 1-800-654-2452 (U.S. and Canada); 314-447-8871 (outside U.S. and Canada). Fax: 314-447-8029. E-mail: journalscustomerservice-usa@elsevier.com (for print support); journalsonlinesupport-usa@elsevier.com (for online support).**

Reprints. For copies of 100 or more, of articles in this publication, please contact the Commercial Reprints Department, Elsevier Inc., 360 Park Avenue South, New York, New York 10010-1710. Tel. 212-633-3874, Fax: 212-633-3820, E-mail: reprints@elsevier.com.

Immunology and Allergy Clinics of North America is covered in MEDLINE/PubMed (Index Medicus), Current Contents/Life Sciences, Science Citation Index, ISI/BIOMED, Chemical Abstracts, and EMBASE/Excerpta Medica.

Contributors

EDITORS

CORINNE A. KEET, MD, PhD
Assistant Professor of Pediatrics, Pediatric Allergy and Immunology, Johns Hopkins School of Medicine, Baltimore, Maryland

PAMELA A. FRISCHMEYER-GUERRERIO, MD, PhD
Chief, Food Allergy Research Unit, Laboratory of Allergic Diseases, National Institute of Allergy and Infectious Diseases (NIAID), Bethesda, Maryland

ROBERT A. WOOD, MD
Professor of Pediatrics and International Health, Chief of Pediatric Allergy and Immunology, Pediatric Allergy and Immunology, Johns Hopkins School of Medicine, Baltimore, Maryland

AUTHORS

SEEMA S. ACEVES, MD, PhD
Associate Professor, Department of Pediatrics and Medicine, Division of Allergy and Immunology, Center for Infection, Inflammation, and Immunology, La Jolla, California

STEPHANIE ALBIN, MD
Clinical Fellow, Division of Allergy and Immunology, Department of Pediatrics, Icahn School of Medicine at Mount Sinai, New York, New York

KATHLEEN C. BARNES, PhD
Professor, Department of Medicine, The Johns Hopkins Asthma and Allergy Center, Baltimore, Maryland

PETER J. GERGEN, MD, MPH
Medical Officer, Allergy, Asthma, Airway Biology Branch (AAABB), Rockville, Maryland

MICHELLE A. GILL, MD, PhD
Associate Professor, Departments of Pediatrics and Immunology, Divisions of Pediatric Infectious Diseases and Pulmonary Vascular Biology, UT Southwestern Medical Center, Dallas, Texas

MICHELLE FOX HUFFAKER, MD
Clinical Instructor in Medicine, Division of Medicine, Brigham and Women's Hospital, Harvard Medical School, Boston, Massachusetts

CHRISTINA B. JOHNS, BA
Division of Rheumatology, Immunology, and Allergy, Brigham and Women's Hospital, Boston, Massachusetts

CHRISTINE COLE JOHNSON, PhD
Department of Public Health Sciences, Henry Ford Hospital, Detroit, Michigan

JACOB D. KATTAN, MD
Assistant Professor of Pediatric Allergy and Immunology, Jaffe Food Allergy Institute, Icahn School of Medicine at Mount Sinai, New York, New York

JOHN M. KELSO, MD
Division of Allergy, Asthma, and Immunology, Scripps Clinic, San Diego, California

STEPHEN F. KEMP, MD
Professor of Medicine and Pediatrics, Division of Clinical Immunology and Allergy, Department of Medicine, The University of Mississippi Medical Center, Jackson, Mississippi

JONATHAN J. LYONS, MD
Assistant Clinical Investigator, Genetics and Pathophysiology of Allergy Section, Laboratory of Allergic Diseases, National Institute of Allergy and Infectious Diseases, National Institutes of Health, Bethesda, Maryland

JOSHUA D. MILNER, MD
Chief, Genetics and Pathophysiology of Allergy Section, Laboratory of Allergic Diseases, National Institute of Allergy and Infectious Diseases, National Institutes of Health, Bethesda, Maryland

ANNA NOWAK-WĘGRZYN, MD
Associate Professor of Pediatrics, Division of Allergy and Immunology, Department of Pediatrics, Kravis Children's Hospital, Jaffe Food Allergy Institute, Icahn School of Medicine at Mount Sinai, New York, New York

ROMINA A. ORTIZ, MS
Department of Medicine, The Johns Hopkins Asthma and Allergy Center, Baltimore, Maryland

WANDA PHIPATANAKUL, MD, MS
Associate Professor of Pediatrics, Division of Immunology, Boston Children's Hospital, Harvard Medical School, Boston, Massachusetts

REGINA K. ROWE, MD, PhD
Pediatric Infectious Diseases Fellowship Program, Department of Pediatrics, UT Southwestern Medical Center, Dallas, Texas

JESSICA SAVAGE, MD, MHS
Instructor of Medicine, Division of Rheumatology, Immunology, and Allergy, Brigham and Women's Hospital, Harvard Medical School, Boston, Massachusetts

HEMANT P. SHARMA, MD, MHS
Acting Chief, Division of Allergy and Immunology, Children's National Medical Center, Children's National Health System; Assistant Professor of Pediatrics, George Washington University School of Medicine, Washington, DC

SCOTT H. SICHERER, MD
Elliot and Roslyn Jaffe Professor of Pediatric Allergy and Immunology, Jaffe Food Allergy Institute, Icahn School of Medicine at Mount Sinai, New York, New York

KELLY D. STONE, MD, PhD
Deputy Chief, Genetics and Pathophysiology of Allergy Section, Laboratory of Allergic Diseases, National Institute of Allergy and Infectious Diseases, National Institutes of Health, Bethesda, Maryland

CHET A. THARPE, MD
Fellow, Allergy and Immunology, The University of Mississippi Medical Center, Jackson, Mississippi

ALKIS TOGIAS, MD
Branch Chief, Allergy, Asthma, Airway Biology Branch (AAABB), Rockville, Maryland

GANESA WEGIENKA, PhD
Department of Public Health Sciences, Henry Ford Hospital, Detroit, Michigan

KELLI W. WILLIAMS, MD, MPH
Allergy and Immunology Clinical Fellow, Laboratory of Clinical Infectious Diseases, National Institute of Allergy and Infectious Diseases, National Institutes of Health, Bethesda, Maryland

EDWARD ZORATTI, MD
Division of Allergy and Immunology, Department of Internal Medicine, Henry Ford Hospital, Detroit, Michigan

BRET A. THARPE, MD
Fellow, Allergy and Immunology, The University of Mississippi Medical Center, Jackson, Mississippi

ALKIS TOGIAS, MD
Branch Chief, Allergy, Asthma, Airway Biology Branch (AAABB), Rockville, Maryland

GANESA WEGIENKA, PhD
Department of Public Health Sciences, Henry Ford Hospital, Detroit, Michigan

KELLI W. WILLIAMS, MD, MPH
Allergy and Immunology Clinical Fellow, Laboratory of Clinical Infectious Diseases, National Institute of Allergy and Infectious Diseases, National Institutes of Health, Bethesda, Maryland

EDWARD ZORATTI, MD
Division of Allergy and Immunology, Department of Internal Medicine, Henry Ford Hospital, Detroit, Michigan

Contents

> A consensus has been reached that the development of allergic disorders is strongly influenced by early-life exposures. An overview of several prenatal and early-life factors that have been investigated for their associations with development of childhood allergy is presented. Delivery mode, the gut microbiome, vitamin D, folate, breastfeeding, pets, antibiotics, environmental tobacco smoke, and airborne traffic pollutants are also discussed. Although many studies suggest an effect, no risk factors clearly increase or reduce the risk of allergic outcomes.

> Genome-wide association studies (GWAS) have been employed in the field of allergic disease, and significant associations have been published for nearly 100 asthma genes/loci. An outcome of GWAS in allergic disease has been the formation of national and international collaborations leading to consortia meta-analyses and an appreciation for the specificity of genetic associations to sub-phenotypes of allergic disease. Molecular genetics has undergone a technological revolution, leading to next-generation sequencing strategies that are increasingly employed to hone in on the causal variants associated with allergic diseases. Unmet needs include the inclusion of diverse cohorts and strategies for managing big data.

> The prevalence of food allergy is rising for unclear reasons, with prevalence estimates in the developed world approaching 10%. Knowledge regarding the natural course of food allergies is important because it can aid the clinician in diagnosing food allergies and in determining when to consider evaluation for food allergy resolution. Many food allergies with onset in early childhood are outgrown later in childhood, although a minority of food allergy persists into adolescence and even adulthood. More research is needed to improve food allergy diagnosis, treatment, and prevention.

> Accurately diagnosing a patient with a possible food allergy is important to avoid unnecessary dietary restrictions and prevent life-threatening

reactions. Routine testing modalities have limited accuracy, and an oral food challenge is often required to make a definitive diagnosis. Given that they are labor intensive and risk inducing an allergic reaction, several alternative diagnostic modalities have been investigated. Testing for IgE antibodies to particular protein components in foods has shown promise to improve diagnostics and has entered clinical practice. Additional modalities show potential, including epitope binding, T-cell studies, and basophil activation.

This article presents an overview of potential treatments of food allergy, with an emphasis on various forms of immunotherapy (including oral immunotherapy, sublingual immunotherapy, epicutaneous immuno-therapy, immunotherapy with modified food antigens, and immunotherapy with a recombinant peanut vaccine). Allergen nonspecific treatments, such as Chinese herbal formulas, probiotics/prebiotics, helminths, monoclonal antibodies, and toll-like receptor agonists, are also summarized.

The inner city has long been recognized as an area of high asthma morbidity and mortality. A wide range of factors interact to create this envi-ronment. These factors include well-recognized asthma risk factors that are not specific to the inner city, the structure and delivery of health care, the location and function of the urban environment, and social ineq-uities. In this article, these facets are reviewed, and successful and unsuc-cessful interventions are discussed, to understand what is needed to solve this problem.

Respiratory viruses and allergens synergistically contribute to disease pathogenesis in asthma. Potential mechanisms underlying this clinically relevant association are the subject of intense investigation. This review summarizes current knowledge and recent advances in this area, with an emphasis on potential mechanisms involving immunoglobulin E, type I interferon antiviral responses, epithelial factors, and the role of dendritic cells and other antigen-presenting cells in linking viral and allergic inflam-matory responses relevant to asthmatic disease.

Over the past several decades, the evidence supporting rational pediatric asthma management has grown considerably. As more is learned about the various phenotypes of asthma, the complexity of management will continue to grow. This article focuses on the evidence supporting the current guidelines-based pediatric asthma management and explores the future of asthma management with respect to phenotypic heterogeneity and biologics.

Eosinophilic esophagitis (EoE) is a clinicopathologic disease of increasing prevalence. Because EoE is a chronic disease, its prevalence will continue to increase. Antigen triggers, including food and aeroallergens, drive eosinophilic and T helper cell type 2 inflammation, resulting in subepithelial fibrosis; this esophageal remodeling is the likely underlying pathogenesis for complications of narrowing, rigidity, and food impactions. Management includes dietary antigen elimination and topical corticosteroids. Long-term therapy and repeated endoscopy are often needed; consideration must be given to maintenance regimens and side effects. This review describes the clinical features, treatment options, epidemiology, and pathogenesis of EoE.

Atopic dermatitis (AD) is a chronic, relapsing, highly pruritic skin condition resulting from disruption of the epithelial barrier and associated immune dysregulation in the skin of genetically predisposed hosts. AD generally develops in early childhood, has a characteristic age-dependent distribution, and is commonly associated with elevated IgE, peripheral eosinophilia, and other allergic diseases. Medications such as antihistamines have demonstrated poor efficacy in controlling AD-associated itch. Education of patients regarding the primary underlying defects and provision of a comprehensive skin care plan is essential for disease maintenance and management of flares.

Allergic rhinitis is a common pediatric problem with significant comorbidities and potential complications. This article is an overview of the epidemiology, pathophysiology, and current therapeutic strategies. Allergic rhinitis management in a specific child is age dependent and influenced by the severity and frequency of the symptoms and the presence of any concurrent conditions. Current strategies permit symptomatic control and improved quality of life for most patients.

Anaphylaxis and urticaria are common presenting allergic complaints. Affecting up to 2% of the population, anaphylaxis is a serious, life-threatening allergic reaction. Although not life-threatening, urticaria is a rash of transient, erythematous, pruritic wheals that can be bothersome and affects up to 25% of the population. All cases of anaphylaxis warrant thorough clinical evaluation by the allergist-immunologist, although most cases of urticaria are self-limited and do not require specialist referral. This article offers an overview of our current knowledge on the epidemiology, pathogenesis, triggers, diagnosis, and treatment of anaphylaxis and urticaria.

Most children with a history of penicillin allergy are labeled allergic and denied treatment with penicillin and sometimes other beta-lactam antibiotics. Most of these children never were or are no longer allergic to penicillin. Penicillin skin testing and oral challenge can identify patients who are not currently allergic, allowing them to be treated with penicillin. Children with egg allergy are often denied influenza vaccination because the vaccine contains a small amount of egg protein. However, recent studies have demonstrated that children with even severe egg allergy can safely receive the vaccine, reducing their risk of the morbidity and mortality associated with influenza.

IMMUNOLOGY AND ALLERGY CLINICS OF NORTH AMERICA

ISSUE OF RELATED INTEREST

Emergency Medicine Clinics, August 2013 (Vol. 31, Issue 3)
Pediatric Emergency Medicine
Le N. Lu, Dale Woolridge, and Ann M. Dietrich, *Editors*
http://www.emed.theclinics.com/

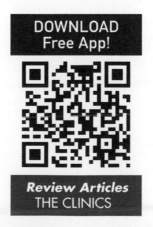

Preface
Pediatric Allergy

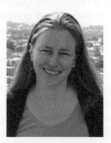
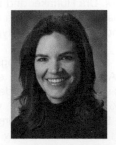
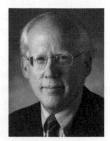

Corinne A. Keet, MD, PhD	Pamela A. Frischmeyer-Guerrerio, MD, PhD *Editors*	Robert A. Wood, MD

Allergic diseases are the most common chronic diseases of childhood, affecting at least one-fourth of US children. In recent years, we have seen great advances in the diagnosis and treatment of these conditions. However, despite major improvements in our understanding of the factors that may contribute to the development of allergic diseases, improved treatments are needed for many conditions, and prevention remains an elusive goal.

In this issue of *Immunology and Allergy Clinics of North America*, our goal is to provide updated reviews on key areas of pediatric allergy by authors who are true experts in the field, many of whom have generated some of the most interesting recent findings in their respective areas. Drs Wegienka, Zoratti, and Johnson start by reviewing the role of the environment in the development of allergic diseases, discussing controversies related to how the microbiome, diet, and other exposures may contribute to—or potentially prevent—the initiation of an allergic phenotype. Ms Ortiz and Dr Barnes then review what we have learned from genome-wide association studies of asthma and other allergic diseases and discuss how newer techniques, including sequencing and other "omics" methods, may help advance our understanding of these diseases.

Food allergy is a topic of increasing clinical importance that has also seen tremendous growth from a research perspective in the past decade. Because of the central role food allergy now plays in the world of pediatric allergy, we devote three articles to advances in this area. Ms Johns and Dr Savage review the epidemiology of food allergy; Drs Kattan and Sicherer review the diagnosis of food allergy, and Drs Albin and Nowak-Węgrzyn present a state-of-the-art review of potential treatment approaches. This trio of reviews highlights both how much we have learned and how far we have to go to optimally care for food allergic patients.

Pediatric asthma remains the third leading cause of hospitalization among children and particularly affects children living in the inner city. Drs Gergen and Togias review what is known about this major health disparity. Although both allergens and

Immunol Allergy Clin N Am 35 (2015) xiii–xiv
http://dx.doi.org/10.1016/j.iac.2014.09.015
immunology.theclinics.com

respiratory viruses have long been associated with the development of asthma, how they interact to promote asthma is only now being elucidated, as discussed by Drs Rowe and Gill. In 2007, the National Heart, Lung, and Blood Institute/National Asthma Education and Prevention Program updated guidelines for asthma management, with an emphasis on asthma control. Drs Huffaker and Phipatanakul review these guidelines, discuss the potential role of biologics in the treatment of asthma, and outline how advances in the understanding of asthma subtypes may change the management of asthma.

Eosinophilic esophagitis is a clinically challenging disease that appears to be increasing in prevalence. Dr Aceves reviews the epidemiology, pathogenesis, and management of this emerging syndrome. Atopic dermatitis is an extremely common condition, affecting up to 20% of young children, with significant effects on quality of life. Drs Lyons, Milner, and Stone review exciting advances in our understanding of the pathophysiology of this condition and how these advances can be used to improve therapy. Finally, Drs Tharpe and Kemp provide a superb review of allergic rhinitis; Drs Willams and Sharma summarize the diagnosis and management of urticaria and anaphylaxis, and Dr Kelso provides an approach to drug and vaccine allergy that will be of value to all clinicians.

Corinne A. Keet, MD, PhD
Pediatric Allergy and Immunology
Johns Hopkins School of Medicine
CMSC 1102
600 N. Wolfe St.
Baltimore, MD 21202, USA

Pamela A. Frischmeyer-Guerrerio, MD, PhD
Food Allergy Research Unit
Laboratory of Allergic Diseases
National Institute of Allergy and Infectious Diseases (NIAID)
4 Memorial Drive
Building 4, Room 228B
MSC0425
Bethesda, MD 20892, USA

Robert A. Wood, MD
Pediatric Allergy and Immunology
Johns Hopkins School of Medicine
CMSC 1102
600 N. Wolfe St.
Baltimore, MD 21202, USA

E-mail addresses:
ckeet1@jhmi.edu (C.A. Keet)
rwood@jhmi.edu (P.A. Frischmeyer-Guerrerio)
pfrisch1@jhmi.edu (R.A. Wood)

The Role of the Early-Life Environment in the Development of Allergic Disease

CrossMark

Ganesa Wegienka, PhD[a],*, Edward Zoratti, MD[b],
Christine Cole Johnson, PhD[a]

KEYWORDS

• Asthma • Allergy • IgE • Prenatal • Eczema • Atopic dermatitis

KEY POINTS

• Brief summaries of several prenatal and early-life risk factors that have been analyzed for potential associations with the development of childhood allergy are presented.

• The results and conclusions from individual studies of a single risk factor are often conflicting and may be caused by considerable variability in the specific allergy-related outcomes evaluated as well as the methods used to measure an individual's exposure to the risk factor.

• Teams of scientists with diverse expertise are needed to work together to have the greatest impact on understanding risk factors for allergic diseases.

INTRODUCTION

The developmental origins of health and disease hypothesis suggests that a child's environment from conception to 1000 days greatly influences the child's risk for chronic disease. Although it is not well tested in association with immunologic diseases such as allergies and asthma, it is believed that this hypothesis is applicable to allergic diseases, and recent studies have focused on early-life risk factors and the development of allergic diseases later in life.[1-3] In this review, studies of prenatal and early postpartum exposures and the subsequent development of allergy-related outcomes are summarized, with a focus on delivery mode, the gut microbiome, nutritional factors, and exposure to animals, medications, and airborne pollutants. Further, these early-life factors are reviewed in the context of disease incidence rather than disease exacerbation or management.

Disclosures: The authors receive research support from the National Institutes of Health (NIH) grants HL113010 and AI089473.
[a] Department of Public Health Sciences, Henry Ford Hospital, Detroit, MI, USA; [b] Division of Allergy and Immunology, Department of Internal Medicine, Henry Ford Hospital, Detroit, MI, USA
* Corresponding author. 1 Ford Place, 3E, Detroit, MI 48202.
E-mail address: gwegien1@hfhs.org

DELIVERY MODE

Birth by cesarean section may increase the risk of allergic disease. The mechanism is not known, but recent research suggests that lack of exposure to beneficial microbes present in the birth canal may affect the colonization of the child's gut microbiome and subsequent immune development.

Comparisons of studies correlating delivery mode and allergy are affected by variability in both type of allergy assessed and outcome definitions (ie, clinical evaluation vs parental report). For eczema, most studies have shown no association between mode of delivery and diagnosis. No association between delivery mode and eczema diagnostic codes was found in the West Midlands General Practice Research Database (n = 24,690)[4] or a Kaiser Permanente Northwestern birth registry cohort (n = 7872).[5] In a Japanese birth cohort,[6] no association was found between delivery mode and maternal report of physician-diagnosed eczema (n = 213). A meta-analysis conducted in 2008 resulted in a similar conclusion,[7] as did the subsequent Finnish SKARP study (n = 4799).[8] However, in the recent Netherlands KOALA study, children born via cesarean section were more likely to have parental-reported eczema.[9]

Stronger associations have been found between mode of delivery and allergic sensitization or food allergy. No association between delivery mode and skin prick test results at age 7 years was found in the English ALSPAC (Avon Longitudinal Study of Parents and Children) cohort.[10] A meta-analysis concluded that children born by cesarean section were more likely to have food allergy/sensitization but not inhalant sensitivity.[7] Similar associations with food allergy were reported in a systematic review[11] and in the KOALA birth cohort.[9] Among offspring of nonallergic parents in the Dutch PIAMA (Prevention and Incidence of Asthma and Mite Allergy) study (n = 2917), children born via cesarean section were more likely to have positive allergen-specific IgE testing.[12] Among Boston children, cesarean section was associated with positive skin prick tests or allergen-specific IgE at age 9 years,[13] as it was among 8-year-old children whose parents were allergic in the Republic of Cyprus.[14]

A meta-analysis concluded that cesarean section is associated with increased asthma risk,[7] although such an association was seen only among girls in the Kaiser Permanente study[5] and restricted to children born by emergency cesarean section in a registry report from Sweden.[15] In contrast, the West Midlands General Practice Research Database report found no association.[4] Several studies using questionnaire data have reported associations between cesarean section and increased asthma frequency,[12,14] whereas others failed to confirm this finding.[8,10] Questionnaire data may not provide sufficient specificity for defining asthma as an outcome; hence, the emergence of conflicting results.

MICROBIOME

Intensive interest in the influence of the human microbiome, in particular the gut microbiome, on the developing immune system and allergy has been ignited with the recent development of culture-independent tools to more comprehensively measure bacterial community composition.[16,17] However, even before these technologies, investigators[18,19] postulated that mechanisms underlying the hygiene hypothesis were linked to alterations in patterns of normal infant intestinal microbial colonization. Small studies[20] using culture-dependent methods indicated differences in the prevalence of intestinal microorganisms between atopic and nonatopic infants, although subsequent studies[21] did not find confirmed differences linked to food sensitization or atopic eczema using culture-dependent assessments. In 2001, Kalliomaki and colleagues[22] assessed fecal samples from a small birth cohort (n = 76), using both culture-dependent and culture-independent bacterial measures. The study reported that culture-independent approaches detected fecal microbial differences that distinguished children who developed allergic sensitization. Murray and colleagues[23] used a similar approach in a case-control study of 33 pairs of children and found that the ratio of bifidobacteria to total fecal bacteria was lower in children with eczema at age 4 years.

The KOALA birth cohort was the first to study selected fecal bacteria phylogroups (n = 5) in a large group of infants (n = 1032) using quantitative real-time polymerase chain reaction. Microbial colonization patterns were associated with several proposed risk factors linked to allergy development, such as mode of delivery, breastfeeding, antibiotic use, and birth order.[24] Another European group reported distinct fecal bacterial composition patterns among populations of children with varied prevalences of allergy.[25] Penders and colleagues[26] later related fecal bacteria in the KOALA study to atopic outcomes at age 2 years and found that both increased Escherichia coli and Clostridium difficile levels were associated with eczema, whereas only C difficile was associated with recurrent wheeze and allergic sensitization. A 2007 review[27] of 17 studies stressed the importance of considering the techniques used to measure the presence of bacteria as well as the timing of measurement.

Other recently reported birth cohort studies[9,28–31] have addressed the relationship of the intestinal microbiome and allergic outcomes, with most suggesting associations. Investigators can now take advantage of advances in 16S ribosomal RNA gene deep sequencing and array technologies, which allow comprehensive detection of microbial communities on a large scale.[32,33] For instance, in a group of 40 Swedish infants,[34] low fecal microbial diversity measured with 16S ribosomal DNA 454-pyrosequencing was associated with atopic eczema. Studies of the infant gut microbiome and atopic outcomes need to appropriately consider other factors, many mentioned in this review, such as mode of delivery, diet and breastfeeding patterns, antibiotic use, and other environmental factors that may affect the maternal and infant gut microbiome (eg, animals, daycare, vitamin D). For example, data from infants in the Canadian CHILD study and the Detroit area WHEALS birth cohort, using these new high-throughput, culture-independent technologies, suggest that pets are associated with distinct infant gut and environmental microbiome signatures, respectively.[35,36]

VITAMIN D

Interest in the role of vitamin D in allergic disease has increased tremendously in recent years, particularly because vitamin D supplementation is perceived as low risk and noninvasive. Overall, the evidence that vitamin D modifies the incidence of allergy-related outcomes is mixed. Studies including a direct measure of vitamin D (25-hydroxyvitamin D [25(OH)D] or 25[OH]D_2 or 25[OH]D_3) that clearly precede childhood allergy are reviewed later. We have excluded studies using food frequency questionnaires, because they approximate dietary vitamin D intake rather than reflect bioavailable levels, which are also influenced by sun exposure, supplement intake, genetic variation in vitamin D metabolism, and variable dietary absorption. Further, early vitamin D levels beyond the prenatal period have not been well studied, so discussion is limited to reports measuring either prenatal maternal or cord blood vitamin D.

Although considered a treatment of atopic dermatitis (AD),[37] there is limited evidence detailing the relationship between early-life vitamin D levels and childhood AD risk. In a birth cohort of 440 English infants (age 9 months), children whose mothers had the highest quartiles of 25(OH)D during pregnancy had an increased risk of AD.[38]

However, there was no association between prenatal 25(OH)D levels and eczema (assessed by questionnaire) among 7-year-old to 8-year-old children in the ALSPAC birth cohort.[39] Considering cord blood, 25(OH)D$_3$ was weakly inversely associated with eczema (by clinical examination or parental report of doctor diagnosis) at 1 year of age in an Australian cohort (n = 231) with at least 1 allergic parent.[40] Cord blood 25(OH)D levels were also inversely associated with AD (assessed by questionnaire) by age 5 years in children in the EDEN birth cohort (n = 239).[41] These conflicting results could be caused by the use of outcomes based on questionnaire versus clinical examination. Also, correlations between prenatal and cord blood vitamin D levels are variable, which could account for some inconsistencies.

Prenatal 25(OH)D levels were not associated with childhood skin prick test results in either the ALSPAC cohort[39] or the Southampton Women's Survey (n = 860).[42] Associations were not found between cord blood 25(OH)D$_3$ and skin prick tests in the Perth cohort[40] or cord blood 25(OH)D and allergic rhinitis in the EDEN cohort.[41]

However, Weisse and colleagues[43] reported that higher prenatal and cord blood 25(OH)D$_3$ were associated with increased risk of food allergy (report of doctor diagnosis) at age 2 years in the German LINA cohort (n = 272), and in the Tucson Infant Immune Study, high cord blood 25(OH)D levels were associated with increased rates of having a positive skin prick test, whereas both high and low 25(OH)D levels were associated with higher levels of total IgE.[44]

In contrast, a study in Southampton, UK,[38] although limited by loss to follow-up, found that higher 25(OH)D levels in late pregnancy were associated with increased frequency of asthma at age 9 years. No association was found between prenatal 25(OH)D level and lung function in the ALSPAC cohort[39] or with childhood asthma in the Southampton Women's Study.[42] Cord blood 25(OH)D was not associated with asthma at age 5 years in the EDEN study[41] or New Zealand Allergy and Asthma cohort (n = 922).[45]

FOLATE

The evidence that folate or its synthetic form (folic acid) is associated with risk of allergy is decidedly mixed. Study of this relationship is complicated, because in parallel with the allergy epidemic, folic acid has been added to numerous foods and recommended for pregnant women to prevent birth defects.[46] In the KOALA birth cohort (n = 837), prenatal erythrocyte folic acid levels were not associated with AD at 2-year examination.[47] However, in children carrying a mutation in the methylenetetra-hydrofolate reductase gene, cord blood folate was associated with a report of physician-diagnosed eczema at ages 4 and 6 years in the Generation R birth cohort in the Netherlands.[48] No association was reported between prenatal or cord folate levels with doctor diagnosis or observation of eczema in an Australian birth cohort (n = 484)[49]; however, higher folate supplement ingestion during the third trimester led to higher risk of eczema by age 1 year. Folic acid–only supplements and prenatal supplements with folic acid, multivitamin supplements, or vitamin D complex were not associated with parental-reported eczema in children up to age 8 years in the PIAMA study.[50] Interpretation is further complicated by the heavy reliance on parental report of AD versus study-specific validated reports or clinical evaluations.

Prenatal intracellular folic acid was not associated with total IgE or sensitization in the KOALA birth cohort.[47] Cord blood folate between 50 and 70 nmol/L was associated with lower risk of positive skin test results at 1 year compared with higher or lower levels in a birth cohort from Western Australia (n = 484),[49] but no association with prenatal folate was evident. Sensitization (surface IgE [sIgE] $\geq$0.70 IU/mL) at age 8 years was not associated with prenatal folic acid supplements in the PIAMA birth cohort.[50] However, higher folate levels up to age 8 years were associated with sensitization (including to foods), in the Wisconsin COAST cohort.[51]

A recent meta-analysis reported a lack of association between maternal folic acid supplementation and risk of asthma in their children.[52] Neither cord blood folate nor prenatal folic acid supplements were associated with recurrent wheeze at age 1 year in Western Australia (n = 484).[49] Maternal folic acid supplementation was associated with wheeze at age 1 year, but not at other time points up to 8 years, or with asthma symptoms at any age in the PIAMA cohort (n = 3786).[50] Cord blood folate was not associated with diagnosed asthma, wheeze, exhaled nitric oxide, or lung function at age 6 years in the Generation R birth cohort (n = 2001).[48] Prenatal intracellular folic acid levels were inversely associated with asthma at age 6 to 7 years in the KOALA birth cohort.[47] Child folate levels were not associated with wheeze in the COAST cohort.[51]

BREASTFEEDING

The American Academy of Pediatrics recommends breastfeeding for at least a year, with exclusive breastfeeding in the first 6 months (with vitamin D supplementation).[53] Although widely investigated regarding a role in allergy prevention, a consensus on breastfeeding remains elusive. Many publications have analyzed different breastfeeding characteristics, including duration of breastfeeding, maternal diet during lactation,[54] or age at complementary food introduction.[55–57] Further complicating study interpretation are the facts that breast milk varies in composition,[58–60] and some women alter their diet while breastfeeding, based on varying recommendations. Among the proposed mechanisms by which breastfeeding might protect from or promote allergy are alteration of the infant's gut microbiome and immune development.[61,62] Breastfeeding may also alter a child's risk of respiratory infections through maternal antibody transfer[61] or affect intake of nutrients, such as vitamin D, during infancy. Recent publications on breastfeeding provide mixed results for commonly investigated allergic outcomes: AD,[56–61,63–65] sensitization/sIgE,[59,61,66–68] and asthma.[56–58,61,68–73]

PETS

Numerous studies have reported that prenatal or early-life exposures to mammals, including pets and livestock, are inversely associated with pediatric allergy. Protective associations have been reported for total IgE, atopic sensitization, and clinical disorders such as AD, allergic rhinitis, and asthma. Most reports on livestock exposure have been based in the Alpine areas of Europe, whereas domestic pet studies have been conducted worldwide. The theory that animal exposure is protective for allergy has been linked to the hygiene hypothesis, with the concept that environments with animals are less hygienic, although studies have not identified which specific animal exposure characteristics might afford protection. Hypotheses implicate high levels of allergen exposure, animal transport of outdoor substances into the home, increased physical activity associated with animal ownership, or even decreased stress levels. Recently, attention has focused on the impact that an animal may have on a child's microbial environment or the microbial population inhabiting the child's gastrointestinal tract, skin, and respiratory tract. Thus, the hygiene hypothesis has evolved into the microbiome hypothesis, or perhaps, better, the microbiome dysbiosis hypothesis.[16] Studies initially were limited to analyzing culturable bacteria,[74] but the Human Microbiome Project and sequencing technology have expanded knowledge and assessment of entire microbial populations consisting of thousands of taxa in samples ranging from environmental residential dust to human stool, skin, and airway samples.

Several reviews and meta-analyses have summarized early-life cat and dog exposure as risk factors for allergic conditions.[75–79] Results have been less consistent for cats than dogs.[76] Dog exposure has been associated with less risk for allergy, especially allergic sensitization.[75–77] A study from the Cincinnati CCAAPS cohort[80] found that infants with dogs were less likely to have an eczema diagnosis at age 1 year (odds ratio [OR] = 0.62, 95% confidence interval (CI) 0.40–0.97) and at age 4 years. Two meta-analyses also suggested inverse relationships between early dog (but not cat) exposure and eczema.[79,81] In the European PASTURE/EFRAIM cohort,[82] prenatal exposure to more farm animals, cats, or dogs was associated with significant or borderline significant decreased ORs for AD by age 2 years. A large Australian study of 5276 infants[83] found that first year exposure to dogs was associated with less egg allergy (OR = 0.72, 95% CI 0.52–0.99), with a similar but nonsignificant risk estimate for cat exposure. The Detroit area Childhood Allergy Study[75] found that early exposure to 2 or more cats or dogs was associated with a lower prevalence of sensitization to all inhalant allergens at age 6 years. A protective effect of pets on asthma has been less evident.

The timing of exposure to pets seems critical, with prenatal or infancy exposure more consistently inversely associated and later exposure sometimes positively associated with allergic outcomes. A recent meta-analysis of 11 European birth cohorts did not find associations between cat exposure and current asthma, allergic asthma, allergic rhinitis, or allergic sensitization in midchildhood.[78] However, dogs were inversely associated with allergic sensitization (OR = 0.65, 95% CI 0.45–0.95), with borderline significant findings for allergic rhinitis (OR = 0.77, 95% CI 0.55–1.07) and current asthma (OR = 0.77, 95% CI 0.58–1.03).

Inconsistent results may relate to differences in study populations with respect to genetic factors, the prevalence of local pet keeping, and unmeasured risk factors associated with pet exposure.[84,85] Therefore, although not settled, there is no consistent evidence that early pet exposure increases the risk for allergic disorders, and some evidence of a protective effect. In recent years, many think that both pet and livestock exposure reflects a complex causal pathway, in which they contribute to normal immune development through their impact on the infant's environmental and human microbiome.[74]

MEDICATIONS

Antibiotic use in the first years of life as a risk factor for allergic disorders is an attractive hypothesis. Use of antibiotics has increased in parallel with the increasing prevalence of allergic conditions, and the 2 can be linked through potential plausible mechanisms. One such mechanism is decreased duration or number of bacterial infections and consequent effects on the immune system; a second is downstream effects on the immune system caused by gastrointestinal dysbiosis resulting from antibiotic use. Numerous studies have addressed this hypothesis with respect to asthma. A recent exquisitely detailed review identified 45 studies up to 2012 that focused on early childhood antibiotics and pediatric asthma.[86] Several meta-analyses and reviews have addressed this topic.[86–90] These reviews all reach similar conclusions: that studies associating early antibiotic use and asthma are typically fraught with biases. A particular challenge is to disentangle early respiratory infections as risk factors or early markers of asthma versus their role as the most common indication for antibiotic use during infancy. Studies that attempt to account for this complicated pathway generally show little or no associations. A large 2011 cross-sectional study[91] distinguished between 3 common asthma phenotypes; transient wheezing, early onset wheezing/asthma, and late onset wheezing/asthma at age 6 to 7 years, but not allergic versus nonallergic disease. This study reported associations between antibiotics and disease younger than age 2 years that were strong but dissipated to a weak, albeit statistically significant, association with disease onset at later time points. These investigators cautioned against the conclusion of a potential causal association. In contrast, a 2014 finding[92] from 62,576 children in a nationwide health insurance plan yielded remarkably similar findings, and the investigators recommended heightened caution regarding unnecessary use of antibiotics in infants. Acetaminophen (paracetamol) use during pregnancy and infancy has also been under investigation as a risk factor for childhood asthma, with parallel results and methodological concerns, because respiratory infections are also linked to acetaminophen use.[86]

Fewer studies have addressed antibiotic use and the outcomes of AD or sensitization in which reverse causation may be of less concern. Jordan and colleagues[93] identified 12 publications focused on antibiotic use during pregnancy and childhood eczema and summarized the results as equivocal. Results from the KOALA birth cohort followed to age 2 years[88,94,95] did not indicate associations of eczema or atopic sensitization with antibiotic use, which they reported as being consistent with other cohort studies. A Belgian birth cohort followed to age 4 years[96] reported that prenatal exposure to antibiotics was associated with AD but not sensitization, but no association of postnatal antibiotic exposure to either outcome was apparent. Even fewer studies address early antibiotic exposure and allergic rhinitis. An early Boston cohort analysis[94] found no evidence of an association, and a 2008 study from a high-risk Australian birth cohort[97] deploying propensity score analyses was also consistent with no associations for allergic rhinitis (or any other allergic outcome).

AIRBORNE EXPOSURES: TOBACCO SMOKE AND TRAFFIC-RELATED AIRBORNE POLLUTION

It is well established that many airborne irritants and pollutants trigger wheezing and exacerbations of asthma as well as upper respiratory tract symptoms. However, the specific impact of early-life pollutant exposure on the development of childhood atopy is less clear. Because many pollutants are airway irritants, studies with outcomes related to airway symptoms are excluded and discussion of potential relationships of early-life exposure pollutants to allergy is limited to 2 of the most extensively studied environmental exposures: environmental tobacco smoke (ETS) and traffic-related air pollutants.

ENVIRONMENTAL TOBACCO SMOKE

Tobacco smoke contains more than 5000 chemical substances, with nearly 100 linked to poor health.[98] Exposure to ETS has been one of the most studied early-life risk factors for allergy and asthma. This section summarizes studies that address the potential impact of early-life passive smoke exposure on the risk for the development of childhood atopy.

In 1998, Strachan and Cook[99] completed a systematic review of ETS and its association with allergy-related outcomes, including a quantitative meta-analysis of 12 qualifying reports of the effects of parental smoking on positive childhood allergen skin prick tests. Parental smoking during pregnancy or infancy was not associated with increased likelihood of allergen skin prick positivity (pooled OR = 0.87, 95% CI 0.62–1.24). Furthermore, the results of subsequent studies potentially linking ETS to allergic rhinitis, eczema, and sensitization have been mixed.[100–102]

However, results from subsequent prospective cohort studies have suggested that early-life ETS may increase allergic sensitization among specific subgroups of children. In the German MAS (Multicenter Allergy Study) cohort, 342 children were assessed for outcomes reported at age 3 years. Compared with unexposed children, those who were prenatally and postnatally exposed to ETS had a higher likelihood of sensitization to food allergens (OR = 2.3, 95% CI 1.1–4.6), with a similar estimate among those exposed only postnatally (OR = 2.2, 95% CI 0.9–5.9). No association with inhalant allergens was evident.[103] Among 1-year-old children in the CCAAPS cohort, those living in homes in which greater than 20 cigarettes/d were consumed had higher risk of allergic rhinitis defined by the combination of previous rhinitis symptoms and a positive skin prick test at 12 months of age to at least 1 of 15 allergens (OR = 2.7,95% CI 1.04–6.8).[104] In a large Swedish cohort, prenatal maternal smoking was not associated with risk for IgE sensitization. However, a dose-response relationship was reported between postnatal ETS exposure during the first several months of life and the likelihood of having a positive specific IgE test among 2534 children at age 4 years (any of 14 allergens: adjusted OR [aOR] = 1.28, 95% CI 1.01–1.62; food allergens only: aOR = 1.46, 95% CI 1.11–1.93; cat allergen aOR = 1.96, 95% CI 1.28–2.99).[105]

Some studies suggest interactions between ETS exposure and inherited predisposition for allergy. Among 10-year-old MAS cohort children with 2 allergic parents,[106] routine maternal smoking during and after pregnancy was associated with increased allergic sensitization (sIgE >0.35 kU/L) to at least 1 of 9 common food or inhalant allergens measured at 7 time points up to age 10 years (aOR = 4.8, 95% CI 1.3–18.2) compared with those not exposed to ETS. Increased risk was still apparent among children with 1 allergic parent (aOR = 1.8, 95% CI 1.1–2.9) but absent among children with 2 nonallergic parents (aOR = 0.7, 95% CI 0.4–1.3). Paternal smoking or occasional maternal smoking was not associated with altered risk of sensitization. In stark contrast to the MAS report, early-life ETS exposure increased childhood allergen sensitization only among children with nonallergic mothers in the WHEALS birth cohort.[107] Several methodological differences may have contributed to these discrepant findings, including different adjustment and exposure classification methodologies.

Few definitive prospective data on potential associations between ETS and allergic diseases (other than asthma) have been published. A large cross-sectional study of nearly 7800 French children at age 10 years[108] that reported no impact on atopy from childhood exposure to parental smoking at any time from pregnancy forward did present evidence of inverse associations between maternal smoking (current and during pregnancy) with eczema and current ETS with hay fever. However, the investigators speculated that reverse causation could provide a plausible explanation for their findings.

TRAFFIC-RELATED AIR POLLUTION

Motor vehicle traffic volume, resultant pollutant exposure, and allergic disease prevalence increased in parallel during the twentieth century. This correlation has stimulated investigators to scrutinize the impact of traffic-related air pollution (TRAP) on the development of allergy-related disorders. TRAP is a complex mixture of inhaled substances, including carbon monoxide, nitrogen oxides (NO), benzene, sulfur dioxides, ozone and particulate matter (PM), with the primary source of vehicular PM being derived from diesel exhaust. The mechanism(s) responsible for potential associations of TRAP to atopy remain uncertain. However, experimental studies have shown that diesel exhaust particle (DEP) exposure can increase symptoms in patients with established disease, enhance allergic inflammation, and induce the development of Th2-driven allergic immune responses.[109–111] Specifically, polyaromatic hydrocarbons (a major component of DEPs) enhance IgE production.[112]

The evidence supporting a role for TRAP in the induction of allergic sensitization is mixed.[113] Several early studies suggested linkage of atopy with exposure to NO,[114,115] ozone,[116] and PM,[117,118] but other studies[119,120] failed to find substantial associations between allergy and these same components. Factors that may explain the discrepant findings include varying and inefficient methods to approximate individual-level exposures and a limited ability to measure key qualitative variations in the composition of particulate air pollution.[121] Recent prospective data from several European birth cohorts are reflective of the overall literature, and these reports are summarized later.

Morgenstern and colleagues[122] reported on data from GINI and LISA, 2 Munich-based birth cohorts. In this report, a complex exposure assessment method combining local air pollution measurement and the geographic proximity of the participant's home to major roads was applied. The exposure variable included evaluating addresses for road proximity at birth and was adjusted with available data at ages 2, 3, and 6 years. At age 6 years, previous exposure to higher concentrations of $PM_{2.5}$ (particles <2.5 μm) was associated with an increased odds of sensitization to any of 9 inhalant allergens (aOR = 1.45, 95% CI 1.12–1.74). This finding was driven by pollen allergen sensitization (aOR = 1.52, 95% CI 1.23–1.87) but not indoor allergens, including cat, dog, dust mite, and mold. In addition, when compared with homes located more than 1000 m from a major road, those living within 250 m showed higher risk for sensitivity to pollens and those within 50 m higher risk of sensitivity to any allergen. These investigators also reported associations between $PM_{2.5}$ exposure and hay fever (aOR = 1.59, 95% CI 1.11–2.27) and NO_2 exposure and physician-diagnosed eczema (aOR = 1.18, 95% CI 1.00–1.39).

Similar findings were found in a large prospective cohort of infants in Sweden, in which TRAP exposure during the first year of life was associated with higher rates of pollen sensitization (sIgE) at age 4 years. This association was noted with both PM_{10} (OR = 2.3, 95% CI 1.23–4.29) and traffic-related NO (OR = 1.67, 95% CI 1.1–2.5).[123] However, when the cohort was evaluated at age 8 years, the impact of these first year exposures on sensitization was no longer present, although new sensitization to food allergens between the ages of 4 and 8 years was associated with exposure to NO (aOR = 2.30, 95% CI 1.10–4.82).[124]

First and second year exposure to NO_2, $PM_{2.5}$, and PM_{10} were analyzed for associations with positive skin tests (10 allergens) among 9-year-old to 10-year-old participants in a Norwegian birth cohort.[125] No associations were found. Although lifetime pollutant exposure was marginally associated with higher rates of dust mite and cat sensitization, the effect appeared to diminish with adjustment for socioeconomic factors. Similarly, among 8-year-old participants in the Dutch PIAMA birth cohort, no altered risk for allergen sensitization or eczema was apparent in association with estimated levels of exposure to soot, $PM_{2.5}$, or NO_2 at their original birth address.[126] However, a higher rate of hay fever was associated with $PM_{2.5}$ exposure in a subpopulation of children who had never moved from their birth address (aOR = 1.43, 95% CI 1.01–2.04).

A soon-to-be-published meta-analysis of 5 large European birth cohorts (including several of the aforementioned studies)[127] does not present any convincing associations between multiple measures of air pollution ($PM_{2.5}$, $PM_{2.5-10}$ PM_{10}, blackness of $PM_{2.5}$ filters, NOs, traffic intensity, and traffic load), measured either cross-sectionally or at birth of the child, to common food or inhalant allergen sensitization among children up to 10 years of age. Thus, there are conflicting data regarding potential associations of early-life exposure to pollutants and the development of allergy. However, recent data suggest that studies may need to consider an individual's genetic variation in response to oxidative stress as well as pollution exposure levels to fully understand the relationship between pollution and allergy.[128]

FUTURE CONSIDERATIONS/SUMMARY

We have summarized reports addressing potential linkage between early-life exposure to several factors and an altered risk for childhood allergy. However, previous and emerging data not discussed also suggest other potential factors that may modulate risk. A partial listing includes viruses, allergens, polyunsaturated fatty acids, antioxidants, a variety of specific medications and non–traffic-related pollutants (eg, bisphenol, endotoxin, phthalates, polychlorinated biphenyls, volatile organic compounds). Other exposures that are more difficult to quantify, such as stress and magnetic field exposure, have also been implicated.

Although existing reports all have methodological limitations, we must properly leverage what we have learned from important epidemiologic studies. Although large cohort and cross-sectional studies based on questionnaire data help us to recognize patterns and associations, future longitudinal epidemiologic cohort studies with enhanced and detailed exposure measurements and outcome classifications based on comprehensive clinical examinations are needed to more precisely assess true relationships. Use of disease phenotypes and endotypes will also improve our understanding of relationships with exposures.[129,130] Challenges will persist in identifying modifiable risk factors; however, teams of scientists with diverse expertise in clinical care, epidemiology, statistics, microbiology, genetics, and molecular science will be needed to work together to have the greatest impact on this critical area of investigation.

REFERENCES

1. Peters JL, Boynton-Jarrett R, Sandel M. Prenatal environmental factors influencing IgE levels, atopy and early asthma. Curr Opin Allergy Clin Immunol 2013;13(2):187–92.
2. Barker D, Barker M, Fleming T, et al. Developmental biology: support mothers to secure future public health. Nature 2013;504(7479):209–11.
3. Wegienka G, Johnson CC, Havstad S, et al. Lifetime dog and cat exposure and dog- and cat-specific sensitization at age 18 years. Clin Exp Allergy 2011;41(7): 979–86.
4. McKeever TM, Lewis SA, Smith C, et al. Mode of delivery and risk of developing allergic disease. J Allergy Clin Immunol 2002;109(5):800–2.
5. Renz-Polster H, David MR, Buist AS, et al. Caesarean section delivery and the risk of allergic disorders in childhood. Clin Exp Allergy 2005;35(11):1466–72.
6. Sugiyama M, Arakawa H, Ozawa K, et al. Early-life risk factors for occurrence of atopic dermatitis during the first year. Pediatrics 2007;119(3):e716–23.
7. Bager P, Wohlfahrt J, Westergaard T. Caesarean delivery and risk of atopy and allergic disease: meta-analyses. Clin Exp Allergy 2008;38(4):634–42.
8. Pyrhonen K, Nayha S, Hiltunen L, et al. Caesarean section and allergic manifestations: insufficient evidence of association found in population-based study of children aged 1 to 4 years. Acta Paediatr 2013;102(10):982–9.
9. van Nimwegen FA, Penders J, Stobberingh EE, et al. Mode and place of delivery, gastrointestinal microbiota, and their influence on asthma and atopy. J Allergy Clin Immunol 2011;128(5):948–55.e1-3.

10. Maitra A, Sherriff A, Strachan D, et al. Mode of delivery is not associated with asthma or atopy in childhood. Clin Exp Allergy 2004;34(9):1349–55.
11. Koplin J, Allen K, Gurrin L, et al. Is caesarean delivery associated with sensitization to food allergens and IgE-mediated food allergy: a systematic review. Pediatr Allergy Immunol 2008;19(8):682–7.
12. Roduit C, Scholtens S, de Jongste JC, et al. Asthma at 8 years of age in children born by caesarean section. Thorax 2009;64(2):107–13.
13. Pistiner M, Gold DR, Abdulkerim H, et al. Birth by cesarean section, allergic rhinitis, and allergic sensitization among children with a parental history of atopy. J Allergy Clin Immunol 2008;122(2):274–9.
14. Kolokotroni O, Middleton N, Gavatha M, et al. Asthma and atopy in children born by caesarean section: effect modification by family history of allergies–a population based cross-sectional study. BMC Pediatr 2012;12:179.
15. Almqvist C, Cnattingius S, Lichtenstein P, et al. The impact of birth mode of delivery on childhood asthma and allergic diseases–a sibling study. Clin Exp Allergy 2012;42(9):1369–76.
16. Fujimura KE, Slusher NA, Cabana MD, et al. Role of the gut microbiota in defining human health. Expert Rev Anti Infect Ther 2010;8(4):435–54.
17. Favier CF, Vaughan EE, De Vos WM, et al. Molecular monitoring of succession of bacterial communities in human neonates. Appl Environ Microbiol 2002;68(1): 219–26.
18. Wold AE. The hygiene hypothesis revised: is the rising frequency of allergy due to changes in the intestinal flora? Allergy 1998;53(Suppl 46):20–5.
19. Rautava S, Ruuskanen O, Ouwehand A, et al. The hygiene hypothesis of atopic disease–an extended version. J Pediatr Gastroenterol Nutr 2004;38(4):378–88.
20. Bjorksten B, Sepp E, Julge K, et al. Allergy development and the intestinal microflora during the first year of life. J Allergy Clin Immunol 2001;108(4): 516–20.
21. Adlerberth I, Strachan DP, Matricardi PM, et al. Gut microbiota and development of atopic eczema in 3 European birth cohorts. J Allergy Clin Immunol 2007; 120(2):343–50.
22. Kalliomaki M, Kirjavainen P, Eerola E, et al. Distinct patterns of neonatal gut microflora in infants in whom atopy was and was not developing. J Allergy Clin Immunol 2001;107(1):129–34.
23. Murray CS, Tannock GW, Simon MA, et al. Fecal microbiota in sensitized wheezy and non-sensitized non-wheezy children: a nested case-control study. Clin Exp Allergy 2005;35(6):741–5.
24. Penders J, Thijs C, Vink C, et al. Factors influencing the composition of the intestinal microbiota in early infancy. Pediatrics 2006;118(2):511–21.
25. Dicksved J, Floistrup H, Bergstrom A, et al. Molecular fingerprinting of the fecal microbiota of children raised according to different lifestyles. Appl Environ Microbiol 2007;73(7):2284–9.
26. Penders J, Thijs C, van den Brandt PA, et al. Gut microbiota composition and development of atopic manifestations in infancy: the KOALA Birth Cohort Study. Gut 2007;56(5):661–7.
27. Penders J, Stobberingh EE, van den Brandt PA, et al. The role of the intestinal microbiota in the development of atopic disorders. Allergy 2007;62(11): 1223–36.
28. Sjogren YM, Jenmalm MC, Bottcher MF, et al. Altered early infant gut microbiota in children developing allergy up to 5 years of age. Clin Exp Allergy 2009;39(4): 518–26.

29. Bisgaard H, Li N, Bonnelykke K, et al. Reduced diversity of the intestinal micro-biota during infancy is associated with increased risk of allergic disease at school age. J Allergy Clin Immunol 2011;128(3):646–652 e1-5.
30. Vael C, Vanheirstraeten L, Desager KN, et al. Denaturing gradient gel electro-phoresis of neonatal intestinal microbiota in relation to the development of asthma. BMC Microbiol 2011;11:68.
31. Johansson MA, Sjogren YM, Persson JO, et al. Early colonization with a group of Lactobacilli decreases the risk for allergy at five years of age despite allergic heredity. PLoS One 2011;6(8):e23031.
32. Vebo HC, Sekelja M, Nestestog R, et al. Temporal development of the infant gut microbiota in immunoglobulin E-sensitized and nonsensitized children determined by the GA-map infant array. Clin Vaccine Immunol 2011;18(8): 1326–35.
33. Nakayama J, Kobayashi T, Tanaka S, et al. Aberrant structures of fecal bacterial community in allergic infants profiled by 16S rRNA gene pyrosequencing. FEMS Immunol Med Microbiol 2011;63(3):397–406.
34. Abrahamsson TR, Jakobsson HE, Andersson AF, et al. Low diversity of the gut microbiota in infants with atopic eczema. J Allergy Clin Immunol 2012;129(2): 434–40.e1-2.
35. Azad MB, Konya T, Maughan H, et al. Gut microbiota of healthy Canadian in-fants: profiles by mode of delivery and infant diet at 4 months. CMAJ 2013; 185(5):385–94.
36. Fujimura KE, Johnson CC, Ownby DR, et al. Man's best friend? The effect of pet ownership on house dust microbial communities. J Allergy Clin Immunol 2010; 126(2):410–2, 412 e1–3.
37. Searing DA, Leung DY. Vitamin D in atopic dermatitis, asthma and allergic dis-eases. Immunol Allergy Clin North Am 2010;30(3):397–409.
38. Gale CR, Robinson SM, Harvey NC, et al. Maternal vitamin D status during preg-nancy and child outcomes. Eur J Clin Nutr 2008;62(1):68–77.
39. Wills AK, Shaheen SO, Granell R, et al. Maternal 25-hydroxyvitamin D and its as-sociation with childhood atopic outcomes and lung function. Clin Exp Allergy 2013;43(10):1180–8.
40. Jones AP, Palmer D, Zhang G, et al. Cord blood 25-hydroxyvitamin D3 and allergic disease during infancy. Pediatrics 2012;130(5):e1128–35.
41. Baiz N, Dargent-Molina P, Wark JD, et al, EDEN Mother-Child Cohort Study Group. Cord serum 25-hydroxyvitamin D and risk of early childhood transient wheezing and atopic dermatitis. J Allergy Clin Immunol 2014;133(1):147–53.
42. Pike KC, Inskip HM, Robinson S, et al. Maternal late-pregnancy serum 25-hy-droxyvitamin D in relation to childhood wheeze and atopic outcomes. Thorax 2012;67(11):950–6.
43. Weisse K, Winkler S, Hirche F, et al. Maternal and newborn vitamin D status and its impact on food allergy development in the German LINA cohort study. Allergy 2013;68(2):220–8.
44. Rothers J, Wright AL, Stern DA, et al. Cord blood 25-hydroxyvitamin D levels are associated with aeroallergen sensitization in children from Tucson, Arizona. J Allergy Clin Immunol 2011;128(5):1093–9.e1-5.
45. Camargo CA Jr, Ingham T, Wickens K, et al. Cord-blood 25-hydroxyvitamin D levels and risk of respiratory infection, wheezing, and asthma. Pediatrics 2011;127(1):e180–7.
46. CDC. Folic Acid Recommendations. Folic Acid. 2012. Available at: http://www.cdc.gov/ncbddd/folicacid/recommendations.html. Accessed 12 March, 2014.

47. Magdelijns FJ, Mommers M, Penders J, et al. Folic acid use in pregnancy and the development of atopy, asthma, and lung function in childhood. Pediatrics 2011;128(1):e135–44.
48. van der Valk RJ, Kiefte-de Jong JC, Sonnenschein-van der Voort AM, et al. Neonatal folate, homocysteine, vitamin B12 levels and methylenetetrahydrofolate reductase variants in childhood asthma and eczema. Allergy 2013;68(6): 788–95.
49. Dunstan JA, West C, McCarthy S, et al. The relationship between maternal folate status in pregnancy, cord blood folate levels, and allergic outcomes in early childhood. Allergy 2012;67(1):50–7.
50. Bekkers MB, Elstgeest LE, Scholtens S, et al. Maternal use of folic acid supplements during pregnancy, and childhood respiratory health and atopy. Eur Respir J 2012;39(6):1468–74.
51. Okupa AY, Lemanske RF Jr, Jackson DJ, et al. Early-life folate levels are associated with incident allergic sensitization. J Allergy Clin Immunol 2013;131(1): 226–8.e1-2.
52. Crider KS, Cordero AM, Qi YP, et al. Prenatal folic acid and risk of asthma in children: a systematic review and meta-analysis. Am J Clin Nutr 2013;98(5): 1272–81.
53. AAP. FAQs. Available at: http://www2.aap.org/breastfeeding/faqsbreastfeeding. html. Accessed 14 March, 2014.
54. Lumia M, Luukkainen P, Kaila M, et al. Maternal dietary fat and fatty acid intake during lactation and the risk of asthma in the offspring. Acta Paediatr 2012; 101(8):e337–43.
55. Joseph CL, Ownby DR, Havstad SL, et al. Early complementary feeding and risk of food sensitization in a birth cohort. J Allergy Clin Immunol 2011;127(5): 1203–10.e5.
56. Nwaru BI, Craig LC, Allan K, et al. Breastfeeding and introduction of complementary foods during infancy in relation to the risk of asthma and atopic diseases up to 10 years. Clin Exp Allergy 2013;43(11):1263–73.
57. Nwaru BI, Takkinen HM, Niemela O, et al. Timing of infant feeding in relation to childhood asthma and allergic diseases. J Allergy Clin Immunol 2013;131(1): 78–86.
58. Lowe AJ, Thien FC, Stoney RM, et al. Associations between fatty acids in colostrum and breast milk and risk of allergic disease. Clin Exp Allergy 2008;38(11): 1745–51.
59. Wijga AH, van Houwelingen AC, Kerkhof M, et al. Breast milk fatty acids and allergic disease in preschool children: the Prevention and Incidence of Asthma and Mite Allergy birth cohort study. J Allergy Clin Immunol 2006;117(2):440–7.
60. Oddy WH, Pal S, Kusel MM, et al. Atopy, eczema and breast milk fatty acids in a high-risk cohort of children followed from birth to 5 yr. Pediatr Allergy Immunol 2006;17(1):4–10.
61. Matheson MC, Allen KJ, Tang ML. Understanding the evidence for and against the role of breastfeeding in allergy prevention. Clin Exp Allergy 2012;42(6):827–51.
62. Azad MB, Becker AB, Guttman DS, et al. Gut microbiota diversity and atopic disease: does breast-feeding play a role? J Allergy Clin Immunol 2013;131(1): 247–8.
63. Patel R, Oken E, Bogdanovich N, et al. Cohort profile: the Promotion of Breastfeeding Intervention Trial (PROBIT). Int J Epidemiol 2014;43(3):679–90.
64. Flohr C, Nagel G, Weinmayr G, et al. Lack of evidence for a protective effect of prolonged breastfeeding on childhood eczema: lessons from the International

Study of Asthma and Allergies in Childhood (ISAAC) Phase Two. Br J Dermatol 2011;165(6):1280–9.

65. Giwercman C, Halkjaer LB, Jensen SM, et al. Increased risk of eczema but reduced risk of early wheezy disorder from exclusive breast-feeding in high-risk infants. J Allergy Clin Immunol 2010;125(4):866–71.

66. Elliott L, Henderson J, Northstone K, et al. Prospective study of breast-feeding in relation to wheeze, atopy, and bronchial hyperresponsiveness in the Avon Longitudinal Study of Parents and Children (ALSPAC). J Allergy Clin Immunol 2008; 122(1):49–54, 54.e1–3.

67. Lee SY, Kang MJ, Kwon JW, et al. Breastfeeding might have protective effects on atopy in children with the CD14C-159T CT/CC genotype. Allergy Asthma Immunol Res 2013;5(4):239–41.

68. Friedman NJ, Zeiger RS. The role of breast-feeding in the development of allergies and asthma. J Allergy Clin Immunol 2005;115(6):1238–48.

69. Silvers KM, Frampton CM, Wickens K, et al. Breastfeeding protects against current asthma up to 6 years of age. J Pediatr 2012;160(6):991–6.e1.

70. Dogaru CM, Strippoli MP, Spycher BD, et al. Breastfeeding and lung function at school age: does maternal asthma modify the effect? Am J Respir Crit Care Med 2012;185(8):874–80.

71. Silvers KM, Frampton CM, Wickens K, et al. Breastfeeding protects against adverse respiratory outcomes at 15 months of age. Matern Child Nutr 2009; 5(3):243–50.

72. Grabenhenrich LB, Gough H, Reich A, et al. Early-life determinants of asthma from birth to age 20 years: a German birth cohort study. J Allergy Clin Immunol 2014;133(4):979–88.

73. Guilbert TW, Stern DA, Morgan WJ, et al. Effect of breastfeeding on lung function in childhood and modulation by maternal asthma and atopy. Am J Respir Crit Care Med 2007;176(9):843–8.

74. Nermes M, Niinivirta K, Nylund L, et al. Perinatal pet exposure, faecal microbiota, and wheezy bronchitis: is there a connection? ISRN Allergy 2013;2013: 827934.

75. Ownby DR, Johnson CC. Does exposure to dogs and cats in the first year of life influence the development of allergic sensitization? Curr Opin Allergy Clin Immunol 2003;3(6):517–22.

76. Simpson A, Custovic A. Pets and the development of allergic sensitization. Curr Allergy Asthma Rep 2005;5(3):212–20.

77. Chen CM, Tischer C, Schnappinger M, et al. The role of cats and dogs in asthma and allergy–a systematic review. Int J Hyg Environ Health 2010; 213(1):1–31.

78. Lodrup Carlsen KC, Roll S, Carlsen KH, et al. Does pet ownership in infancy lead to asthma or allergy at school age? Pooled analysis of individual participant data from 11 European birth cohorts. PLoS One 2012;7(8):e43214.

79. Pelucchi C, Galeone C, Bach JF, et al. Pet exposure and risk of atopic dermatitis at the pediatric age: a meta-analysis of birth cohort studies. J Allergy Clin Immunol 2013;132(3):616–22.e7.

80. Epstein TG, Bernstein DI, Levin L, et al. Opposing effects of cat and dog ownership and allergic sensitization on eczema in an atopic birth cohort. J Pediatr 2011;158(2):265–71.e1-5.

81. Langan SM, Flohr C, Williams HC. The role of furry pets in eczema: a systematic review. Arch Dermatol 2007;143(12):1570–7.

82. Roduit C, Wohlgensinger J, Frei R, et al. Prenatal animal contact and gene expression of innate immunity receptors at birth are associated with atopic dermatitis. J Allergy Clin Immunol 2011;127(1):179–85, 185.e1.

83. Koplin JJ, Dharmage SC, Ponsonby AL, et al. Environmental and demographic risk factors for egg allergy in a population-based study of infants. Allergy 2012; 67(11):1415–22.

84. Lau S, Illi S, Platts-Mills TA, et al. Longitudinal study on the relationship between cat allergen and endotoxin exposure, sensitization, cat-specific IgG and development of asthma in childhood–report of the German Multicentre Allergy Study (MAS 90). Allergy 2005;60(6):766–73.

85. Smallwood J, Ownby D. Exposure to dog allergens and subsequent allergic sensitization: an updated review. Curr Allergy Asthma Rep 2012;12(5):424–8.

86. Heintze K, Petersen KU. The case of drug causation of childhood asthma: antibiotics and paracetamol. Eur J Clin Pharmacol 2013;69(6):1197–209.

87. Penders J, Kummeling I, Thijs C. Infant antibiotic use and wheeze and asthma risk: a systematic review and meta-analysis. Eur Respir J 2011;38(2):295–302.

88. Kummeling I, Thijs C. Reverse causation and confounding-by-indication: do they or do they not explain the association between childhood antibiotic treatment and subsequent development of respiratory illness? Clin Exp Allergy 2008;38(8):1249–51.

89. Murk W, Risnes KR, Bracken MB. Prenatal or early-life exposure to antibiotics and risk of childhood asthma: a systematic review. Pediatrics 2011;127(6): 1125–38.

90. Marra F, Lynd L, Coombes M, et al. Does antibiotic exposure during infancy lead to development of asthma?: a systematic review and metaanalysis. Chest 2006; 129(3):610–8.

91. Rusconi F, Gagliardi L, Galassi C, et al. Paracetamol and antibiotics in childhood and subsequent development of wheezing/asthma: association or causation? Int J Epidemiol 2011;40(3):662–7.

92. Ong MS, Umetsu DT, Mandl KD. Consequences of antibiotics and infections in infancy: bugs, drugs, and wheezing. Ann Allergy Asthma Immunol 2014;112(5): 441–5.e1.

93. Jordan S, Storey M, Morgan G. Antibiotics and allergic disorders in childhood. Open Nurs J 2008;2:48–57.

94. Celedon JC, Litonjua AA, Ryan L, et al. Lack of association between antibiotic use in the first year of life and asthma, allergic rhinitis, or eczema at age 5 years. Am J Respir Crit Care Med 2002;166(1):72–5.

95. McKeever TM, Lewis SA, Smith C, et al. Early exposure to infections and antibiotics and the incidence of allergic disease: a birth cohort study with the West Midlands General Practice Research Database. J Allergy Clin Immunol 2002; 109(1):43–50.

96. Dom S, Droste JH, Sariachvili MA, et al. Pre- and post-natal exposure to antibiotics and the development of eczema, recurrent wheezing and atopic sensitization in children up to the age of 4 years. Clin Exp Allergy 2010;40(9):1378–87.

97. Kusel MM, de Klerk N, Holt PG, et al. Antibiotic use in the first year of life and risk of atopic disease in early childhood. Clin Exp Allergy 2008;38(12):1921–8.

98. Talhout R, Schulz T, Florek E, et al. Hazardous compounds in tobacco smoke. Int J Environ Res Public Health 2011;8(2):613–28.

99. Strachan DP, Cook DG. Health effects of passive smoking. 5. Parental smoking and allergic sensitisation in children. Thorax 1998;53(2):117–23.

100. Murray CS, Woodcock A, Smillie FI, et al. Tobacco smoke exposure, wheeze, and atopy. Pediatr Pulmonol 2004;37(6):492–8.
101. Ciaccio CE, DiDonna AC, Kennedy K, et al. Association of tobacco smoke exposure and atopic sensitization. Ann Allergy Asthma Immunol 2013;111(5):387–90.
102. Ciaccio CE, Gentile D. Effects of tobacco smoke exposure in childhood on atopic diseases. Curr Allergy Asthma Rep 2013;13(6):687–92.
103. Kulig M, Luck W, Lau S, et al. Effect of pre- and postnatal tobacco smoke exposure on specific sensitization to food and inhalant allergens during the first 3 years of life. Multicenter Allergy Study Group, Germany. Allergy 1999;54(3):220–8.
104. Biagini JM, LeMasters GK, Ryan PH, et al. Environmental risk factors of rhinitis in early infancy. Pediatr Allergy Immunol 2006;17(4):278–84.
105. Lannero E, Wickman M, van Hage M, et al. Exposure to environmental tobacco smoke and sensitisation in children. Thorax 2008;63(2):172–6.
106. Keil T, Lau S, Roll S, et al. Maternal smoking increases risk of allergic sensitization and wheezing only in children with allergic predisposition: longitudinal analysis from birth to 10 years. Allergy 2009;64(3):445–51.
107. Havstad SL, Johnson CC, Zoratti EM, et al. Tobacco smoke exposure and allergic sensitization in children: a propensity score analysis. Respirology 2012;17(7):1068–72.
108. Raherison C, Penard-Morand C, Moreau D, et al. In utero and childhood exposure to parental tobacco smoke, and allergies in schoolchildren. Respir Med 2007;101(1):107–17.
109. Riedl M, Diaz-Sanchez D. Biology of diesel exhaust effects on respiratory function. J Allergy Clin Immunol 2005;115(2):221–8 [quiz: 229].
110. Diaz-Sanchez D, Proietti L, Polosa R. Diesel fumes and the rising prevalence of atopy: an urban legend? Curr Allergy Asthma Rep 2003;3(2):146–52.
111. Ghio AJ, Smith CB, Madden MC. Diesel exhaust particles and airway inflammation. Curr Opin Pulm Med 2012;18(2):144–50.
112. Polosa R, Salvi S, Di Maria GU. Allergic susceptibility associated with diesel exhaust particle exposure: clear as mud. Arch Environ Health 2002;57(3):188–93.
113. Braback L, Forsberg B. Does traffic exhaust contribute to the development of asthma and allergic sensitization in children: findings from recent cohort studies. Environ Health 2009;8:17.
114. Kramer U, Koch T, Ranft U, et al. Traffic-related air pollution is associated with atopy in children living in urban areas. Epidemiology 2000;11(1):64–70.
115. Janssen NA, Brunekreef B, van Vliet P, et al. The relationship between air pollution from heavy traffic and allergic sensitization, bronchial hyperresponsiveness, and respiratory symptoms in Dutch schoolchildren. Environ Health Perspect 2003;111(12):1512–8.
116. Penard-Morand C, Charpin D, Raherison C, et al. Long-term exposure to background air pollution related to respiratory and allergic health in schoolchildren. Clin Exp Allergy 2005;35(10):1279–87.
117. Annesi-Maesano I, Moreau D, Caillaud D, et al. Residential proximity fine particles related to allergic sensitisation and asthma in primary school children. Respir Med 2007;101(8):1721–9.
118. Brauer M, Hoek G, Smit HA, et al. Air pollution and development of asthma, allergy and infections in a birth cohort. Eur Respir J 2007;29(5):879–88.
119. Nicolai T, Carr D, Weiland SK, et al. Urban traffic and pollutant exposure related to respiratory outcomes and atopy in a large sample of children. Eur Respir J 2003;21(6):956–63.

120. Hirsch T, Weiland SK, von Mutius E, et al. Inner city air pollution and respiratory health and atopy in children. Eur Respir J 1999;14(3):669–77.
121. Heinrich J, Wichmann HE. Traffic related pollutants in Europe and their effect on allergic disease. Curr Opin Allergy Clin Immunol 2004;4(5):341–8.
122. Morgenstern V, Zutavern A, Cyrys J, et al. Atopic diseases, allergic sensitization, and exposure to traffic-related air pollution in children. Am J Respir Crit Care Med 2008;177(12):1331–7.
123. Nordling E, Berglind N, Melen E, et al. Traffic-related air pollution and childhood respiratory symptoms, function and allergies. Epidemiology 2008;19(3):401–8.
124. Gruzieva O, Bellander T, Eneroth K, et al. Traffic-related air pollution and development of allergic sensitization in children during the first 8 years of life. J Allergy Clin Immunol 2012;129(1):240–6.
125. Oftedal B, Brunekreef B, Nystad W, et al. Residential outdoor air pollution and allergen sensitization in schoolchildren in Oslo, Norway. Clin Exp Allergy 2007;37(11):1632–40.
126. Gehring U, Wijga AH, Brauer M, et al. Traffic-related air pollution and the development of asthma and allergies during the first 8 years of life. Am J Respir Crit Care Med 2010;181(6):596–603.
127. Gruzieva O, Gehring U, Aalberse R, et al. Meta-analysis of air pollution exposure association with allergic sensitization in European birth cohorts. J Allergy Clin Immunol 2014;133(3):767–76.e7.
128. Carlsten C, Melen E. Air pollution, genetics, and allergy: an update. Curr Opin Allergy Clin Immunol 2012;12(5):455–60.
129. Prosperi MC, Sahiner UM, Belgrave D, et al. Challenges in identifying asthma subgroups using unsupervised statistical learning techniques. Am J Respir Crit Care Med 2013;188(11):1303–12.
130. Havstad S, Johnson CC, Kim H, et al. Atopic phenotypes identified with latent class analyses at age 2 years. J Allergy Clin Immunol 2014;134(3):722–7.e2.

Genetics of Allergic Diseases

Romina A. Ortiz, MS, Kathleen C. Barnes, PhD*

KEYWORDS

- Allergic disease • Genetics • Single nucleotide polymorphism
- Genome-wide association study • Next-generation sequencing • Epigenetics
- Transcriptome

KEY POINTS

- Nearly 100 asthma genes/loci in addition to multiple genes/loci for atopic dermatitis, allergic rhinitis, and immunoglobulin E have been identified by genome-wide association studies.
- Next-generation sequencing strategies are increasingly being used to hone in on the causal variants associated with allergic diseases.
- A goal of the genetics of allergic disease is to better match individualized treatments to specific genotypes to improve therapeutic outcomes and minimize adverse effects.

INTRODUCTION

Coca and Cooke were the first to describe asthma, atopic dermatitis (AD), allergic rhinitis (AR), food allergy, and urticaria as "phenomena of hypersensitiveness" at the annual meeting of the American Association of Immunologists in 1922.[1] Just prior to and following this discourse, there was considerable focus on the relative influence of the environment versus hereditary factors on allergic diseases, with family-based twin and migration studies providing the earliest and most compelling evidence for genetic contributions.[2–6] Studies on the prevalence of allergic traits in relation to family history demonstrated incremental increases in risk of developing asthma, AR, or AD with the presence of at least 1 parent with allergic disease, and greater than 3 times the risk if allergic disease occurred in more than 1 first-degree relative.[7] To date, and despite the dramatic technological advances that have led to the identification of hundreds of genetic variants in genes associated

Disclosure Statement: The authors have nothing to disclose.
K.C. Barnes was supported in part by the Mary Beryl Patch Turnbull Scholar Program; R.A. Ortiz was supported by NHLBI Diversity Supplement 3R01HL104608-02S1.
Department of Medicine, The Johns Hopkins Asthma and Allergy Center, 5501 Hopkins Bayview Circle, Room 3A.62, Baltimore, MD 21224, USA
* Corresponding author.
E-mail address: kbarnes@jhmi.edu

with asthma, AD remains one of the most reliable tools for prognosis of allergic disease.

Approaches for disentangling the genetic basis for the allergic diseases have evolved as technological tools for the field of molecular genetics have progressed. With the introduction of the polymerase chain reaction (PCR) in the 1980s, DNA fragments in the human genome could be amplified and then studied for variable fragment lengths of repeats, or genetic fingerprinting. With a catalog of microsatellite markers spanning the human genome, genome-wide linkage studies emerged as a robust approach for identifying genetic hot spots associated with complex traits. Nearly a dozen genome-wide linkage screens were performed on asthma and its associated phenotypes,[8-18] for which multiple chromosomal regions provided significant evidence for linkage. From several of these family-based linkage genome-wide screens, 6 novel asthma genes were identified by positional cloning.[18-23] Similarly, multiple linkage studies were performed for AD[24] and AR.[25-29] It was frequently observed that loci overlapped across associated traits; for example, Daniels and colleagues[8] observed overlapping linkage peaks with quantitative traits associated with asthma including total serum IgE, skin test index, and eosinophil counts, as well as atopy as a qualitative trait. Alternatively, the multiethnic *Collaborative Study on the Genetics of Asthma* reported linkage peaks that were specific to different racial and ethnic groups.[9]

With the publication of initial efforts in sequencing the human genome,[30,31] the opportunity to genotype markers directly in genes of interest was greatly expanded as polymorphisms were identified in the approximately 20,000 to 25,000 genes across the 3 billion chemical base pairs that make up human DNA. Relying upon one of the simplest of these polymorphisms, single nucleotide polymorphisms (SNPs), and relatively simple structural variants, such as insertions/deletions and repeats, this advancement allowed researchers to expand genetic studies beyond linkage toward the genetic association study design. For asthma alone, literally hundreds of candidate genes have been elucidated, and summarized elsewhere,[32-35] representing the relative success of this approach.

THE GENOME-WIDE ASSOCIATION STUDIES ERA

Following completion of the Human Genome Project, the International HapMap Project[36-38] cataloged genomes representing 4 biogeographical groups (whites from the United States with northern and western European ancestry; Yorubans from Ibadan, Nigeria [YRI]; Han Chinese from Beijing, China [CHB]; and Japanese from Tokyo, Japan [JPT]) to advance the development of new analytical methods and investigating patterns of genetic variation. Simultaneously, the technological capacity to rapidly (and cheaply) genotype more than 1 million common (>5%) SNPs on thousands of DNA samples from patients phenotyped for various complex clinical traits took the spotlight, and the GWAS era took off. The content of commercially available GWAS chips grew exponentially with expansion of the human genome catalog through the Thousand Genomes Project (TGP),[39] and the capacity for discovery of genetic associations has likewise increased with the development of SNP genotype imputation methodologies,[40,41] whereby genotyped content from the chip can be combined with the more than 35 million sequenced variants cataloged in the TGP. In the span of only 7 years, over 1924 publications and 13,403 SNPs associated with various complex and quantitative traits[42,43] have been generated by GWAS (**Fig. 1A**).

GWAS have been widely employed in the field of allergic disease. Although the precise number of GWAS are difficult to determine, approximately 40 asthma, 3 atopy,

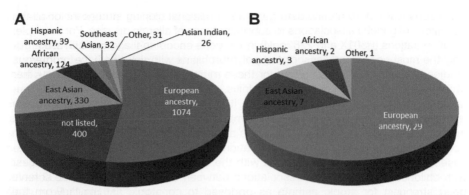

Fig. 1. Published GWAS to date according to ethnicity and race for all cataloged GWAS (*A*) and asthma GWAS (*B*). (*Data from* the National Human Genome Research Institute's GWAS catalog Web site. Accessed June 16, 2014. Available at: http://www.genome.gov/gwastudies/.)

and 3 AD GWAS (plus a study of >30,000 AD patients genotyped on the Immunochip[44]) have been reported in the *Catalog of Published Genome-Wide Association Studies* (see **Fig. 1**B and summarized in Appendix A).[42,43] A major outcome of GWAS in allergic disease has been the formation of national and international collaborations leading to consortia meta-analyses, which have greatly facilitated gene discovery owed to the increased power generated from larger sample sizes (which are necessary to detect true associations while adjusting for the multiple comparisons). For example, the first asthma GWAS only showed a significant association between childhood onset asthma and markers near the *ORMDL3* gene on chromosome 17q21 ($P<10^{-12}$) among European populations.[45] When the study was expanded to include more than 26,000 cases and unaffected controls (eg, the European-based GABRIEL Consortium[46]), five additional genes plus the 17q locus were strongly associated with asthma.[47] Following completion of 8 US-based, independent asthma GWAS, the National Heart Lung and Blood Institute (NHLBI)-supported EVE Consortium was established, comprising more than 12,000 European American, African American, and Hispanic cohorts plus more than 12,000 independent samples for replication.[48] More recently, the Transnational Asthma Genetics Consortium (TAGC) was formed to perform a global meta-analysis for asthma, and to date TAGC includes 67 cohorts representing nearly 20 studies spanning the globe, representing data on over 100,000 asthma cases, controls, and family members (Demenais and colleagues, unpublished data, 2014).

It can be argued that the huge research efforts and expense committed to GWAS on allergic disease have confirmed suspected genes and pathways, some of which were the focus following linkage study discoveries and a result of the many candidate gene studies undertaken. However, GWAS has, for the most part, generated novel candidate genes and a new appreciation for the role of innate as well as adaptive immune-response genes in allergic disease. In the European-based GABRIEL Consortium, 6 genes were strongly associated with asthma,[47] of which 3 genes (*IL33*, *ST2*, and the *IKZF3-ZPBP2-GSDMB-ORMDL3* region on chromosome 17q21) were replicated in the EVE Consortium.[48] Independent GWAS have provided further support for these same loci.[49–51] One of the strongest signals from the combined meta-analysis was for *IL1RL1*,[48] even though the peak SNP differed across ethnic groups. The association between *IL1RL1 SNPs* among African samples was marginal, and might have been overlooked, but in light of evidence for association in other cohorts, *IL1RL1* showed the strongest association overall ($P = 1.4 \times 10^{-8}$).

Lessons learned from candidate gene and positional cloning studies included the specificity of genetic associations to subphenotypes of allergic disease. For example, 2 null mutations (R501X and 2282del4) in the gene encoding filaggrin *(FLG)* are arguably the most consistently associated polymorphisms with risk of AD, but numerous studies have also implicated a role for these mutations in the development of other atopic diseases, such as asthma and rhinitis, suggesting generalizability of *FLG* mutations to the allergic diathesis. However, it has been argued that the atopic march (eg, the tendency for AD to precede asthma, food allergy, and AR) and the fact that approximately 70% of severe AD patients also have asthma and AR later in life can account for this overlap.[52] Similar observations have come from GWAS of allergic diseases. For example, the associations with the *ORMDL3* locus have been strongest with childhood asthma,[53] and associations between SNPs in *IL1RL1* and *IL33* have been strongest for atopic asthma as opposed to nonatopic asthma.[49] From the GWAS performed total serum IgE levels, there has been relatively little overlap with genes contributing to risk of asthma (see Appendix A).

THE NEXT GENERATION OF ASTHMA GENETICS

Despite its success, discoveries from GWAS have contributed relatively little to the understanding of the specific causal genetic mechanisms underlying allergic disease. For example, the cumulative genetic risk of the variants identified to date for asthma through GWAS (for which, among the allergic diseases, the most GWAS have been performed) is less than 15%.[35] This is thought to be due, at least in part, to the fact that the most strongly associated SNPs in GWAS are generally not directly causal, but most likely tag SNPs in linkage disequilibrium (LD) with the true unobserved disease-causing SNPs. Moreover, the vast proportion of GWAS associations (>85%) involve variants in intergenic or intronic regions,[54] which is likely a consequence of the array design (ie, GWAS arrays are based on tag SNPs for common variants, and coding/exonic variation tends in general to be rare and therefore poorly tagged by a common variant, in contrast to intronic and intergenic regions that have a spectrum of variation that is common). Disappointment in GWAS is compounded by a paradigm shift away from the common disease—common variant hypothesis[55] toward the role of rare variants (unlikely to be identified by GWAS[56]) in non-Mendelian diseases,[57] particularly with the appreciation that rare variation constitutes the majority of polymorphisms across human populations.[39,58]

Resequencing genes in individuals with well-characterized phenotypes is an alternative approach to assess the contribution that both rare and common variants make to disease and overcome the limitations of GWAS. Until recently, Sanger termination sequencing[59] was the only option for interrogating rare variants, but this approach is costly and cannot be done on a large scale. The emergence of massively parallel, second-generation DNA sequencing in 2005[60] has made resequencing an affordable tool to study genetic variation, and in the past several years has been increasingly used either as a targeted approach to follow-up on specific genetic regions or as an unbiased approach toward gene discovery either by whole-exome (WES; ~30 Mb total) or whole-genome sequencing (WGS).[61] Although rare coding variants may have a greater functional impact than common variants, their analysis must consider the low frequency of any variant, since it will reduce the power to infer statistical associations (ie, insufficient numbers of copies of the rare variant allele in a typical dataset). However, this can be overcome by evaluating the collective frequency of rare, nonsynonymous variants within one or more genes, or for a pathway(s), or the functional impact of the discovered variations, such as nonsense substitutions, frameshifts, and splice-site disruptions, that have important a priori evidence compared with other types of changes.[61]

To date, there are limited examples of the application of next-generation sequencing (NGS) technology to identify variants associated with risk of allergic disease, although efforts are underway. A recent example of success combined targeted array-based and in-solution enrichment with the sequencing by oligonucleotide ligation and detection (SOLiD) sequencing platform to accurately and simultaneously detect 161 of 170 mutations and deletions associated with primary immunodeficiency (PID) disorders.[62] NGS has also been applied to the study of airway inflammation, including asthma. A study by Leung and colleagues[63] utilized the NGS technique called Roche 454 pyrosequencing on peak asthma association signals found in a large consortium-based study in European white subjects and a small group of Chinese children, and found substantial variation in haplotype structures across the populations, thus supporting the notion of potential sequence variations of asthma loci across different ethnic populations. WES has been applied to a small family-based study[64] as well as asthmatics selected at both ends of a phenotype distribution (those with extreme severity phenotypes)[65] with limited success, and a large WGS (>1000 genomes) on asthma is underway.[66]

MEASURING THE TRANSCRIPTOME IN ALLERGIC DISEASE AND ITS APPLICATION TO GENETIC STUDIES

Whole-genome gene expression profiling, or transcriptomics, is a robust approach toward the quantitative and qualitative characterization of RNA expressed in a biological system. Since the development of synthetic oligonucleotide microarray platforms in 2003,[67] transcriptomic profiling has been widely applied in allergic disease. For asthma and its associated traits alone, dozens of studies focusing on whole blood and target cells of the immune system and tissue from the upper and lower airways have been performed using these conventional platforms.[68]

The same robust NGS technology that has recently advanced genetics has similarly transformed transcriptomics. RNA-Sequencing (RNA-Seq) is a more powerful approach to interrogate the transcriptome compared with older microarray technology because of its smaller technical variation[69] and higher correlation with protein expression.[70] RNA-Seq has virtually unlimited dynamic range and permits digital quantification of transcript abundance, assessment of transcript isoforms, and alternative splicing,[71–73] and it allows for unbiased assembly of transcripts without relying on previous annotation (including noncoding RNAs). To date there are limited examples of applying RNA-Seq technology to allergic disease, but successes include the identification of transcriptomic changes in human airway smooth muscle (ASM) in asthmatics compared with nonasthmatics[74] and the identification of genes differentially expressed in response to glucocorticosteroid exposure (CRISPLD2,[75] FAM129A and SYNPO2[76]).

Although it is ideal to measure the transcriptome of a primary cell specific to the disease of interest (ie, cells from lung tissue in asthma), this is challenging when considering the large number of samples required given the demands of power. Recently, however, studies have demonstrated the value of focusing on surrogate target tissues/cells in predicting gene expression in tissues/cells that are challenging to access in large numbers (ie, lung tissue), which have the potential to significantly move the field forward. For example, Poole and colleagues[77] used whole-transcriptome sequencing (RNA-Seq) to demonstrate that the nasal airway epithelium mirrors the bronchial airway, and subsequent RNA sequencing of candidate airway biomarkers confirmed that children with asthma have an altered nasal airway transcriptome compared with healthy controls, and these changes are reflected by differential expression in the bronchial airway.

Differential gene expression in people is heritable,[78,79] and GWAS of gene expression is an innovative approach for mapping functional noncoding variation. Referred to as expression quantitative trait locus (eQTL) mapping, this approach is predicated on the notion that abundance of a gene transcript (a quantitative trait) is directly modified by genetic polymorphisms in regulatory elements. The added value of eQTL is the ability to identify disease markers identified in GWAS that are also associated with gene transcripts, and several studies have integrated findings from asthma GWAS with cataloged genome-wide gene expression data,[80,81] which can result in a gain in power.[82] Because of limited access to human primary cell types from large populations, many of the human eQTL studies have focused on convenient and immortalized Epstein-Barr virus transformed lymphoblastoid cell lines (LCLs),[83–85] but this approach has had limited success in mapping eQTLs for more than a few of the known asthma genes. In one of the first asthma eQTL studies, SNPs associated with asthma in a subset of the GABRIEL sample were consistently and strongly associated ($P<10^{-22}$) with transcript levels of ORMDL3.[45] Hao and colleagues[81] performed an eQTL analysis using lung samples from transplant patients to identify variants affecting gene expression in human lung tissue, then integrated their lung eQTLs with GWAS data from GABRIEL to determine that one of their strongest eQTLs was, similar to the eQTL in LCLs study, an SNP in the chr. 17q21 region. Murphy and colleagues[86] identified common genetic variants influencing expression of 1585 genes in peripheral blood CD4+ T cells from 200 asthmatics using conventional microarrays, but they acknowledged power was a major limitation. In mining a catalog of 285 published GWAS, however, they identified significant associations with variants in the ORMDL3 region. When performing tests for association on 6706 cis-acting expression-associated variants (eSNPs) from a genome-wide eQTL survey of CD4+ T cells from asthmatics, the ORMDL3/GSDMB locus held up ($P = 2.9 \times 10^{-8}$).[87]

COMMON GENES IN COMMON DISEASES

Several reports have found that allergic diseases such as asthma, rhinitis, conjunctivitis, and dermatitis, as well as allergic reactions to drugs and foods, are more common in patients with the autoimmune disease systemic lupus erythematosus (SLE).[88–91] Furthermore, bronchial asthma was found to be the most common cause of cough in a small cohort of SLE patients from Bangladesh[92] and Taiwan.[93] In addition, the inflammatory gene tumor necrosis factor α (TNFα) was found to be a common genetic risk factor for asthma, and autoimmune diseases juvenile rheumatoid arthritis (JRA) and SLE.[94] In a more recent study, PCR-based genotyping identified 4 FCRL3 single nucleotide polymorphisms associated with protection in either JRA or asthma, but no association was observed with childhood-onset SLE in male Mexican patients. The gene NRF2 has also been associated with various immunologic pathologies including RA, acute lung injury, asthma, and emphysema,[95] among others. There is a long-standing observation of common genetic determinants for both asthma and chronic obstructive pulmonary disease (COPD) identified both through candidate gene studies as well as GWAS.[96,97] Recently, Hardin and colleagues[98] performed a GWAS focusing specifically on patients from the COPD Gene Study with both asthma and COPD, referred to as the COPD-asthma overlap syndrome, and identified associations with variants in genes (ie, GPR65) unique to this subphenotype. Finally, there is a large body of research associated with the hygiene hypothesis[99] addressing the potential beneficial role of microbial exposures for later development of asthma and allergies. Specifically, the underlying immunologic mechanisms and the type of infectious/microbial stimuli relevant to helminth infection (ie, schistosomiasis) are the same mechanisms that promote the Th2-mediated response in allergic disease,[100,101] and common genetic mechanisms that underlie both schistosomiasis and asthma have been reported from linkage and candidate gene studies.[101]

OTHER OMICS AND ALLERGIC DISEASE

Omics refers to an experimental design in which large-scale datasets are acquired from a complete class of biomolecules with the aim of identifying the functional or pathologic mechanisms of disease.[102] Such data-dense technologies include: DNA in the context of complete genomics; gene regulation technologies (epigenomics); global protein and/or post-transcriptional modifications (proteomics); and all cellular metabolites (metabolomics).[103]

Transcriptomics extended to micro-RNA is another burgeoning field. Several micro-RNA have been identified as distinct profiles for the development and status of asthma, as well as other allergic phenotypes.[104,105] Approximately 200 micro-RNA are known to be altered in steroid-naïve asthmatics, establishing a link between abnormal micro-RNA expression in asthmatic patients and inflammation.[106–108] High-throughput data combined with sequence-based micro-RNA predictions have been successfully applied,[109–113] and more recently, a transcriptome study on micro-RNA-long noncoding RNA interactions suggested better understanding of lung disease regulation and progression.[114] NGS has been utilized to study microRNA expression and interactions with the phosphoinositide 3-kinase (PI3K) pathway in primary human airway smooth muscle (HASM) cells.[115]

Concordance rates for asthma and allergies of only approximately 50% among monozygotic twins suggest differences in exposure to environmental triggers are critical in disease expression,[2,116,117] and it has been demonstrated that genes and environmental factors contribute equally to asthma and its associated traits such as total Immunoglobulin E (tIgE).[3] Similar to the other allergic diseases, the prevalence of asthma has increased dramatically within the 20 to 30 years in relation to the deterioration of the environment, favoring a significant contribution of environmental factors.[118] Added to this complexity is the observation that associations with alleles at candidate genes and interactions between these genes might only be observed among certain subpopulations despite nearly identical environmental exposures and similar genetic backgrounds. For example, the CD14(-260)C>T variant was associated with low tIgE in school children living in urban/suburban Tucson, Arizona,[119] but the opposite association was reported in a farming community.[120] Alternatively, it has been shown that this same variant depends on the dose of endotoxin from household dust among African-ancestry asthmatics living in the tropics,[121] suggesting the role of endotoxin in allergic disease may be caused by the combination of susceptibility genes and exposure. A large body of evidence implicates in utero and early life environmental tobacco smoke (ETS) exposure leads to impaired lung function and increased risk of asthma,[122–125] and ETS exposure increases strength of the association between markers in candidate genes and atopic asthma.[126–128] Indeed, environmental exposures such as smoking, air pollution, and stress have been shown to cause changes in epigenetic modifications of genes as well as altered microRNA expression.[129]

Immune responses in allergic disease are dominantly initiated by the release of cytokines such as interleukin-4 (IL4), IL5, and IL13, which activate type 2 helper T cells

(TH2), resulting in a decrease of TH1 cytokines and impaired regulatory T cell function, and up- or down-regulation of DNA methylation on Th-1/Th-2 cytokine genes may affect the sensitization of experimental asthma.[130] In addition, epigenetic changes in immune cells such as T cells, B cells, mast cells, and dendritic cells exposed to environmental factors have also been shown to be associated with asthma.[131] A recent study found that DNA methylation in the β-2 adrenergic receptor (*ADRB2*) gene is associated with decreased asthma severity.[132] In addition, an asthma mouse model found that microRNAs targeted genes involved in inflammatory responses and tissue remodeling, and demethylation status in the promoter of the IFN-γ, changed in response to chronic antigen sensitization.[133]

Environmental stimuli have been shown to directly influence epigenetic modifications, and thus epigenetic regulation may play a role in immune-mediated lung diseases like asthma. Epigenetic regulation maintains tolerance to self-antigens. Thus, abnormal epigenetic activity may lead to a deregulated immune response and thus an immune disorder.[134] Epigenomics allows for the study of gene regulation at the chromosomal level using DNA methylation and chromatin immunoprecipitation (CHIP) technologies. As an example, 870 genes are differentially methylated in idiopathic pulmonary fibrosis (IPF) tissues,[135] and changes in micro-RNA and fibroblast signature for genes are known to regulate the extracellular matrix in IPF.[136,137] While methylation decreases gene expression, acetylation of histones relaxes chromatin, facilitating gene transcription and increasing expression. A recent study has implicated histone modifications in the decrease of *Fas* expression as well as resistance to apoptosis in fibrotic lung fibroblasts.[138]

A novel example of this technology is a study in which methylated DNA immunoprecipitation-next generation sequencing (MeDIP-seq) on lung tissue DNA from saline and house dust mite (HDM)-exposed mice was performed, and researchers found that chronic exposure to HDM increased airway reactivity and inflammation, as interpreted through increases in IL-4, IL-5 and serum immunoglobulin E (IgE) levels, resulting in structural remodeling and hyper-responsiveness consistent with allergic disease. In addition, mice that received HDM exposure had global changes in methylation and hydroxymethylation of approximately 213 genes, with *TGFβ2* and *SMAD3* having the most connected network.[139] These findings demonstrate how allergen exposure could trigger epigenetic changes in the lung genome.

CLINICAL IMPLICATIONS AND PERSONALIZED MEDICINE

Arguably the ultimate goal of genetic studies of allergic disease is to better match individualized treatments to specific genotypes to improve therapeutic outcomes and minimize adverse effects. For example, despite the relative success of conventional asthma therapies such as inhaled beta agonists and glucocorticoids, most cause adverse side effects[140–142] and a subset of asthmatics are refractory to anti-asthma therapies resulting in significant morbidity as well as a significant financial burden.[143–145] Genetic variation determines drug response through various mechanisms including pharmacodynamics mechanisms, which determine drug metabolism.[146]

Recent GWAS and studies of candidate genes related to the β2-adrenergic receptor pathway have attempted to identify specific variants associated with the response to inhaled beta agonists.[147–149] The Arg[16] allele in *ADRB2* has been associated with greater postbronchodilator forced expiratory volume in 1 minute (FEV1) response to short-acting beta agonists (SABA) asthma therapy in asthmatic children,[150,151] while the Gly[16] variant has been associated with changes in peak flow rate (PEFR).[152–154]

In contrast, the Arg[16] allele has been associated with worsening asthma symptom scores with long-acting beta agonist (LABA) therapy compared with Gly[16] homozygotes.[155] Other studies show no difference between the *ADRB2* alleles and asthma symptoms after LABA therapy.[156,157] Further pharmacogenetic studies may achieve a more definitive characterization of the role of Gly[16]Arg after beta agonist exposure and determine whether receptor kinetics or proinflammatory effects play a role in the contrasting effects of the genotypes. Additional candidate genes found to be associated with altered beta agonist response in asthmatic children include *ADCY9*[149] and *ARG1*[158] with FEV1 change, and *CRH2*[147] and *SPATS2L*[148] with bronchodilator response. Additional candidate gene studies have also demonstrated altered asthma phenotypes in response to glucocorticoid therapies including *CRH1*,[159] *STIP1*,[160] *TBX21*,[161,162] *ADCY9*,[149,163] and *ORDML3*.[164]

FUTURE CONSIDERATIONS/SUMMARY

Although GWAS has yielded promising results in the field of allergic disease, association does not imply biological functionality, and follow-up studies are needed to translate initial findings into the biological insights that ultimately will advance prognostics, diagnostics and therapeutics. Although the vast amount of genomic data that are now available for a plethora of complex diseases, including allergic disease, have facilitated follow-up association analyses to explore new hypotheses, meta-analyses, and replication of novel findings,[165] the scientific community is facing a big data crisis,[166] as the size of genomic data sets today has begun to overwhelm the existing infrastructure and resources that allow researchers to share or use these data. For the genetics of allergic diseases specifically, there is increasing awareness of the need to design studies that are more inclusive of racially and ethnically diverse study participants.[167] Consider that, in the field of pharmacogenetics, it has been demonstrated that, as an example, African American asthmatics have an increased likelihood for treatment failures and overall differential response to treatment that may be caused by genetic variants specific to their ancestry.[168,169] Each of these needs will undoubtedly be addressed as clinicians and scientists in the field continue to move in a direction of collaboration and an appreciation for a multidisciplinary approach, attributes that have already pushed the genetics of allergic disease into the genomic revolution, with promises of improved outcome for the patient.

ACKNOWLEDGMENTS

The authors are grateful for technical assistance from Pat Oldewurtel and Joseph Potee.

REFERENCES

1. Coca AF, Cooke RA. On the classification of the phenomena of hypersensitiveness. J Immunol 1923;8:163–71.
2. Duffy DL, Martin NG, Battistutta D, et al. Genetics of asthma and hay fever in Australian twins. Am Rev Respir Dis 1990;142:1351–8.
3. Palmer LJ, Burton PR, James AL, et al. Familial aggregation and heritability of asthma-associated quantitative traits in a population-based sample of nuclear families. Eur J Hum Genet 2000;8(11):853–60.
4. Manolio TA, Barnes KC, Beaty TH, et al. Sex differences in heritability of sensitization to Blomia tropicalis in asthma using regression of offspring on midparent (ROMP) methods. Hum Genet 2003;113(5):437–46.

5. Davis LR, Marten RH, Sarkany I. Atopic eczema in European and Negro West Indian infants in London. Br J Dermatol 1961;73:410–4.
6. Cooke RA, VanderVeer VA. Human sensitisation. J Immunol 1916;1:201–5.
7. Dold S, Wjst M, Mutius EV, et al. Genetic risk for asthma, allergic rhinitis, and atopic dermatitis. Arch Dis Child 1992;67:1018–22.
8. Daniels SE, Bhattacharrya S, James A, et al. A genome-wide search for quantitative trait loci underlying asthma. Nature 1996;383:247–50.
9. CSGA. The Collaborative Study on the Genetics of Asthma: a genome-wide search for asthma susceptibility loci in ethnically diverse populations. Nat Genet 1997;15(4):389–92.
10. Ober C, Cox NJ, Abney M, et al. Genome-wide search for asthma susceptibility loci in a founder population. The Collaborative Study on the Genetics of Asthma. Hum Mol Genet 1998;7(9):1393–8.
11. Malerba G, Trabetti E, Patuzzo C, et al. Candidate genes and a genome-wide search in Italian families with atopic asthmatic children. Clin Exp Allergy 1999; 29(Suppl 4):27–30.
12. Wjst M, Fischer G, Immervoll T, et al. A genome-wide search for linkage to asthma. German Asthma Genetics Group. Genomics 1999;58(1):1–18.
13. Dizier MH, Besse-Schmittler C, Guilloud-Bataille M, et al. Genome screen for asthma and related phenotypes in the French EGEA study. Am J Respir Crit Care Med 2000;162(5):1812–8.
14. Ober C, Tsalenko A, Parry R, et al. A second-generation genomewide screen for asthma-susceptibility alleles in a founder population. Am J Hum Genet 2000; 67(5):1154–62.
15. Yokouchi Y, Nukaga Y, Shibasaki M, et al. Significant evidence for linkage of mite-sensitive childhood asthma to chromosome 5q31-q33 near the interleukin 12 B locus by a genome-wide search in Japanese families. Genomics 2000; 66(2):152–60.
16. Laitinen T, Daly MJ, Rioux JD, et al. A susceptibility locus for asthma-related traits on chromosome 7 revealed by genome-wide scan in a founder population. Nat Genet 2001;28(1):87–91.
17. Hakonarson H, Bjornsdottir US, Halapi E, et al. A major susceptibility gene for asthma maps to chromosome 14q24. Am J Hum Genet 2002;71(3):483–91.
18. Van Eerdewegh P, Little RD, Dupuis J, et al. Association of the ADAM33 gene with asthma and bronchial hyperresponsiveness. Nature 2002;418(6896): 426–30.
19. Allen M, Heinzmann A, Noguchi E, et al. Positional cloning of a novel gene influencing asthma from chromosome 2q14. Nat Genet 2003;35(3):258–63.
20. Laitinen T, Polvi A, Rydman P, et al. Characterization of a common susceptibility locus for asthma-related traits. Science 2004;304(5668):300–4.
21. Nicolae D, Cox NJ, Lester LA, et al. Fine mapping and positional candidate studies identify HLA-G as an asthma susceptibility gene on chromosome 6p21. Am J Hum Genet 2005;76:349–57.
22. Noguchi E, Yokouchi Y, Zhang J, et al. Positional identification of an asthma susceptibility gene on human chromosome 5q33. Am J Respir Crit Care Med 2005; 172(2):183–8.
23. Zhang Y, Leaves NI, Anderson GG, et al. Positional cloning of a quantitative trait locus on chromosome 13q14 that influences immunoglobulin E levels and asthma. Nat Genet 2003;34(2):181–6.
24. Barnes KC. An update on the genetics of atopic dermatitis: scratching the surface in 2009. J Allergy Clin Immunol 2009;125(1):16–29.e1-11 [quiz: 30–11].

25. Haagerup A, Bjerke T, Schoitz PO, et al. Allergic rhinitis—a total genome-scan for susceptibility genes suggests a locus on chromosome 4q24-q27. Eur J Hum Genet 2001;9(12):945–52.
26. Yokouchi Y, Shibasaki M, Noguchi E, et al. A genome-wide linkage analysis of orchard grass-sensitive childhood seasonal allergic rhinitis in Japanese families. Genes Immun 2002;3(1):9–13.
27. Kurz T, Altmueller J, Strauch K, et al. A genome-wide screen on the genetics of atopy in a multiethnic European population reveals a major atopy locus on chromosome 3q21.3. Allergy 2005;60(2):192–9.
28. Dizier MH, Bouzigon E, Guilloud-Bataille M, et al. Genome screen in the French EGEA study: detection of linked regions shared or not shared by allergic rhinitis and asthma. Genes Immun 2005;6(2):95–102.
29. Kruse LV, Nyegaard M, Christensen U, et al. A genome-wide search for linkage to allergic rhinitis in Danish sib-pair families. Eur J Hum Genet 2012;20(9):965–72.
30. Venter JC, Adams MD, Myers EW, et al. The sequence of the human genome. Science 2001;291(5507):1304–51.
31. Lander ES, Linton LM, Birren B, et al. Initial sequencing and analysis of the human genome. Nature 2001;409(6822):860–921.
32. Ober C, Hoffjan S. Asthma genetics 2006: the long and winding road to gene discovery. Genes Immun 2006;7(2):95–100.
33. Vercelli D. Discovering susceptibility genes for asthma and allergy. Nat Rev Immunol 2008;8(3):169–82.
34. Ober C, Yao TC. The genetics of asthma and allergic disease: a 21st century perspective. Immunol Rev 2011;242(1):10–30.
35. Mathias RA. Introduction to genetics and genomics in asthma: genetics of asthma. Adv Exp Med Biol 2014;795:125–55.
36. The International HapMap Consortium. The International HapMap Project. Nature 2003;426(6968):789–96.
37. International HapMap Consortium. A haplotype map of the human genome. Nature 2005;437(7063):1299–320.
38. Thorisson GA, Smith AV, Krishnan L, et al. The International hapmap project web site. Genome Res 2005;15(11):1592–3.
39. Abecasis GR, Auton A, Brooks LD, et al. An integrated map of genetic variation from 1,092 human genomes. Nature 2012;491(7422):56–65.
40. Howie B, Fuchsberger C, Stephens M, et al. Fast and accurate genotype imputation in genome-wide association studies through pre-phasing. Nature Genetics 2012;44(8):955–99.
41. Auer PL, Johnsen JM, Johnson AD, et al. Imputation of exome sequence variants into population- based samples and blood-cell-trait-associated loci in African Americans: NHLBI GO Exome Sequencing Project. Am J Hum Genet 2012; 91(5):794–808.
42. Hindorff LA, MacArthur J, Morales J, et al. A catalog of published genome-wide association studies, 2012. Available at: http://www.genome.gov/gwastudies.
43. Welter D, Macarthur J, Morales J, et al. The NHGRI GWAS catalog, a curated resource of SNP-trait associations. Nucleic Acids Res 2014;42(1):D1001–6.
44. Trynka G, Hunt KA, Bockett NA, et al. Dense genotyping identifies and localizes multiple common and rare variant association signals in celiac disease. Nat Genet 2011;43(12):1193–201.
45. Moffatt MF, Kabesch M, Liang L, et al. Genetic variants regulating ORMDL3 expression are determinants of susceptibility to childhood asthma. Nature 2007;448(7152):470–3.

46. Gabriel A. GABRIEL Consortium large-scale genome-wide association study of asthma. 2014. Available at: http://www.cng.fr/gabriel/index.html.
47. Moffatt MF, Gut IG, Demenais F, et al. A large-scale, consortium-based genome-wide association study of asthma. N Engl J Med 2010;363(13):1211–21.
48. Torgerson DG, Ampleford EJ, Chiu GY, et al. Meta-analysis of genome-wide association studies of asthma in ethnically diverse North American populations. Nat Genet 2011;43(9):887–92.
49. Gudbjartsson DF, Bjornsdottir US, Halapi E, et al. Sequence variants affecting eosinophil numbers associate with asthma and myocardial infarction. Nat Genet 2009;41(3):342–7.
50. Ferreira MA, McRae AF, Medland SE, et al. Association between ORMDL3, IL1RL1 and a deletion on chromosome 17q21 with asthma risk in Australia. Eur J Hum Genet 2010;19(4):458–64.
51. Ferreira MA, Matheson MC, Duffy DL, et al. Identification of IL6R and chromosome 11q13.5 as risk loci for asthma. Lancet 2011;378(9795):1006–14.
52. Weidinger S, O'Sullivan M, Illig T, et al. Filaggrin mutations, atopic eczema, hay fever, and asthma in children. J Allergy Clin Immunol 2008;121(5):1203–9.e1.
53. Ono JG, Worgall TS, Worgall S. 17q21 locus and ORMDL3: an increased risk for childhood asthma. Pediatr Res 2014;75(1–2):165–70.
54. Brown CD, Mangravite LM, Engelhardt BE. Integrative modeling of eQTLs and cis-regulatory elements suggests mechanisms underlying cell type specificity of eQTLs. PLoS Genet 2013;9(8):e1003649.
55. Reich DE, Lander ES. On the allelic spectrum of human disease. Trends Genet 2001;17(9):502–10.
56. Manolio TA, Collins FS, Cox NJ, et al. Finding the missing heritability of complex diseases. Nature 2009;461(7265):747–53.
57. Gorlov IP, Gorlova OY, Frazier ML, et al. Evolutionary evidence of the effect of rare variants on disease etiology. Clin Genet 2011;79(3):199–206.
58. Marth GT, Yu F, Indap AR, et al. The functional spectrum of low-frequency coding variation. Genome Biol 2011;12(9):R84.
59. Sanger F, Nicklen S, Coulson AR. DNA sequencing with chain-terminating inhibitors. Proc Natl Acad Sci U S A 1977;74(12):5463–7.
60. Shendure J, Porreca GJ, Reppas NB, et al. Accurate multiplex polony sequencing of an evolved bacterial genome. Science 2005;309(5741):1728–32.
61. Panoutsopoulou K, Tachmazidou I, Zeggini E. In search of low-frequency and rare variants affecting complex traits. Hum Mol Genet 2013;22(R1):R16–21.
62. Nijman IJ, van Montfrans JM, Hoogstraat M, et al. Targeted next-generation sequencing: a novel diagnostic tool for primary immunodeficiencies. J Allergy Clin Immunol 2014;133(2):529–34.
63. Leung TF, Ko FW, Sy HY, et al. Differences in asthma genetics between Chinese and other populations. J Allergy Clin Immunol 2014;133(1):42–8.
64. DeWan AT, Egan KB, Hellenbrand K, et al. Whole-exome sequencing of a pedigree segregating asthma. BMC Med Genet 2012;13:95.
65. Fu W, O'Connor TD, Jun G, et al. Analysis of 6,515 exomes reveals the recent origin of most human protein-coding variants. Nature 2013;493(7431):216–20.
66. Mathias RA, Huang L, O'Connor TD, et al. Patterns of genetic variation in populations of African ancestry observed in whole genome sequencing of 691 individuals from CAAPA. Am J Hum Genet 2013.
67. Shaikh TH. Oligonucleotide arrays for high-resolution analysis of copy number alteration in mental retardation/multiple congenital anomalies. Genet Med 2007;9(9):617–25.

68. Sordillo J, Raby BA. Gene expression profiling in asthma. Adv Exp Med Biol 2014;795:157–81.
69. Marioni JC, Mason CE, Mane SM, et al. RNA-seq: an assessment of technical reproducibility and comparison with gene expression arrays. Genome Res 2008;18(9):1509–17.
70. Fu X, Fu N, Guo S, et al. Estimating accuracy of RNA-Seq and microarrays with proteomics. BMC Genomics 2009;10:161.
71. Cullum R, Alder O, Hoodless PA. The next generation: using new sequencing technologies to analyse gene regulation. Respirology 2011;16(2):210–22.
72. Cloonan N, Grimmond SM. Transcriptome content and dynamics at single-nucleotide resolution. Genome Biol 2008;9(9):234.
73. Wang Z, Gerstein M, Snyder M. RNA-Seq: a revolutionary tool for transcriptomics. Nat Rev Genet 2009;10(1):57–63.
74. Yick CY, Zwinderman AH, Kunst PW, et al. Gene expression profiling of laser microdissected airway smooth muscle tissue in asthma and atopy. Allergy 2014; 69:1233–40.
75. Himes BE, Jiang X, Wagner P, et al. RNA-Seq transcriptome profiling identifies CRISPLD2 as a glucocorticoid responsive gene that modulates cytokine function in airway smooth muscle cells. PLoS One 2014;9:e99625.
76. Yick CY, Zwinderman AH, Kunst PW, et al. Glucocorticoid-induced changes in gene expression of airway smooth muscle in patients with asthma. Am J Respir Crit Care Med 2013;187(10):1076–84.
77. Poole A, Urbanek C, Eng C, et al. Dissecting childhood asthma with nasal transcriptomics distinguishes subphenotypes of disease. J Allergy Clin Immunol 2014;133(3):670–8.e2.
78. Schadt EE, Monks SA, Drake TA, et al. Genetics of gene expression surveyed in maize, mouse and man. Nature 2003;422(6929):297–302.
79. Cheung VG, Spielman RS. Genetics of human gene expression: mapping DNA variants that influence gene expression. Nat Rev Genet 2009;10(9): 595–604.
80. Li B, Leal SM. Methods for detecting associations with rare variants for common diseases: application to analysis of sequence data. Am J Hum Genet 2008; 83(3):311–21.
81. Hao K, Bosse Y, Nickle DC, et al. Lung eQTLs to help reveal the molecular underpinnings of asthma. PLoS Genet 2012;8(11):e1003029.
82. Li L, Kabesch M, Bouzigon E, et al. Using eQTL weights to improve power for genome-wide association studies: a genetic study of childhood asthma. Front Genet 2013;4:103.
83. Dixon AL, Liang L, Moffatt MF, et al. A genome-wide association study of global gene expression. Nat Genet 2007;39(10):1202–7.
84. Stranger BE, Nica AC, Forrest MS, et al. Population genomics of human gene expression. Nat Genet 2007;39(10):1217–24.
85. Min JL, Taylor JM, Richards JB, et al. The use of genome-wide eQTL associations in lymphoblastoid cell lines to identify novel genetic pathways involved in complex traits. PLoS One 2011;6(7):e22070.
86. Murphy A, Chu JH, Xu M, et al. Mapping of numerous disease-associated expression polymorphisms in primary peripheral blood CD4+ lymphocytes. Hum Mol Genet 2010;19(23):4745–57.
87. Sharma S, Zhou X, Thibault DM, et al. A genome-wide survey of CD4 lymphocyte regulatory genetic variants identifies novel asthma genes. J Allergy Clin Immunol 2014.

88. Goldman JA, Klimek GA, Ali R. Allergy in systemic lupus erythematosus. IgE levels and reaginic phenomenon. Arthritis Rheum 1976;19(4):669–76.
89. Diumenjo MS, Lisanti M, Valles R, et al. Allergic manifestations of systemic lupus erythematosus. Allergol Immunopathol (Madr) 1985;13(4):323–6 [in Spanish].
90. Sequeira JF, Cesic D, Keser G, et al. Allergic disorders in systemic lupus erythematosus. Lupus 1993;2(3):187–91.
91. Shahar E, Lorber M. Allergy and SLE: common and variable. Isr J Med Sci 1997; 33(2):147–9.
92. Azad AK, Islam N, Islam MA, et al. Cough in systemic lupus erythematosus. Mymensingh Med J 2013;22(2):300–7.
93. Shen TC, Tu CY, Lin CL, et al. Increased risk of asthma in patients with systemic lupus erythematosus. Am J Respir Crit Care Med 2014;189(4):496–9.
94. Jimenez-Morales S, Velazquez-Cruz R, Ramirez-Bello J, et al. Tumor necrosis factor-alpha is a common genetic risk factor for asthma, juvenile rheumatoid arthritis, and systemic lupus erythematosus in a Mexican pediatric population. Hum Immunol 2009;70(4):251–6.
95. Rangasamy T, Guo J, Mitzner WA, et al. Disruption of Nrf2 enhances susceptibility to severe airway inflammation and asthma in mice. J Exp Med 2005;202(1): 47–59.
96. Postma DS, Kerkhof M, Boezen HM, et al. Asthma and chronic obstructive pulmonary disease: common genes, common environments? Am J Respir Crit Care Med 2011;183(12):1588–94.
97. Yao TC, Du G, Han L, et al. Genome-wide association study of lung function phenotypes in a founder population. J Allergy Clin Immunol 2014;133: 248–55.e1-10.
98. Hardin M, Cho M, McDonald ML, et al. The clinical and genetic features of COPD-asthma overlap syndrome. Eur Respir J 2014;44:341–50.
99. Strachan DP. Hay fever, hygiene, and household size. BMJ 1989;299(6710): 1259–60.
100. Pearce EJ, MacDonald AS. The immunobiology of schistosomiasis. Nat Rev Immunol 2002;2(7):499–511.
101. Barnes KC, Grant AV, Gao P. A review of the genetic epidemiology of resistance to parasitic disease and atopic asthma: common variants for common phenotypes? Curr Opin Allergy Clin Immunol 2005;5(5):379–85.
102. Wheelock CE, Goss VM, Balgoma D, et al. Application of 'omics technologies to biomarker discovery in inflammatory lung diseases. Eur Respir J 2013;42(3): 802–25.
103. Derks KW, Hoeijmakers JH, Pothof J. The DNA damage response: the omics era and its impact. DNA Repair (Amst) 2014;19:214–20.
104. Donaldson A, Natanek SA, Lewis A, et al. Increased skeletal muscle-specific microRNA in the blood of patients with COPD. Thorax 2013;68(12):1140–9.
105. Tan Z, Randall G, Fan J, et al. Allele-specific targeting of microRNAs to HLA-G and risk of asthma. Am J Hum Genet 2007;81(4):829–34.
106. Jardim MJ, Dailey L, Silbajoris R, et al. Distinct microRNA expression in human airway cells of asthmatic donors identifies a novel asthma-associated gene. Am J Respir Cell Mol Biol 2012;47(4):536–42.
107. Solberg OD, Ostrin EJ, Love MI, et al. Airway epithelial miRNA expression is altered in asthma. Am J Respir Crit Care Med 2012;186(10):965–74.
108. Plank M, Maltby S, Mattes J, et al. Targeting translational control as a novel way to treat inflammatory disease: the emerging role of microRNAs. Clin Exp Allergy 2013;43(9):981–99.

109. Huang JC, Babak T, Corson TW, et al. Using expression profiling data to identify human microRNA targets. Nat Methods 2007;4(12):1045–9.
110. Sales G, Coppe A, Bisognin A, et al. MAGIA, a web-based tool for miRNA and Genes Integrated Analysis. Nucleic Acids Res 2010;38(Web Server Issue): W352–9.
111. Elkan-Miller T, Ulitsky I, Hertzano R, et al. Integration of transcriptomics, proteomics, and microRNA analyses reveals novel microRNA regulation of targets in the mammalian inner ear. PLoS One 2011;6(4):e18195.
112. Beck D, Ayers S, Wen J, et al. Integrative analysis of next generation sequencing for small non-coding RNAs and transcriptional regulation in Myelodysplastic Syndromes. BMC Med Genomic 2011;4:19.
113. Muniategui A, Pey J, Planes FJ, et al. Joint analysis of miRNA and mRNA expression data. Brief Bioinform 2013;14(3):263–78.
114. Jalali S, Bhartiya D, Lalwani MK, et al. Systematic transcriptome wide analysis of lncRNA-miRNA interactions. PLoS One 2013;8(2):e53823.
115. Hu R, Pan W, Fedulov AV, et al. MicroRNA-10a controls airway smooth muscle cell proliferation via direct targeting of the PI3 kinase pathway. FASEB J 2014; 28(5):2347–57.
116. Marsh DG, Meyers DA, Bias WB. The epidemiology and genetics of atopic allergy. N Engl J Med 1981;305(26):1551–9.
117. Nystad W, Roysamb E, Magnus P, et al. A comparison of genetic and environmental variance structures for asthma, hay fever and eczema with symptoms of the same diseases: a study of Norwegian twins. Int J Epidemiol 2005;34(6):1302–9.
118. Norman RE, Carpenter DO, Scott J, et al. Environmental exposures: an underrecognized contribution to noncommunicable diseases. Rev Environ Health 2013;28(1):59–65.
119. Baldini M, Lohman IC, Halonen M, et al. A Polymorphism* in the 5' flanking region of the CD14 gene is associated with circulating soluble CD14 levels and with total serum immunoglobulin E. Am J Respir Cell Mol Biol 1999;20(5): 976–83.
120. Ober C, Tselenko A, Cox NJ. Searching for asthma and atopy genes in the Hutterites: genome-wide studies using linkage and association. Am J Respir Crit Care Med 2000;161(3):A600.
121. Zambelli-Weiner A, Ehrlich A, Stockton ML, et al. Evaluation of the CD14/-260 polymorphism and house dust endotoxin exposure in the Barbados asthma genetics study. J Allergy Clin Immunol 115(6):1203-9.
122. Magnusson LL, Olesen AB, Wennborg H, et al. Wheezing, asthma, hayfever, and atopic eczema in childhood following exposure to tobacco smoke in fetal life. Clin Exp Allergy 2005;35(12):1550–6.
123. Li YF, Gilliland FD, Berhane K, et al. Effects of in utero and environmental tobacco smoke exposure on lung function in boys and girls with and without asthma. Am J Respir Crit Care Med 2000;162(6):2097–104.
124. Moshammer H, Hoek G, Luttmann-Gibson H, et al. Parental smoking and lung function in children: an international study. Am J Respir Crit Care Med 2006; 173(11):1255–63.
125. Raherison C, Penard-Morand C, Moreau D, et al. In utero and childhood exposure to parental tobacco smoke, and allergies in schoolchildren. Respir Med 2007;101(1):107–17.
126. Colilla S, Nicolae D, Pluzhnikov A, et al. Evidence for gene–environment interactions in a linkage study of asthma and smoking exposure. J Allergy Clin Immunol 2003;111(4):840–6.

127. Choudhry S, Avila PC, Nazario S, et al. CD14 tobacco gene-environment inter-action modifies asthma severity and immunoglobulin E levels in Latinos with asthma. Am J Respir Crit Care Med 2005;172(2):173–82.

128. Meyers DA, Postma DS, Stine OC, et al. Genome screen for asthma and bron-chial hyperresponsiveness: interactions with passive smoke exposure. J Allergy Clin Immunol 2005;115(6):1169–75.

129. Lovinsky-Desir S, Miller RL. Epigenetics, asthma, and allergic diseases: a re-view of the latest advancements. Curr Allergy Asthma Rep 2012;12(3):211–20.

130. Brand S, Kesper DA, Teich R, et al. DNA methylation of TH1/TH2 cytokine genes affects sensitization and progress of experimental asthma. J Allergy Clin Immu-nol 2012;129(6):1602–10.e6.

131. Mikhaylova L, Zhang Y, Kobzik L, et al. Link between epigenomic alterations and genome-wide aberrant transcriptional response to allergen in dendritic cells conveying maternal asthma risk. PLoS One 2013;8(8):e70387.

132. Gaffin JM, Raby BA, Petty CR, et al. beta-2 adrenergic receptor gene methyl-ation is associated with decreased asthma severity in inner-city schoolchildren: asthma and rhinitis. Clin Exp Allergy 2014;44(5):681–9.

133. Collison A, Siegle JS, Hansbro NG, et al. Epigenetic changes associated with disease progression in a mouse model of childhood allergic asthma. Dis Model Mech 2013;6(4):993–1000.

134. Durham A, Chou PC, Kirkham P, et al. Epigenetics in asthma and other inflam-matory lung diseases. Epigenomics 2010;2(4):523–37.

135. Sanders YY, Ambalavanan N, Halloran B, et al. Altered DNA methylation profile in idiopathic pulmonary fibrosis. Am J Respir Crit Care Med 2012;186(6):525–35.

136. Pandit KV, Milosevic J, Kaminski N. MicroRNAs in idiopathic pulmonary fibrosis. Transl Res 2011;157(4):191–9.

137. Dakhlallah D, Batte K, Wang Y, et al. Epigenetic regulation of miR-17~92 con-tributes to the pathogenesis of pulmonary fibrosis. Am J Respir Crit Care Med 2013;187(4):397–405.

138. Huang SK, Scruggs AM, Donaghy J, et al. Histone modifications are responsible for decreased Fas expression and apoptosis resistance in fibrotic lung fibro-blasts. Cell Death Dis 2013;4:e621.

139. Cheng RY, Shang Y, Limjunyawong N, et al. Alterations of the lung methylome in allergic airway hyper-responsiveness. Environ Mol Mutagen 2014;55(3):244–55.

140. Castle W, Fuller R, Hall J, et al. Serevent nationwide surveillance study: compar-ison of salmeterol with salbutamol in asthmatic patients who require regular bronchodilator treatment. BMJ 1993;306(6884):1034–7.

141. Nelson HS, Weiss ST, Bleecker ER, et al. The Salmeterol Multicenter Asthma Research Trial: a comparison of usual pharmacotherapy for asthma or usual pharmacotherapy plus salmeterol. Chest 2006;129(1):15–26.

142. Salpeter SR, Buckley NS, Ormiston TM, et al. Meta-analysis: effect of long-acting beta-agonists on severe asthma exacerbations and asthma-related deaths. Ann Intern Med 2006;144(12):904–12.

143. Adel-Patient K, Creminon C, Bernard H, et al. Evaluation of a high IgE-responder mouse model of allergy to bovine beta-lactoglobulin (BLG): development of sandwich immunoassays for total and allergen-specific IgE, IgG1 and IgG2a in BLG-sensitized mice. J Immunol Methods 2000;235(1–2):21–32.

144. Chan MT, Leung DY, Szefler SJ, et al. Difficult-to-control asthma: clinical charac-teristics of steroid-insensitive asthma. J Allergy Clin Immunol 1998;101(5):594–601.

145. Serra-Batlles J, Plaza V, Morejon E, et al. Costs of asthma according to the degree of severity. Eur Respir J 1998;12(6):1322–6.
146. Miller SM, Ortega VE. Pharmacogenetics and the development of personalized approaches for combination therapy in asthma. Curr Allergy Asthma Rep 2013; 13(5):443–52.
147. Poon AH, Tantisira KG, Litonjua AA, et al. Association of corticotropin-releasing hormone receptor-2 genetic variants with acute bronchodilator response in asthma. Pharmacogenet Genomics 2008;18(5):373–82.
148. Himes BE, Jiang X, Hu R, et al. Genome-wide association analysis in asthma subjects identifies SPATS2L as a novel bronchodilator response gene. PLoS Genet 2012;8(7):e1002824.
149. Tantisira KG, Small KM, Litonjua AA, et al. Molecular properties and pharmacogenetics of a polymorphism of adenylyl cyclase type 9 in asthma: interaction between beta-agonist and corticosteroid pathways. Hum Mol Genet 2005;14(12):1671–7.
150. Silverman EK, Kwiatkowski DJ, Sylvia JS, et al. Family-based association analysis of beta2-adrenergic receptor polymorphisms in the childhood asthma management program. J Allergy Clin Immunol 2003;112(5):870–6.
151. Martinez FD, Graves PE, Baldini M, et al. Association between genetic polymorphisms of the beta2-adrenoceptor and response to albuterol in children with and without a history of wheezing. J Clin Invest 1997;100(12):3184–8.
152. Taylor DR, Drazen JM, Herbison GP, et al. Asthma exacerbations during long term beta agonist use: influence of beta(2) adrenoceptor polymorphism. Thorax 2000;55(9):762–7.
153. Israel E, Drazen JM, Liggett SB, et al. The effect of polymorphisms of the beta(2)-adrenergic receptor on the response to regular use of albuterol in asthma. Am J Respir Crit Care Med 2000;162(1):75–80.
154. Israel E, Chinchilli VM, Ford JG, et al. Use of regularly scheduled albuterol treatment in asthma: genotype-stratified, randomised, placebo-controlled cross-over trial. Lancet 2004;364(9444):1505–12.
155. Wechsler ME, Lehman E, Lazarus SC, et al. beta-Adrenergic receptor polymorphisms and response to salmeterol. Am J Respir Crit Care Med 2006;173(5): 519–26.
156. Bleecker ER, Postma DS, Lawrance RM, et al. Effect of ADRB2 polymorphisms on response to longacting beta2-agonist therapy: a pharmacogenetic analysis of two randomised studies. Lancet 2007;370(9605):2118–25.
157. Bleecker ER, Yancey SW, Baitinger LA, et al. Salmeterol response is not affected by beta2-adrenergic receptor genotype in subjects with persistent asthma. J Allergy Clin Immunol 2006;118(4):809–16.
158. Litonjua AA, Lasky-Su J, Schneiter K, et al. ARG1 is a novel bronchodilator response gene: screening and replication in four asthma cohorts. Am J Respir Crit Care Med 2008;178(7):688–94.
159. Tantisira KG, Lake S, Silverman ES, et al. Corticosteroid pharmacogenetics: association of sequence variants in CRHR1 with improved lung function in asthmatics treated with inhaled corticosteroids. Hum Mol Genet 2004;13(13):1353–9.
160. Hawkins GA, Lazarus R, Smith RS, et al. The glucocorticoid receptor heterocomplex gene STIP1 is associated with improved lung function in asthmatic subjects treated with inhaled corticosteroids. J Allergy Clin Immunol 2009; 123(6):1376–83.e7.
161. Tantisira KG, Hwang ES, Raby BA, et al. TBX21: a functional variant predicts improvement in asthma with the use of inhaled corticosteroids. Proc Natl Acad Sci U S A 2004;101(52):18099–104.

162. Ye YM, Lee HY, Kim SH, et al. Pharmacogenetic study of the effects of NK2R G231E G>A and TBX21 H33Q C>G polymorphisms on asthma control with inhaled corticosteroid treatment. J Clin Pharm Ther 2009;34(6): 693–701.

163. Kim SH, Ye YM, Lee HY, et al. Combined pharmacogenetic effect of ADCY9 and ADRB2 gene polymorphisms on the bronchodilator response to inhaled combination therapy. J Clin Pharm Ther 2011;36(3):399–405.

164. Berce V, Kozmus CE, Potocnik U. Association among ORMDL3 gene expression, 17q21 polymorphism and response to treatment with inhaled corticosteroids in children with asthma. Pharmacogenomics J 2013;13(6):523–9.

165. Wooten EC, Huggins GS. Mind the dbGAP: the application of data mining to identify biological mechanisms. Mol Interv 2011;11(2):95–102.

166. O'Driscoll A, Daugelaite J, Sleator RD. 'Big data', Hadoop and cloud computing in genomics. J Biomed Inform 2013;46(5):774–81.

167. Barnes KC. Genomewide association studies in allergy and the influence of ethnicity. Curr Opin Allergy Clin Immunol 2010;10(5):427–33.

168. Lemanske RF Jr, Mauger DT, Sorkness CA, et al. Step-up therapy for children with uncontrolled asthma receiving inhaled corticosteroids. N Engl J Med 2010;362(11):975–85.

169. Wechsler ME, Castro M, Lehman E, et al. Impact of race on asthma treatment failures in the asthma clinical research network. Am J Respir Crit Care Med 2011;184(11):1247–53.

APPENDIX A: A SUMMARY OF GENOME-WIDE ASSOCIATION STUDIES (GWAS) PERFORMED ON ALLERGIC DISEASES (*P*-VALUES ON THE DISCOVERY SAMPLE *P*<10^{-5})

Population	Location	Reported Gene	Adjacent Gene (L, R)	References
Asthma				
European	1p13.1	*IGSF3*	*CD58, MIR320B1*	Ding et al,[1] 2013
European	1q25.3	*XPR1*	*ACBD6, KIAA1614*	Ding et al,[1] 2013
European	1q44	*C1orf100*	*CEP170, HNRNPU*	Forno et al,[2] 2012
European	1q21.3	*IL6R*	*SHE, LOC101928101*	Ferreira et al,[3] 2011
Mixed ethnicities	1q23.1	*PYHIN1*	*IFI16, LOC646377*	Torgerson et al,[4] 2011
Mixed ethnicities	1q21.3	*CRCT1*	*LCE5A, LCE3E*	Torgerson et al,[4] 2011
European	1q31.3	*DENND1B*	*CRB1, C1orf53*	Sleiman et al,[5] 2010
Korean	2p22.2	*CRIM1*	*LOC10028911, FEZ2*	Kim et al,[6] 2013
Korean	2q36.2	*DOCK10*	*CUL3, MIR4439*	Kim et al,[6] 2013
European	2p22.1	*Intergenic*	*THUMPD2, SLC8A1-AS1*	Ding et al,[1] 2013
European	2q34	*CPS1*	*LOC102724820, ERBB4*	Melen et al,[7] 2013
European	2p23.3	*ADCY3*	*NCOA1, DNAJC27-AS1*	Melen et al,[7] 2013
European	2p23.3	*ADCY3*	*PTRHD1, DNAJC27*	Melen et al,[7] 2013
European	2p23.3	*EFR3B*	*DNAJC27, DNMT3A*	Melen et al,[7] 2013
European	2p23.3	*Intergenic*	*ADCY3, DNAJC27*	Melen et al,[7] 2013
European	2q12.1	*IL1RL1*	*IL1R1, IL18RAP*	Ramasamy et al,[8] 2012
European	2q33.1	*SPATS2L*	*TYW5, SGOL2*	Himes et al,[9] 2012
European	2q12.1	*IL1RL1, IL18R1*	*IL1R2, IL18RAP*	Wan et al,[10] 2012
Mixed ethnicities	2q12.1	*IL1RL1*	*IL1R1, IL18RAP*	Torgerson et al,[4] 2011
European	2q12.1	*IL18R1*	*IL1RL1, IL18RAP*	Moffatt et al,[11] 2010
European	3q13.2	*ATG3*	*BTLA, SLC3A5*	Ding et al,[1] 2013
European	3p22.3	*Intergenic*	*LOC101928135, ARPP21*	Ding et al,[1] 2013
European	3q26.32	*Intergenic*	*LOC102724550, KCNB2*	Ding et al,[1] 2013
European	3q12.2	*ABI3BP*	*TFG, IMPG2*	Ding et al,[1] 2013
European	3p26.2	*IL5RA*	*CNTN4, LRRN1*	Forno et al,[2] 2012
Korean	4q26	*SYNPO2*	*SEC24D, MYOZ2*	Kim et al,[6] 2013
European	4q12	*Intergenic*	*IGFBP7, LPHN3*	Ding et al,[1] 2013
European	4p14	*KLHL5*	*TMEM156, WDR19*	Ding et al,[1] 2013
European	4p15.1	*Intergenic*	*PCDH7, ARAP2*	Melen et al,[7] 2013
Japanese	4q31.21	*LOC729675*	*INPP4B, USP38*	Hirota et al,[12] 2011
Japanese	4q31.21	*GAB1*	*USP38, SMARCA5*	Hirota et al,[12] 2011
European	5q31.1	*C5orf56*	*SLC22A5, IRF1*	Wan et al,[10] 2012
European	5q31.3	*NDFIP1*	*GNPDA1, NDFIP1*	Wan et al,[10] 2012
Japanese	5q22.1	*TSLP*	*SLC25A46, WDR36*	Hirota et al,[12] 2011
Mixed ethnicities	5q22.1	*TSLP*	*SLC25A46, WDR36*	Torgerson et al,[4] 2011

(continued on next page)

(continued)

Population	Location	Reported Gene	Adjacent Gene (L, R)	References
European	5q31.1	SLC22A5	LOC553103, C5orf56	Moffatt et al,[11] 2010
European	5q31.1	IL13	RAD50, IL4	Moffatt et al,[11] 2010
European	5q31.1	RAD50	IL5, IL13	Li et al,[13] 2010
European	5q12.1	PDE4D	RAB3C, PART1	Himes et al,[14] 2009
European	6p21.1	Intergenic	CDC5L, SUPT3H	Ding et al,[1] 2013
European	6q21	Intergenic	RFPL4B, LINC01268	Ding et al,[1] 2013
European	6p12.3	AL139097.1	TFA2B, PKHD1	Melen et al,[7] 2013
European	6p21.32	HLA-DQA1	HLA-DRB1, HLA-DQB1	Lasky-Su et al,[15] 2012
Korean	6p21.32	HLA-DPB1	HLA-DPA1, HLA-DPB2	Park et al,[16] 2013
European	6p21.32	BTNL2	HCG23, HLA-DRA	Ramasamy et al,[8] 2012
European	6q27	T	LINC00602, PRR18	Tantisira et al,[17] 2012
Japanese	6p21.32	PBX2	AGER, GPSM3	Hirota et al,[12] 2011
Japanese	6p21.32	NOTCH4	GPSM2, C6orf10	Hirota et al,[12] 2011
Japanese	6p21.32	C6orf10	NOTCH4, HCG23	Hirota et al,[12] 2011
Japanese	6p21.32	BTNL2	HCG23, HLA-DRA	Hirota et al,[12] 2011
Japanese	6p21.32	HLA-DRA	BTNL2, HLA-DRB5	Hirota et al,[12] 2011
Japanese	6p21.32	HLA-DQB1	HLA-DQA1, HLA-DQA2	Hirota et al,[12] 2011
Japanese	6p21.32	HLA-DQA2	HLA-DQB1, HLA-DQB2	Hirota et al,[12] 2011
Japanese	6p21.32	HLA-DOA	BRD2, HLA-DPA1	Hirota et al,[12] 2011
Japanese	6p21.32	HLA-DPB1	HLA-DPA1, HLA-DPB2	Noguchi et al,[18] 2011
European	6p21.32	HLA-DQB1	HLA-DQA1, HLA-DQA2	Moffatt et al,[11] 2010
European	7p15.3	Intergenic	NPY, STK31	Ding et al,[1] 2013
European	7q32.3	MKLN1	LINC-PINT, PODXL	Ding et al,[1] 2013
Korean	8q11.23	OPRK1	NPBWR1, ATP6V1H	Kim et al,[6] 2013
European	8p12	Intergenic	DUSP26, UNC5D	Ding et al,[1] 2013
European	8q24.23	COL22A1	FAM135B, KCNK9	Duan et al,[19] 2014
Japanese	8q24.11	SLC30A8	AARD, MED30	Noguchi et al,[18] 2011
Korean	9p13.3	TLN1	TPM2, MIR6852	Kim et al,[6] 2013
European	9p23	Intergenic	PTPRD-AS2, TYRP1	Ding et al,[1] 2013
European	9q21.33	Intergenic	ZCCHC6, GAS1	Ding et al,[1] 2013
European	9p22.1	SLC24A2	ACER2, MLLT3	Melen et al,[7] 2013
European	9q33.3	DENND1A	CRB2, LHX2	Melen et al,[7] 2013
European	9p21.1	ACO1	LINX01242, DDX58	Wan et al,[10] 2012
Mixed ethnicities	9p24.1	IL33	RANBP6, TPD52L3	Torgerson et al,[4] 2011
European	9p24.1	IL33	RANBP6, TPD52L3	Moffatt et al,[11] 2010
Mexican	9q21.31	TLE4, CHCHD9	LOC101927450, LOC101927477	Hancock et al,[20] 2009
Korean	9p21.3	Intergenic	SLC24A2, MLLT3	Kim et al,[21] 2009
European	10q24.2	HPSE2	HPS1, CNNM1	Ding et al,[1] 2013
European	10q22.1	PSAP	CDH23, CHST3	Ding et al,[1] 2013
European	10p15.1	PRKCQ	LOC399715, PRKCQ-AS1	Melen et al,[7] 2013

(continued on next page)

(continued)

Population	Location	Reported Gene	Adjacent Gene (L, R)	References
European	10q26.11	EMX2	PDZD8, RAB11FIP2	Li et al,[22] 2013
European	10p15.1	PRKCQ	LOC101927964, LINC00702	Duan et al,[19] 2014
European	10q21.1	PRKG1	A1CF, PRKG1-AS1	Ferreira et al,[3] 2011
Japanese	10p14	LOC338591	LINC00708, LOC101928272	Hirota et al,[12] 2011
Korean	10q21.3	CTNNA3	LOC101928913, LRRTM3	Kim et al,[21] 2009
Korean	11q24.1	OR6X1	ZNF202, OR6M1	Kim et al,[6] 2013
European	11q13.4	P2RY2	FCHSD2, P2RY2	Melen et al,[7] 2013
European	11q24.2	NR	LOC101929497, ETS1	Forno et al,[2] 2012
European	11q13.5	LRRC32	C11orf30, GUCY2EP	Ferreira et al,[3] 2011
Mixed ethnicities	11q23.2	C11orf71	LOC101928940, RBM7	Torgerson et al,[4] 2011
Japanese	12q13.2	CDK2	PMEL, RAB5B	Hirota et al,[12] 2011
Japanese	12q13.2	IKZF4	SUOX, RPS26	Hirota et al,[12] 2011
European	13q13.1	STARD13, RP11-81F11.3	KL, RFC3	Melen et al,[7] 2013
European	13q13.3	NR	MIR548F5, DCLK1	Forno et al,[2] 2012
European	13q21.31	PCDH20	MIR3169, LINC00358	Ferreira et al,[3] 2011
Korean	13q12.13	Intergenic	GPR12, USP12	Kim et al,[21] 2009
Korean	14q32.2	LOC730217	C14orf64, C14orf177	Kim et al,[6] 2013
European	15q22.33	SMAD3	SMAD6, AAGAB	Moffatt et al,[11] 2010
European	15q22.2	RORA	LOC101928784, VPS13C	Moffatt et al,[11] 2010
European	15q21.2	SCG3	DMXL2, LYSMD2	Li et al,[13] 2010
Korean	16q23.3	CDH13	MPH0SPH6, MLYCD	Kim et al,[6] 2013
European	17q21.32	Intergenic	MIR196A1, PRAC1	Melen et al,[7] 2013
European	17q21.32	Intergenic	MIR196A1, PRAC1	Melen et al,[7] 2013
European	17q12	ORMDL3	GSDMB, LRRC3C	Wan et al,[10] 2012
European	17p12	NR	HS3ST3A1, COX10-AS1	Forno et al,[2] 2012
Mixed ethnicities	17q12	GSDMB	ZPBP2, ORMDL3	Torgerson et al,[4] 2011
European	17q12	ORMDL3	GSDMB, LRRC3C	Ferreira et al,[23] 2011
European	17q12	GSDMB	ZPBP2, ORMDL3	Moffatt et al,[11] 2010
European	17q21.1	GSDMA	LRRC3C, PSMD3	Moffatt et al,[11] 2010
European	17q12	ORMDL3	GSDMB, LRRC3C	Moffatt et al,[11] 2010
European	18p11.31	LPIN2	EMILIN2, MYOM1	Melen et al,[7] 2013
European	18p11.32	YES1	ENOSF1, ADCYAP1	Li et al,[22] 2013
Korean	19q13.43	ZNF71	ZNF470, SMIM17	Kim et al,[6] 2013
European	19p13.11	IL12RB1	AARDC2, MAST3	Li et al,[22] 2013
European	19q13.42	ZNF665	ZNF347, ZNF818P	Wan et al,[10] 2012
European	20p12.3	Intergenic	MIR8062, HA01	Ding et al,[1] 2013

(continued on next page)

(continued)

Population	Location	Reported Gene	Adjacent Gene (L, R)	References
European	20q13.2	*Intergenic*	*LOC101927700, TSHZ2*	Melen et al,[7] 2013
European	20p13	*KIAA1271*	*AP5S1, MAVS*	Li et al,[13] 2010
European	22q13.31	*UPK3A*	*NUP50, FAM118A*	Li et al,[22] 2013
European	22q12.3	*IL2RB*	*TMPRSS6, C1QTNF6*	Moffatt et al,[11] 2010
European	NR	*Intergenic*		Wan et al,[10] 2012
Atopic Dermatitis				
European	1q21.3	*FLG*	*HRNR, FLG2*	Weidinger et al,[24] 2013
Chinese	1q21.3	*FLG*	*HRNR, FLG2*	Sun et al,[25] 2011
Japanese	2q12.1	*IL1RL1, IL18R1, IL18RAP*	*IL1R1, IL18RAP, IL1R2*	Hirota et al,[26] 2012
Japanese	2q13	*LOC100505634*	*BCL2L11, MIR4435-1*	Hirota et al,[26] 2012
Japanese	3p22.3	*GLB1*	*CCR4, SUSD5*	Hirota et al,[26] 2012
Japanese	3q13.2	*CCDC80*	*LINC01279, LOC101929694*	Hirota et al,[26] 2012
European	5q31.1	*IL13*	*RAD50, IL4*	Weidinger et al,[24] 2013
Japanese	5q31.1	*IL13*	*RAD50, IL4*	Hirota et al,[26] 2012
European	5q31.1	*IL13*	*RAD50, IL4*	Paternoster et al,[27] 2012
European	6p21.33	*TNXB*	*CYP21A2, ATF6B*	Weidinger et al,[24] 2013
Japanese	6p21.33	*HLA-C*	*HCG27, HLA-B*	Hirota et al,[26] 2012
Japanese	6p21.32	*GPSM3*	*PBX2, NOTCH4*	Hirota et al,[26] 2012
Japanese	6p21.32	*C6orf10*	*NOTCH4, HCG23*	Hirota et al,[26] 2012
European	6p21.33	*BAT1*	*MCCD1, DDX39B*	Paternoster et al,[27] 2012
Japanese	7p22.2	*CARD11*	*GNA12, SDK1*	Hirota et al,[26] 2012
Japanese	8q24.21	*MIR1208*	*PVT1, LINC00977*	Hirota et al,[26] 2012
European	8q21.13	*ZBTB10*	*MIR5708, ZNF704*	Paternoster et al,[27] 2012
Japanese	10q21.2	*ZNF365*	*LOC283045, EGR2*	Hirota et al,[26] 2012
Japanese	10q21.3	*ADO, EGR2*	*ZNF365, NRBF2*	Hirota et al,[26] 2012
European	11q13.5	*C11orf30*	*LOC100506127, LRRC32*	Weidinger et al,[24] 2013
Japanese	11p15.4	*OR10A3, NLRP10*	*OR10A3, NLRP10*	Hirota et al,[26] 2012
Japanese	11q13.5	*C11orf30*	*LOC100506127, LRRC32*	Hirota et al,[26] 2012
Japanese	11q13.1	*OVOL1*	*AP5B1, SNX32*	Hirota et al,[26] 2012
European	11q13.1	*OVOL1*	*AP5B1, SNX32*	Paternoster et al,[27] 2012
European	11q13.5	*C11orf30*	*LOC100506127, LRRC32*	Esparza-Gordillo et al,[28] 2009
Japanese	16p13.13	*CLEC16A*	*DEXI, SOCS1*	Hirota et al,[26] 2012
European	19p13.2	*ACTL9*	*ADAMTS10, OR2Z1*	Paternoster et al,[27] 2012
Japanese	20q13.2	*CYP24A1, PFDN4*	*CYP24A1, PFDN4*	Hirota et al,[26] 2012
European	22q12.3	*NCF4*	*PVALB, CSF2RB*	Paternoster et al,[27] 2012

(continued on next page)

(continued)

Population	Location	Reported Gene	Adjacent Gene (L, R)	References
Atopy				
European	2p21	*SGK493*	*C2orf91, PKDCC*	Castro-Giner et al,[29] 2009
Allergic Rhinitis				
European	1p36.13	*CROCC*	*MIR3675, MFAP2*	Ramasamy et al,[30] 2011
European	5q22.1	*TMEM232, SLCA25A46*	*LOC100289673, TSLP*	Ramasamy et al,[30] 2011
European	5q22.1	*TSLP*	*SLC25A46, WDR36*	Ramasamy et al,[30] 2011
European	5q23.1	*SEMA6A*	*LOC101927190, LOC102467223*	Ramasamy et al,[30] 2011
European	7p14.1	*GLI3*	*INHBA-AS1, LINC01448*	Ramasamy et al,[30] 2011
European	11q13.5	*C11orf30, LRRC32*	*LOC100506127, GUCY2EP*	Ramasamy et al,[30] 2011
European	14q23.1	*PPM1A, DHRS7*	*PCNXL4, C14orf39*	Ramasamy et al,[30] 2011
European	16p13.13	*CLEC16A*	*DEXI, SOCS1*	Ramasamy et al,[30] 2011
European	20p11.21	*ENTPD6*	*LOC101926889, PYGB*	Ramasamy et al,[30] 2011
Total and Specific Immunoglobulin E				
European	1p32.3	*EPS15*	*TTC39A, OSBPL9*	Ramasamy et al,[30] 2011
European	1q23.2	*DARC*	*CADM3-AS1, ACKR1*	Granada et al,[31] 2012
European	1q23.2	*FCER1A*	*ACKR1, OR10J3*	Weidinger et al,[32] 2008
European	1q23.2	*FCER1A*	*Mus Olfr418-ps1, OR10J3*	Granada et al,[31] 2012
European	1q23.2	*OR10J3*	*FCER1A, OR10J1*	Granada et al,[31] 2012
European	1q25.2	*ABL2*	*TOR3A, SOAT1*	Ramasamy et al,[30] 2011
Korean	2p22.2	*CRIM1*	*LOC100288911, FEZ2*	Kim et al,[6] 2013
European	2p25.1	*ID2*	*LOC100506299, MBOAT2*	Granada et al,[31] 2012
Korean	2q36.2	*DOCK10*	*CUL3, NYAP2*	Kim et al,[6] 2013
Mixed ethnicities	3p14.1	*SUCLG2*	*MIR4272, SUCLG2-AS1*	Levin et al,[33] 2013
European	3q22.1	*TMEM108*	*NPHP3-AS1, BFSP2*	Ramasamy et al,[30] 2011
European	3q28	*LPP*	*BCL6, TPRG1-AS1*	Granada et al,[31] 2012
Korean	4q26	*SYNPO2*	*SEC240, MYOZ2*	Kim et al,[6] 2013
European	4q27	*IL2*	*ADAD1, IL21*	Ramasamy et al,[30] 2011
European	5p15.2	*DNAH5*	*LINC01194, TRIO*	Ramasamy et al,[30] 2011
European	5q22.1	*TMEM232, SLCA25A46*	*LOC100289673, TSLP*	Ramasamy et al,[30] 2011
European	5q31.1	*IL13*	*BC042122, IL4*	Granada et al,[31] 2012
European	5q31.1	*RAD50*	*IL5, IL13*	Weidinger et al,[32] 2008
European	6p21.32	*HLA region*	*HLA-DQB1, HLADQA2*	Ramasamy et al,[30] 2011
European	6p21.32	*HLA-DQA2*	*HLA-DQB1, HLA-DQB2*	Granada et al,[31] 2012
Mixed ethnicities	6p21.32	*HLA-DQA2*	*HLA-DQB1, HLA-DQB2*	Levin et al,[33] 2013

(continued on next page)

Population	Location	Reported Gene	Adjacent Gene (L, R)	References
(continued)				
Mixed ethnicities	6p21.32	*HLA-DQB1*	*HLA-DQA1, HLADQA2*	Levin et al,[33] 2013
European	6p22.1	*HLA-G*	*LOC554223, HLA-H*	Granada et al,[31] 2012
European	6p22.1	*HLA-A*	*HCG4B, HCG9*	Granada et al,[31] 2012
Korean	8q11.23	*OPRK1*	*NPBWR1, ATP6V1H*	Kim et al,[6] 2013
Korean	9p13.3	*TLN1*	*TPM2, CREB3*	Kim et al,[6] 2013
Korean	11q24.1	*OR6X1*	*ZNF202, ORM1*	Kim et al,[6] 2013
European	12q13.3	*STAT6, NAB2*	*TMEM194A, LRP1*	Granada et al,[31] 2012
Korean	14q32.2	*LOC730217*	*C14orf64, C14orf177*	Kim et al,[6] 2013
European	16p12.1	*IL4R*	*FLJ21408, IL21R*	Granada et al,[31] 2012
European	16p13.2	*Intergenic*	*MIR548X, MIR7641-2*	Ramasamy et al,[30] 2011
Mixed ethnicities	16q22.1	*WWP2*	*NOB1, PDXDC2P*	Levin et al,[33] 2013
Korean	16q23.3	*CDH13*	*MPHOSPH6, LOC102724163*	Kim et al,[6] 2013
Korean	19q13.43	*ZNF71*	*ZNF470, SMIM17*	Kim et al,[6] 2013
Airway Hyper-responsiveness				
European	2q36.3	*AGFG1*	*TM4SF20, C2orf83*	Himes et al,[34] 2013

Mixed ethnicities = African American/African Caribbean, Latino, European ancestry

REFERENCES FOR APPENDIX A

1. Ding L, Abebe T, Beyene J, et al. Rank-based genome-wide analysis reveals the association of ryanodine receptor-2 gene variants with childhood asthma among human populations. Hum Genomics 2013;7:16.
2. Forno E, Lasky-Su J, Himes B, et al. Genome-wide association study of the age of onset of childhood asthma. J Allergy Clin Immunol 2012;130:83–90.e4.
3. Ferreira MA, Matheson MC, Duffy DL, et al. Identification of IL6R and chromosome 11q13.5 as risk loci for asthma. Lancet 2011;378:1006–14.
4. Torgerson DG, Ampleford EJ, Chiu GY, et al. Meta-analysis of genome-wide association studies of asthma in ethnically diverse North American populations. Nat Genet 2011;43:887–92.
5. Sleiman PM, Flory J, Imielinski M, et al. Variants of DENND1B associated with asthma in children. N Engl J Med 2010;362:36–44.
6. Kim JH, Cheong HS, Park JS, et al. A genome-wide association study of total serum and mite-specific IgEs in asthma patients. PLoS One 2013;8:e71958.
7. Melen E, Granell R, Kogevinas M, et al. Genome-wide association study of body mass index in 23 000 individuals with and without asthma. Clin Exp Allergy 2013;43:463–74.
8. Ramasamy A, Kuokkanen M, Vedantam S, et al. Genome-wide association studies of asthma in population-based cohorts confirm known and suggested loci and identify an additional association near HLA. PLoS One 2012;7:e44008.
9. Himes BE, Jiany X, Hu R, et al. Genome-wide association analysis in asthma subjects identifies SPATS2L as a novel bronchodilator response gene. PLoS Genet 2012;8:e1002824.

10. Wan YI, Shrine NR, Soler Artigas M, et al. Genome-wide association study to identify genetic determinants of severe asthma. Thorax 2012;67:762–8.
11. Moffatt MF, Gut IG, Demenais F, et al. A large-scale, consortium-based genome-wide association study of asthma. N Engl J Med 2010;363:1211–21.
12. Hirota T, Takahashi A, Kubo M, et al. Genome-wide association study identifies three new susceptibility loci for adult asthma in the Japanese population. Nat Genet 2011;43:893–6.
13. Li X, Howard TD, Zheng SL, et al. Genome-wide association study of asthma identifies RAD50-IL13 and HLA-DR/DQ regions. J Allergy Clin Immunol 2010; 125:328–35.e11.
14. Himes BE, Hunninghake GM, Baurley JW, et al. Genome-wide association analysis identifies PDE4D as an asthma-susceptibility gene. Am J Hum Genet 2009;84:581–93.
15. Lasky-Su J, Himes BE, Raby BA, et al. HLA-DQ strikes again: genome-wide association study further confirms HLA-DQ in the diagnosis of asthma among adults. Clin Exp Allergy 2012;42:1724–33.
16. Park BL, Kim TH, Kim JH, et al. Genome-wide association study of aspirin-exacerbated respiratory disease in a Korean population. Hum Genet 2013;132: 313–21.
17. Tantisira KG, Damask A, Szefler SJ, et al. Genome-wide association identifies the T gene as a novel asthma pharmacogenetic locus. Am J Respir Crit Care Med 2012;185:1286–91.
18. Noguchi E, Sakamoto H, Hirota T, et al. Genome-wide association study identifies HLA-DP as a susceptibility gene for pediatric asthma in Asian populations. PLoS Genet 2011;7:e1002170.
19. Duan QL, Lasky-Su J, Himes BE, et al. A genome-wide association study of bronchodilator response in asthmatics. Pharmacogenomics J 2014;14:41–7.
20. Hancock DB, Romieu I, Shi M, et al. Genome-wide association study implicates chromosome 9q21.31 as a susceptibility locus for asthma in mexican children. PLoS Genet 2009;5:e1000623.
21. Kim SH, Cho BY, Park CS, et al. Alpha-T-catenin (CTNNA3) gene was identified as a risk variant for toluene diisocyanate-induced asthma by genome-wide association analysis. Clin Exp Allergy 2009;39:203–12.
22. Li X, Hawkins GA, Ampleford EJ, et al. Genome-wide association study identifies TH1 pathway genes associated with lung function in asthmatic patients. J Allergy Clin Immunol 2013;132:313–20.e15.
23. Ferreira MA, McRae AF, Medland SE, et al. Association between ORMDL3, IL1RL1 and a deletion on chromosome 17q21 with asthma risk in Australia. Eur J Hum Genet 2011;19:458–64.
24. Weidinger S, Willis-Owen SA, Kamatani Y, et al. A genome-wide association study of atopic dermatitis identifies loci with overlapping effects on asthma and psoriasis. Hum Mol Genet 2013;22:4841–56.
25. Sun LD, Xiao FL, Li Y, et al. Genome-wide association study identifies two new susceptibility loci for atopic dermatitis in the Chinese Han population. Nat Genet 2011; 43:690–4.
26. Hirota T, Takahashi A, Kubo M, et al. Genome-wide association study identifies eight new susceptibility loci for atopic dermatitis in the Japanese population. Nat Genet 2012;44:1222–6.
27. Paternoster L, Standl M, Chen CM, et al. Meta-analysis of genome-wide association studies identifies three new risk loci for atopic dermatitis. Nat Genet 2012; 44:187–92.

28. Esparza-Gordillo J, Weidinger S, Folster-Hoist R, et al. A common variant on chromosome 11q13 is associated with atopic dermatitis. Nat Genet 2009;41:596–601.

29. Castro-Giner F, Bustamante M, Ramon Gonzalez J, et al. A pooling-based genome-wide analysis identifies new potential candidate genes for atopy in the European Community Respiratory Health Survey (ECRHS). BMC Med Genet 2009;10:128.

30. Ramasamy A, Curjuric I, Coin LJ, et al. A genome-wide meta-analysis of genetic variants associated with allergic rhinitis and grass sensitization and their interaction with birth order. J Allergy Clin Immunol 2011;128:996–1005.

31. Granada M, Wilk JB, Tuzova M, et al. A genome-wide association study of plasma total IgE concentrations in the Framingham Heart Study. J Allergy Clin Immunol 2012;129:840–5.e21.

32. Weidinger S, Gieger C, Rodriquez E, et al. Genome-wide scan on total serum IgE levels identifies FCER1A as novel susceptibility locus. PLoS Genet 2008;4: e1000166.

33. Levin AM, Mathias RA, Huang L, et al. A meta-analysis of genome-wide association studies for serum total IgE in diverse study populations. J Allergy Clin Immunol 2013;131:1176–84.

34. Himes BE, Qiu W, Klanderman B, et al. ITGB5 and AGFG1 variants are associated with severity of airway responsiveness. BMC Med Genet 2013;14:86.

Food Allergy
Epidemiology and Natural History

Jessica Savage, MD, MHS[a,b,*], Christina B. Johns, BA[a]

KEYWORDS

• Food allergy • Epidemiology • Natural history • Peanut • Milk • Egg

KEY POINTS

• Food allergy prevalence is between 5% and 10% throughout the developed world, and is rising at an alarming rate, for unclear reasons.

• The natural history of childhood food allergy varies by food, and can guide the clinician in determining when it may be safe to introduce a food that was previously not tolerated.

• Further research is needed on the optimum time to introduce complimentary allergenic foods, and methods for prevention and treatment of food allergy.

INTRODUCTION

This article reviews the epidemiology and natural history of immunoglobulin (Ig)E-mediated food allergy with emphasis on recent advances in these areas. For several years, it has been suggested that the prevalence of food allergy is rising, and we review the most recent literature to provide supportive evidence including trends by race/ethnicity and geography. The natural history of food allergy refers to both the acquisition of clinical allergy and its resolution or persistence. The timing of the onset of allergy and likelihood and timing of tolerance development varies depending on the food in question and, therefore, the natural history section is organized by specific food allergen (**Table 1**). We review the development of food allergy and the natural history of food allergy with an emphasis on when it is appropriate to assess for resolution of the allergy with a physician-supervised oral food challenge (OFC),[1,2] the gold standard for diagnosis of food allergy.

The majority of studies of the epidemiology and natural history of food allergy have inherent limitations in their design. Precise evaluation of the prevalence and natural

[a] Division of Rheumatology, Immunology, and Allergy, Brigham and Women's Hospital, Harvard Medical School, 1 Jimmy Fund Way, Smith Building, Room 516c, Boston, MA 02115, USA; [b] Division of Rheumatology, Immunology, and Allergy, Brigham and Women's Hospital, Harvard Medical School, 1 Jimmy Fund Way, Smith Building, Room 626, Boston, MA 02215, USA
* Division of Rheumatology, Immunology, and Allergy, Brigham and Women's Hospital, Harvard Medical School, 1 Jimmy Fund Way, Smith Building, Room 516c, Boston, MA 02115.
E-mail address: jrsavage@partners.org

Immunol Allergy Clin N Am 35 (2015) 45–59
http://dx.doi.org/10.1016/j.iac.2014.09.004   **immunology.theclinics.com**

Table 1
Common allergenic foods with general age of onset of clinical allergy and resolution

Food	Age of Onset	Age of Resolution
Egg	Infant/toddler	Early to late childhood
Milk	Infant/toddler	Early to late childhood
Peanut	Infant/toddler Adulthood	Early to late childhood—uncommon Unknown
Tree nuts	Toddler/early childhood Adulthood	Early to late childhood—uncommon Unknown
Soy	Infant/toddler Adulthood (rare)	Early to late childhood Unknown
Wheat	Infant/toddler	Early to late childhood

history of food allergy on a population level requires prospective ascertainment with confirmatory OFCs of a representative sample of infants and young children at predetermined intervals over time. Studies such as this are rarely performed in the United States owing to feasibility and ethical issues. However, recent efforts in Australia have begun to meet this need. Generally speaking, however, it is important to recognize that much of the currently available data on the epidemiology and natural course of food allergy are necessarily imprecise. Furthermore, published studies typically come from selected populations, such as from a particular clinic or referral population, and may not be representative of the general population with food allergies. These limitations are highlighted in this article.

EPIDEMIOLOGY
Prevalence

Estimates of food allergy prevalence vary widely, likely because of differences in study methodology, including use of different definitions of food allergy, and different geographic area studied. In the United States, prevalence estimates range from 1% to 2% to 10%, and most are derived from self-report or parent report of allergy.[3] A recent study reporting on a nationally representative, population-based survey (the National Health and Nutrition Examination Survey [NHANES]), found the prevalence of self-reported food allergy in children to be 6.53%[4] from 2007 to 2010. The most common childhood food allergies reported were to milk (1.94% of children surveyed), peanut (1.16%), and shellfish (0.87%). Another United States, population-based study reported a slightly higher estimate of childhood food allergy prevalence (8%).[5] This survey was internet based, which may have resulted in selection bias, contributing to the higher prevalence estimate. Nonetheless, the most commonly reported food allergies were similar.[5] The importance of the method of ascertaining food allergy in generating prevalence estimates was highlighted by a recent meta-regression using only US survey data from 1988 to 2011. Roughly one half of between-study variability was explained by method of identifying food allergy alone, and because of this and other sources of heterogeneity, the authors were unable to provide a point estimate for current food allergy prevalence in the United States.[6]

In other developed countries, overall prevalence estimates are in general within the range of US estimates. The overall rate of food allergy was estimated at 6.7% in Canada (7.1% for children and 6.6% for adults) in a population-based self-report study using random digit telephone sampling and adjusting for nonresponse, with cow's milk, peanut, and tree nut allergy being the most common allergens among children.[7] A recent meta-analysis of European food allergy prevalence found an overall prevalence of self-reported food allergy of 5.9% from 2000 to 2012, although many of the primary studies had at a least moderate potential for bias.[8]

Estimates relying on self-report are of course limited in part by the subjective nature of the data. Other, more objective methods include measuring sensitization using food allergen-specific serum IgE. In a US-based study, again using NHANES data, prevalence estimates for sensitization were 7.6% to peanut, 5.9% to shrimp, 4.8% to milk, and 3.4% to egg in the overall population aged 6 and over, and 6.8% to peanut, 21.8% to milk, and 14.2% to egg in children aged 1 to 5. These are certainly overestimates of true clinical food allergy prevalence, but are valuable because they provide some objectivity.[9]

The gold standard for food allergy diagnosis is the OFC, but prevalence of OFC-confirmed allergy has not been widely studied on a population level, and there are no US studies using OFC to determine food allergy prevalence. A population-based study of 12-month-old Australian infants using predetermined challenge criteria identified prevalence estimates of 3.0% to peanut, 8.9% to raw egg, and 0.8% to sesame based on OFC. Overall, more than 10% of subjects had allergy to peanut, egg, or sesame.[10] This is moderately greater than recent prevalence estimates from the United States that rely on self-report, suggesting either variation in food allergy prevalence throughout the developed world, perhaps owing to different exposures, or higher than previously estimated levels of transient food allergy.

Changes Over Time

Although the overall prevalence of food allergy seems to be increasing, objective data on this are scarce. Because many estimates of food allergy prevalence are derived from self-report, assessment of changes over time is limited by the potential for increased food allergy awareness in the media and other sources influencing responses over time. Several well-designed studies of self-reported food allergy have supported a worrisome increase in food allergy prevalence over a recent time period. Using meta-regression of 20 US-based surveys conducted by the US Centers for Disease Control representing nearly 400,000 children between 1988 and 2011, Keet and colleagues[6] estimated an overall increase in childhood prevalence of self-reported food allergy of 1.2% points per decade. Interestingly, the increase in food allergy prevalence was nearly twice as high among non-Hispanic Black children (2.1% points per decade) compared with White children (1.0% points) and Hispanic children (1.2% points). Several US and international studies suggest that peanut allergy diagnoses are increasing: in a United States telephone-based population survey that was repeated three times between 1997 and 2008, estimates of the prevalence of peanut allergy increased significantly from 0.4% to 1.4% and estimates of tree nut allergy prevalence increased from 0.2% to 1.1%.[11] Similar trends have been reported from the UK.[12] Hospitalizations for food-induced anaphylaxis are also increasing.[13,14] Overall, these results support a concerning trend over time and by race/ethnicity, and reasons for these increases should be identified, so that prevention strategies can be developed.

Risk Factors

Many risk factors for food allergy have been identified, although it is not clear what is driving the observed increase in prevalence. As in other atopic diseases, a family history of atopy is a strong risk factor. In a population-based study of 1-year-old infants diagnosed via OFC with food allergy (primarily egg or peanut), the risk of food allergy was increased by 40% in patients with one immediate family member with any allergic disease and by 80% in patients with two immediate family members with any allergic disease compared with children without a family history of allergy.[15] Race/ethnicity and other demographic characteristics are also associated with food allergy: Non-Hispanic Black ethnicity,[4,5,16,17] Asian ethnicity,[5] and male sex in children[16,18] have all been associated with higher risk of food allergy. Overall, these findings suggest a genetic predisposition; however, the genetic determinants of food allergy are largely undefined.

Although there is some evidence implicating specific genes in food allergy susceptibility, studies have not been replicated on a wide scale. Loss-of-function mutations in the filaggrin gene have been associated with peanut allergy independent of atopic dermatitis, implicating the skin as a potential route of sensitization.[3] Filaggrin mutations have also been associated with self-reported allergy to eggs, milk, wheat, and fish in a Danish population and with positive specific IgE levels to milk.[19] However, another study reported that although filaggrin mutations do increase the likelihood of sensitization to food-specific IgE in children in the first year of life, they are not associated with an increased risk of clinical allergy among children already sensitized.[20] Polymorphisms in the STAT6 gene have been associated with an increase in the age of tolerance in cow's milk allergy,[21] food sensitization,[22] and risk for nut allergy.[23] Although it seems likely that there is a genetic basis to food allergy development, further studies are needed to identify the specific loci involved.

Environmental factors are also associated with food allergy risk.[3] Children with older siblings[24] and pets in the home may be at lower risk of egg allergy at age 12 months, supporting the hypothesis that increased microbial stimulation in infancy may have a protective effect in terms of developing allergy.[18] Parental nativity has also been implicated: in a study of the 2005 and 2006 NHANES, US-born children and children immigrating to the United States in early childhood had greater odds of sensitization to milk, peanut, or egg than foreign-born children, and among children born in the United States, those children born to immigrant parents had higher odds of sensitization.[25] Vitamin D insufficiency has been associated with an increased risk of food allergy[26–28]; however, these associations are controversial and need further exploration because vitamin D sufficiency has also been associated with an increased risk of allergic sensitization.[29] Increased food diversity in infancy may have a protective effect on food sensitization as well as clinical food allergy later in childhood.[30] Atopy, including co-morbid atopic dermatitis and doctor-diagnosed asthma,[16] has also been associated with an increased risk of food allergy. Whether this represents a more severe allergic phenotype or food allergy arises owing to impaired barrier function is unknown.

NATURAL COURSE

Knowledge about the natural history of food allergy is important for the allergist to guide use of elimination diets and when it may be appropriate to consider liberalizing the diet to include a food that previously caused allergic symptoms. Herein we discuss the clinical and laboratory factors associated with the natural history of food allergy, the natural history of the most common food allergens, and strategies to assess for resolution of food allergy.

Clinical and Laboratory Factors Associated with the Natural History of Food Allergy

Several clinical and laboratory factors have been associated with development of tolerance or persistence of an allergy to an allergenic food. These have been most studied in association with egg, milk, and peanut allergies the most common childhood food allergens. Factors associated with the timing of resolution of allergy to these foods include severity of symptoms on ingestion,[31-35] skin prick test (SPT) size,[31,33,35,36] age at diagnosis,[31,37] comorbid allergic disease[38-41] and severity,[31,33] food-specific IgE levels,[21,31-33,36,38,42-44] rate of change of food-specific IgE levels[37] or SPT sizes,[36] IgE epitope specificity,[45] IgE/IgG$_4$ ratio,[46] and specific IgA and IgA2 levels.[47] Although these were identified in children with egg, milk, or peanut allergies, it is likely that these principles are generalizable to other food allergens, and this warrants further study. Unfortunately, IgE-based methods are imprecise, and OFC is usually necessary to confirm resolution of allergy. New methods such as allergen component testing—determination of individual allergens to which a patient's IgE is directed—or cellular based studies, may help to improve the diagnosis of food allergy,[48,49] but their role in assessing resolution of allergy is not clear.

Egg Allergy

Egg allergy is among the most common IgE-mediated childhood food allergies with a reported prevalence of 1.3% to 1.6%.[50,51] Most egg allergy develops in the first year of life.[52] Several prospective studies have attempted to address the natural history of egg allergy.[32,35,43,53-55] Although families have generally been advised that most children will outgrow their allergy by the early school-age years,[56] recent studies suggest that this is not the current case.

In a retrospective review of 881 patients with egg allergy, the median age at egg allergy resolution was 9 years, when tolerance was defined as passing an egg challenge or having a last recorded egg IgE level of <2 kUA/L and no reported symptomatic accidental ingestions in the last year.[38] However, this study was limited by its retrospective design and its focus on a highly allergic referral population. Further, it was conducted at a time before it was common to introduce baked egg into the diet of children who could tolerate baked egg but not concentrated egg (see below), which has been hypothesized to affect the natural history of egg allergy. In a more recent prospective study of egg-allergic children recruited from primary care offices, the median age of resolution (defined by OFC and successful home introduction of whole egg) was 6 years with a rate of resolution of nearly 50%. Of those children with unresolved allergy, 38.1% were able to tolerate some baked egg products.[33] These studies highlight the importance of the study population in influencing the observed natural history of food allergy.

Although most consumers of egg generally eat cooked eggs, the length and degree of heating can reduce the allergenicity of egg.[57] A majority of children (>70% in some series) who react to concentrated egg (lightly heated egg such as French toast or scrambled egg) can tolerate baked egg in the form of a muffin or waffle.[10,58,59] However, the role of baked egg consumption in the resolution of egg allergy is unknown. One prospective study that assessed tolerance to both baked and concentrated egg demonstrated a median age at baked egg allergy resolution of 5.6 years, and after introduction of baked egg into the diet, a median age at concentrated egg allergy resolution of 10.6 years, suggesting that introduction of baked egg may not hasten the resolution of egg allergy.[53] Similarly, a retrospective chart review demonstrated that the rate of decline of SPT size was not associated with frequency of baked egg consumption.[60] However, other recent prospective studies have shown increased likelihood of[61] and accelerated development of concentrated egg tolerance with frequent ingestion of baked egg.[42]

Milk Allergy

Milk is the most common childhood food allergy, with a prevalence of up to 2.5% when both IgE- and non–IgE-mediated reactions are considered,[62-65] and accounts for about one fifth of all childhood food allergy, according to a national cross-sectional survey of parents.[66] Most milk allergy typically presents in the first year of life.[52,67] Like egg allergy, most studies have shown the prognosis of developing tolerance to cow's milk to be favorable, with the majority outgrowing their allergy throughout childhood and early adolescence.[43,54,62,63,68–73] However, a minority of milk-allergic children become milk-allergic adults.

Data from a large, population-based cohort in Israel demonstrated that only 57% of children with milk allergy resolved their allergy before the study completion by age 4 to 5 years, and the majority of these did so by age 2.[39] However, clinic-based studies, which may include children at greater risk for allergic disease, suggest a worse prognosis. In a recent prospective study from Europe, only 43% had outgrown their allergy by the age of 10, when food challenges were performed after the SPT size to milk had decreased.[74] These data are consistent with a retrospective study of milk allergy in a referral population demonstrating that the median age to outgrow milk allergy is 10 years when allergy is defined as passing an open food challenge, or having a milk-specific IgE of less than 3 kUA/L at the last visit, and no reported symptomatic accidental ingestions in the last year,[40] consistent with the possibility that the natural history of food allergy may be lengthening over time.

Similar to egg allergy, baked milk is tolerated in a majority (75%) of children who are reactive to uncooked milk. Baked milk consumption may affect the natural history of milk allergy. Ingestion of baked milk for 3 months led to significantly decreased milk SPT size and increase in casein IgG$_4$.[75] A follow-up study suggested that ingestion of baked milk accelerated the resolution of milk allergy, because patients who incorporated baked milk into their diet were more likely to become milk tolerant compared with children who underwent clinic standard of care with strict avoidance of milk.[76] Ingestion of extensively hydrolyzed casein formula as opposed to rice hydrolyzed formula, soy formula, and amino acid-based formula has also been demonstrated to increase the rate of milk tolerance acquisition, although other smaller studies have not found such an association.[77] Although it is often incredibly helpful to food-allergic patients and families to introduce foods when they are safely tolerated, larger studies are needed to determine whether ingestion of baked milk is solely a marker of transient milk allergy, or an effective treatment to induce tolerance.

Peanut Allergy

The prevalence of childhood peanut allergy is estimated around 2%,[78] and studies from North America and Europe suggest it is increasing rapidly.[12,79] Interestingly, peanut allergy seems to be more common in Western-born children than in Asian children, according to a population survey of both local and Western-born Singapore and Philippine schoolchildren.[80] Although risk factors for peanut allergy are not well-defined outside of the aforementioned risk factors for general food allergy, the Learning Early About Peanut Allergy (LEAP) study, based in the UK, has recently associated egg allergy and severe atopic dermatitis, or both, with an increased risk of peanut sensitization in infancy.[17] The most common age for the presentation of peanut allergy is 18 months, although peanut allergy can present later in childhood or adulthood, most often as part of the pollen–food allergy syndrome.[81–83]

Unlike the previously discussed foods, the majority of childhood-onset peanut allergy is not outgrown before adulthood.[84] Estimates of tolerance development rates vary with study design.[81,84] The largest study to date reported that 21.5% of patients had become peanut tolerant when patients aged 4 to 20 years with a history of peanut allergy and peanut-specific IgE of less than 20 kUA/L were offered a food challenge.[85] Another study demonstrated a similar rate of tolerance acquisition (20% by age 5) in preschool-aged children by offering an oral challenge to children whose peanut SPT size had decreased to less than of the 95% positive predictive value for peanut allergy.[36] The timing of peanut allergy resolution is not clearly defined, but cases of resolution in adulthood have been reported,[83] suggesting that patients can benefit from long-term follow-up for peanut allergy. In rare cases, symptomatic peanut allergy has been demonstrated to recur after passing an open challenge. This has been seen especially in patients who do not introduce peanut into their diets after a negative peanut challenge.[86,87]

Tree Nut Allergy

Relatively little is known about the natural course of tree nut allergy, but it can present in both childhood and adulthood. One OFC-based study on children and young adults with tree nut IgE levels below 10 kUA/L found that 9% of 101 patients with prior reactions to tree nuts had resolved their allergy, whereas 74% of 19 patients who had never ingested tree nuts but were diagnosed on the basis of an elevated tree nut IgE passed a challenge.[88] They also found that no subject who was allergic to more than two tree nuts outgrew their allergy. Adult tree nut allergy is presumed to represent a mixture of late-onset, IgE-mediated allergy to tree nuts as well as allergy owing to cross-reactivity with inhalant allergens (pollen–food allergy syndrome), although little is known about its natural course.

Soy Allergy

Soy is another common childhood allergen[89] and may be more common in children with concomitant peanut allergy. Soy allergy is typically considered to have its onset in infancy. One study reported a peak incidence of soy sensitization around age 2.[52] Early prospective studies of children with soy allergy and concomitant eczema demonstrated a relatively good prognosis, with a 50% rate of resolution at 1 year of follow-up and 67% rate at 2 years of follow-up.[54,90] However, a retrospective study conducted on soy-allergic patients at a tertiary referral center reported that the allergy was outgrown in 45% of children by age 6, suggesting a less promising prognosis. Soy IgE level was a useful predictor of the speed of tolerance acquisition: By age 6, 59% of children with a peak soy IgE level of less than 5 kUA/L were soy tolerant compared with only 18% of children with a peak soy IgE level of greater than 50 kUA/L.[91]

A phenotype of late-onset soy allergy has been described where some patients develop typical IgE-mediated symptoms to soy after tolerating it as a regular part of their diet. This phenomenon may be more common in patients with persistent peanut allergy[91] or may be related to pollen–food allergy syndrome owing to cross-reactivity with birch pollen.[92]

Wheat Allergy

Wheat is another common childhood food allergen, but little is known about its natural history. Studies on the prognosis of patients with wheat allergy and concomitant atopic dermatitis suggest that 25% to 33% of patients become tolerant by follow-up 1 to 2 years later.[54,90] In a prospective study of 50 Polish children with positive wheat-specific IgE and food challenge results along with predominant gastrointestinal symptoms, 20% of children had resolved allergy by age 4, 52% by age 8, 66% by age 12, and 76% by age 18. Similar results have been obtained by retrospective studies. One such study of children with OFC-proven wheat allergy indicated that 84% had gained tolerance by age 10 when wheat allergy cases included both IgE-mediated and non–IgE-mediated reactions.[93] A larger retrospective study estimated a median age at resolution of wheat allergy of 6.5 years, but 35% of patients remained allergic into their teens.[94] Peak wheat-specific IgE is somewhat useful in determining the age at which tolerance develops, and higher levels may be related to allergy persistence.[95] However, high levels of wheat IgE do not preclude resolution of the allergy.[94]

Other Foods

The natural history of other foods such as sesame and other seeds, seafood, meats, and fruits has not been well described. These food allergies can present both in childhood and adulthood. In general, childhood-onset allergy to seeds, seafood, and meats has a poor prognosis, with the minority outgrowing their food allergies during childhood.[43,96–98] Adult-onset allergy to these foods is thought to be persistent. Recently, a syndrome of delayed allergy to meats caused by reactivity to galactose-alpha-1,3-galactose has been described.[99] The natural history of this entity is currently unknown.

Allergic reactions to fruits and vegetables can also have their onset at any age. In early childhood, adverse reactions to fruits and vegetables are common and are typically short lived, although some children do have IgE-mediated allergies to these foods.[43,62,63] Later in childhood and into adulthood, some proportion of fruit and vegetable reactions are most certainly associated with pollen–food allergy syndrome secondary to cross-reactivity with inhalant allergens, which can develop after clinical sensitivity to seasonal inhalants has developed. The natural history of pollen–food allergy syndrome has not been investigated.

Assessing for Resolution of Food Allergy

Once the diagnosis of food allergy is confirmed, the role of the allergist becomes to guide the assessment for resolution of food allergy. Some food allergens are difficult to avoid and fortunately have a generally high likelihood of resolution (eg, milk and egg). Safely liberalizing the diet to include these foods has important nutritional and quality-of-life benefits.

In general, we recommend yearly evaluation by food-specific IgE or SPT. We prefer to use specific IgE testing because it provides more prognostic information regarding the long-term timing of tolerance acquisition[38] and the short-term likelihood of passing a food challenge. In general, we use a specific IgE cutoff that provides a 50% positive predictive value of passing a food challenge. Values have been published for some foods (**Table 2**), but these should be interpreted with caution because studies are small and other factors beside IgE influence the outcome of a

Table 2
Specific Immunoglobulin E (sIgE) levels associated with a 50% positive predictive value for clinical allergy

Food Allergen	50% Positive Predictive Value	
	Age, if Investigated	sIgE Value (kUA/L)
Egg	—	2^{100}
Milk	—	2^{100}
Peanut	—	2^{100}
Wheat	<1	1
	>1	20^{101}
Soy	—	$20–30^{101}$
Tree nuts	—	N/A

In general, we use the 50% positive predictive value to guide the timing of an oral food challenge, but caution should always be used in considering when to perform a food challenge.

challenge. In patients without a history of previous reaction whose diagnosis was made on the basis of sensitization alone, higher IgE cutoffs may be appropriate.[100] In patients with persistent allergy with unchanged specific IgE levels for several years, testing can be performed less frequently over time.[102] Factors to consider before deciding to pursue an OFC include the chance of success, the potential for risk, and the preferences of the patient and family, including the importance of the food to the diet.[103] Other important considerations may include patient age, history of reactions, family characteristics, and comorbidities (eg, severe atopic dermatitis or eosinophilic esophagitis).

Current Controversies

The observation that children with milk and egg allergy may tolerate extensively heated forms of these allergens has challenged previous food allergy dogma of strict allergen avoidance. Fortunately, this has allowed many patients to safely incorporate these foods into their diets, where just a decade ago strict avoidance of even cooked forms would have been recommended. However, this breakthrough, combined with observations that delayed introduction of food may actually increase the rate of food allergy[80,85,86,100,104] has complicated the management of food allergy. The optimal time to introduce allergenic foods during infancy is not known, and the American Academy of Pediatrics currently does not recommend delaying the introduction of highly allergenic complimentary foods to prevent the development of food allergy. A committee from the American Academy of Allergy, Asthma and Immunology has published advice for complimentary food introduction, including scenarios where allergy evaluation may be helpful.[104] In general, they recommend introduction of complementary foods between the ages of 4 and 6 months, with highly allergenic foods introduced in small quantities at home, once other foods are tolerated. However, young infants may demonstrate clinical allergy to foods on their first exposure. This was highlighted in a recent study that sought to determine whether early egg introduction in children with moderate to severe eczema could prevent the development of egg allergy. Although they were able to show that early egg exposure was associated with a nonsignificant reduction in egg allergy defined by failing an OFC at 1 year, one third of subjects reacted to early egg exposure, including one case of anaphylaxis.[105] More research is certainly needed to better identify those infants who may benefit from early allergen exposure, and those in whom clinical allergy has already developed.

FUTURE DIRECTIONS

Despite the dismal observation that food allergy prevalence is rising rapidly, several interventions are on the horizon that may favorably impact the natural history of food allergy. Small-scale studies have demonstrated that it is possible to induce desensitization to specific foods using oral and sublingual immunotherapy, with tolerance induced in a subset.[106–109] These treatments are still under active research investigation and will hopefully be available widely in the next several years. Improved diagnostic testing for food allergy with epitope specific testing,[110] component-resolved diagnostics,[111] or cellular methods[112] will allow for more precise identification of young patients with food allergy, and will ideally provide insight into the natural course of food allergy on an individual level. Although these efforts are promising for established disease, primary and secondary prevention efforts have had limited success and are needed to stem the rapid rise in food allergy prevalence worldwide.

REFERENCES

1. Boyce JA, Assa'ad A, Burks AW, et al. Guidelines for the diagnosis and management of food allergy in the United States: report of the NIAID-sponsored expert panel. J Allergy Clin Immunol 2010;126(Suppl 6):S1–58.
2. Bindslev-Jensen C, Ballmer-Weber BK, Bengtsson U, et al. Standardization of food challenges in patients with immediate reactions to foods–position paper from the European Academy of Allergology and Clinical Immunology. Allergy 2004;59(7):690–7.
3. Sicherer SH, Sampson HA. Food allergy: epidemiology, pathogenesis, diagnosis, and treatment. J Allergy Clin Immunol 2014;133(2):291–307.e5.
4. McGowan EC, Keet CA. Prevalence of self-reported food allergy in the National Health and Nutrition Examination Survey (NHANES) 2007-2010. J Allergy Clin Immunol 2013;132(5):1216–9.e5.
5. Gupta RS, Springston EE, Warrier MR, et al. The prevalence, severity, and distribution of childhood food allergy in the United States. Pediatrics 2011;128(1):e9–17.
6. Keet CA, Savage JH, Seopaul S, et al. Temporal trends and racial/ethnic disparity in self-reported pediatric food allergy in the United States. Ann Allergy Asthma Immunol 2014;112(3):222–9.e3.
7. Soller L, Ben-Shoshan M, Harrington DW, et al. Overall prevalence of self-reported food allergy in Canada. J Allergy Clin Immunol 2012;130(4):986–8.
8. Nwaru BI, Hickstein L, Panesar SS, et al. The epidemiology of food allergy in Europe: a systematic review and meta-analysis. Allergy 2014;69(1):62–75.
9. Salo PM, Arbes SJ Jr, Jaramillo R, et al. Prevalence of allergic sensitization in the United States: results from the National Health and Nutrition Examination Survey (NHANES) 2005-2006. J Allergy Clin Immunol 2014;134(2):350–9.
10. Osborne NJ, Koplin JJ, Martin PE, et al. Prevalence of challenge-proven IgE-mediated food allergy using population-based sampling and predetermined challenge criteria in infants. J Allergy Clin Immunol 2011;127(3):668–76.e1-2.
11. Sicherer SH, Munoz-Furlong A, Godbold JH, et al. US prevalence of self-reported peanut, tree nut, and sesame allergy: 11-year follow-up. J Allergy Clin Immunol 2010;125(6):1322–6.
12. Kotz D, Simpson CR, Sheikh A. Incidence, prevalence, and trends of general practitioner-recorded diagnosis of peanut allergy in England, 2001 to 2005. J Allergy Clin Immunol 2011;127(3):623–30.e1.
13. Poulos LM, Waters AM, Correll PK, et al. Trends in hospitalizations for anaphylaxis, angioedema, and urticaria in Australia, 1993-1994 to 2004-2005. J Allergy Clin Immunol 2007;120(4):878–84.
14. Lin RY, Anderson AS, Shah SN, et al. Increasing anaphylaxis hospitalizations in the first 2 decades of life: New York State, 1990 -2006. Ann Allergy Asthma Immunol 2008;101(4):387–93.
15. Koplin JJ, Allen KJ, Gurrin LC, et al. The impact of family history of allergy on risk of food allergy: a population-based study of infants. Int J Environ Res Public Health 2013;10(11):5364–77.
16. Liu AH, Jaramillo R, Sicherer SH, et al. National prevalence and risk factors for food allergy and relationship to asthma: results from the National Health and Nutrition Examination Survey 2005-2006. J Allergy Clin Immunol 2010;126(4):798–806.e13.
17. Du Toit G, Roberts G, Sayre PH, et al. Identifying infants at high risk of peanut allergy: the learning early about peanut allergy (LEAP) screening study. J Allergy Clin Immunol 2013;131(1):135–43.e1-12.

18. Koplin JJ, Dharmage SC, Ponsonby AL, et al. Environmental and demographic risk factors for egg allergy in a population-based study of infants. Allergy 2012; 67(11):1415–22.

19. Linneberg A, Fenger RV, Husemoen LL, et al. Association between loss-of-function mutations in the filaggrin gene and self-reported food allergy and alcohol sensitivity. Int Arch Allergy Immunol 2013;161(3):234–42.

20. Tan HT, Ellis JA, Koplin JJ, et al. Filaggrin loss-of-function mutations do not predict food allergy over and above the risk of food sensitization among infants. J Allergy Clin Immunol 2012;130(5):1211–3.e3.

21. Yavuz ST, Buyuktiryaki B, Sahiner UM, et al. Factors that predict the clinical reactivity and tolerance in children with cow's milk allergy. Ann Allergy Asthma Immunol 2013;110(4):284–9.

22. Hancock DB, Romieu I, Chiu GY, et al. STAT6 and LRP1 polymorphisms are associated with food allergen sensitization in Mexican children. J Allergy Clin Immunol 2012;129(6):1673–6.

23. Amoli MM, Hand S, Hajeer AH, et al. Polymorphism in the STAT6 gene encodes risk for nut allergy. Genes Immun 2002;3(4):220–4.

24. Kusunoki T, Mukaida K, Morimoto T, et al. Birth order effect on childhood food allergy. Pediatr Allergy Immunol 2012;23(3):250–4.

25. Keet CA, Wood RA, Matsui EC. Personal and parental nativity as risk factors for food sensitization. J Allergy Clin Immunol 2012;129(1):169–75.e1-5.

26. Keet CA, Matsui EC, Savage JH, et al. Potential mechanisms for the association between fall birth and food allergy. Allergy 2012;67(6):775–82.

27. Sharief S, Jariwala S, Kumar J, et al. Vitamin D levels and food and environmental allergies in the United States: results from the National Health and Nutrition Examination Survey 2005-2006. J Allergy Clin Immunol 2011;127(5):1195–202.

28. Allen KJ, Koplin JJ, Ponsonby AL, et al. Vitamin D insufficiency is associated with challenge-proven food allergy in infants. J Allergy Clin Immunol 2013; 131(4):1109–16, 1116.e1–6.

29. Weisse K, Winkler S, Hirche F, et al. Maternal and newborn vitamin D status and its impact on food allergy development in the German LINA cohort study. Allergy 2013;68(2):220–8.

30. Roduit C, Frei R, Depner M, et al. Increased food diversity in the first year of life is inversely associated with allergic diseases. J Allergy Clin Immunol 2014; 133(4):1056–64.

31. Wood RA, Sicherer SH, Vickery BP, et al. The natural history of milk allergy in an observational cohort. J Allergy Clin Immunol 2013;131(3):805–12.

32. Ford RP, Taylor B. Natural history of egg hypersensitivity. Arch Dis Child 1982; 57(9):649–52.

33. Sicherer SH, Wood RA, Vickery BP, et al. The natural history of egg allergy in an observational cohort. J Allergy Clin Immunol 2014;133(2):492–9.e8.

34. Spergel JM, Beausoleil JL, Pawlowski NA. Resolution of childhood peanut allergy. Ann Allergy Asthma Immunol 2000;85(6 Pt 1):473–6.

35. Boyano-Martinez T, Garcia-Ara C, Diaz-Pena JM, et al. Prediction of tolerance on the basis of quantification of egg white-specific IgE antibodies in children with egg allergy. J Allergy Clin Immunol 2002;110(2):304–9.

36. Ho MH, Wong WH, Heine RG, et al. Early clinical predictors of remission of peanut allergy in children. J Allergy Clin Immunol 2008;121(3):731–6.

37. Shek LPC, Soderstrom L, Ahlstedt S, et al. Determination of food specific IgE levels over time can predict the development of tolerance in cow's milk and hen's egg allergy. J Allergy Clin Immunol 2004;114(2):387–91.

38. Savage JH, Matsui E, Skripak JM, et al. The natural history of egg allergy. J Allergy Clin Immunol 2007;120(6):1413.
39. Elizur A, Rajuan N, Goldberg MR, et al. Natural course and risk factors for persistence of IgE-mediated cow's milk allergy. J Pediatr 2012;161(3):482–7.e1.
40. Skripak JM, Matsui EC, Mudd K, et al. The natural history of IgE-mediated cow's milk allergy. J Allergy Clin Immunol 2007;120(5):1172–7.
41. Cantani A, Micera M. Natural history of cow's milk allergy. An eight-year follow-up study in 115 atopic children. Eur Rev Med Pharmacol Sci 2004;8(4):153–64.
42. Leonard SA, Sampson HA, Sicherer SH, et al. Dietary baked egg accelerates resolution of egg allergy in children. J Allergy Clin Immunol 2012;130(2): 473–80.e1.
43. Dannaeus A, Inganas M. A follow-up study of children with food allergy. Clinical course in relation to serum IgE- and IgG-antibody levels to milk, egg and fish. Clin Allergy 1981;11(6):533–9.
44. Kaczmarski M, Wasilewska J, Cudowska B, et al. The natural history of cow's milk allergy in north-eastern Poland. Adv Med Sci 2013;58(1):22–30.
45. Urisu A, Yamada K, Tokuda R, et al. Clinical significance of IgE-binding activity to enzymatic digests of ovomucoid in the diagnosis and the prediction of the outgrowing of egg white hypersensitivity. Int Arch Allergy Immunol 1999; 120(3):192–8.
46. Caubet JC, Bencharitiwong R, Moshier E, et al. Significance of ovomucoid- and ovalbumin-specific IgE/IgG(4) ratios in egg allergy. J Allergy Clin Immunol 2012; 129(3):739–47.
47. Konstantinou GN, Nowak-Wegrzyn A, Bencharitiwong R, et al. Egg-white-specific IgA and IgA2 antibodies in egg-allergic children: is there a role in tolerance induction? Pediatr Allergy Immunol 2014;25(1):64–70.
48. Nicolaou N, Murray C, Belgrave D, et al. Quantification of specific IgE to whole peanut extract and peanut components in prediction of peanut allergy. J Allergy Clin Immunol 2011;127(3):684–5.
49. Keet CA, Johnson K, Savage JH, et al. Evaluation of Ara h2 IgE thresholds in the diagnosis of peanut allergy in a clinical population. JACI in Practice, Jan 2013; 1(1):101–3.
50. Eggesbo M, Botten G, Halvorsen R, et al. The prevalence of allergy to egg: a population-based study in young children. Allergy 2001;56(5):403–11.
51. Nickel R, Kulig M, Forster J, et al. Sensitization to hen's egg at the age of twelve months is predictive for allergic sensitization to common indoor and outdoor allergens at the age of three years. J Allergy Clin Immunol 1997;99(5):613–7.
52. Kulig M, Bergmann R, Klettke U, et al. Natural course of sensitization to food and inhalant allergens during the first 6 years of life. J Allergy Clin Immunol 1999; 103(6):1173–9.
53. Clark A, Islam S, King Y, et al. A longitudinal study of resolution of allergy to well-cooked and uncooked egg. Clin Exp Allergy 2011;41(5):706–12.
54. Sampson HA, Scanlon SM. Natural history of food hypersensitivity in children with atopic dermatitis. J Pediatr 1989;115:23–7.
55. Kim J, Chung Y, Han Y, et al. The natural history and prognostic factors of egg allergy in Korean infants with atopic dermatitis. Asian Pac J Allergy Immunol 2009;27(2–3):107–14.
56. Wood RA. The natural history of food allergy. Pediatrics 2003;111(6):1631–7.
57. Nowak-Wegrzyn A, Fiocchi A. Rare, medium, or well done? The effect of heating and food matrix on food protein allergenicity. Curr Opin Allergy Clin Immunol 2009;9(3):234–7.

58. Lemon-Mule H, Sampson HA, Sicherer SH, et al. Immunologic changes in children with egg allergy ingesting extensively heated egg. J Allergy Clin Immunol 2008;122(5):977–83.e1.
59. Konstantinou GN, Giavi S, Kalobatsou A, et al. Consumption of heat-treated egg by children allergic or sensitized to egg can affect the natural course of egg allergy: hypothesis-generating observations. J Allergy Clin Immunol 2008;122(2):414–5.
60. Tey D, Dharmage SC, Robinson MN, et al. Frequent baked egg ingestion was not associated with change in rate of decline in egg skin prick test in children with challenge confirmed egg allergy. Clin Exp Allergy 2012;42(12):1782–90.
61. Peters RL, Dharmage SC, Gurrin LC, et al. The natural history and clinical predictors of egg allergy in the first 2 years of life: a prospective, population-based cohort study. J Allergy Clin Immunol 2014;133(2):485–91.
62. Bock SA. Prospective appraisal of complaints of adverse reactions to foods in children during the first 3 years of life. Pediatrics 1987;79(5):683–8.
63. Host A, Halken S. A prospective study of cow milk allergy in Danish infants during the first 3 years of life. Clinical course in relation to clinical and immunological type of hypersensitivity reaction. Allergy 1990;45(8):587–96.
64. Hide DW, Guyer BM. Cows milk intolerance in Isle of Wight infants. Br J Clin Pract 1983;37(9):285–7.
65. Schrander JJ, van den Bogart JP, Forget PP, et al. Cow's milk protein intolerance in infants under 1 year of age: a prospective epidemiological study. Eur J Pediatr 1993;152(8):640–4.
66. Warren CM, Jhaveri S, Warrier MR, et al. The epidemiology of milk allergy in US children. Ann Allergy Asthma Immunol 2013;110(5):370–4.
67. Sampson HA. Food allergy. Part 1: immunopathogenesis and clinical disorders. J Allergy Clin Immunol 1999;103(5 Pt 1):717–28.
68. Hill DJ, Firer MA, Ball G, et al. Natural history of cows' milk allergy in children: immunological outcome over 2 years. Clin Exp Allergy 1993;23(2):124–31.
69. Saarinen KM, Pelkonen AS, Makela MJ, et al. Clinical course and prognosis of cow's milk allergy are dependent on milk-specific IgE status. J Allergy Clin Immunol 2005;116(4):869–75.
70. Bishop JM, Hill DJ, Hosking CS. Natural history of cow milk allergy: clinical outcome. J Pediatr 1990;116(6):862–7.
71. Hill DJ, Davidson GP, Cameron DJ, et al. The spectrum of cow's milk allergy in childhood. Clinical, gastroenterological and immunological studies. Acta Paediatr Scand 1979;68(6):847–52.
72. James JM, Sampson HA. Immunologic changes associated with the development of tolerance in children with cow milk allergy. J Pediatr 1992;121(3):371–7.
73. Levy Y, Segal N, Garty B, et al. Lessons from the clinical course of IgE-mediated cow milk allergy in Israel. Pediatr Allergy Immunol 2007;18(7):589–93.
74. Santos A, Dias A, Pinheiro JA. Predictive factors for the persistence of cow's milk allergy. Pediatr Allergy Immunol 2010;21(8):1127–34.
75. Nowak-Wegrzyn A, Bloom KA, Sicherer SH, et al. Tolerance to extensively heated milk in children with cow's milk allergy. J Allergy Clin Immunol 2008;122(2):342–7, 347.e1–2.
76. Kim JS, Nowak-Wegrzyn A, Sicherer SH, et al. Dietary baked milk accelerates the resolution of cow's milk allergy in children. J Allergy Clin Immunol 2011;128(1):125–31.e2.
77. Berni Canani R, Nocerino R, Terrin G, et al. Formula selection for management of children with cow's milk allergy influences the rate of acquisition of tolerance: a prospective multicenter study. J Pediatr 2013;163(3):771–7.e1.

78. Nicolaou N, Poorafshar M, Murray C, et al. Allergy or tolerance in children sensitized to peanut: prevalence and differentiation using component-resolved diagnostics. J Allergy Clin Immunol 2010;125(1):191–7.e1-13.
79. Rinaldi M, Harnack L, Oberg C, et al. Peanut allergy diagnoses among children residing in Olmsted County, Minnesota. J Allergy Clin Immunol 2012;130(4): 945–50.
80. Shek LP, Cabrera-Morales EA, Soh SE, et al. A population-based questionnaire survey on the prevalence of peanut, tree nut, and shellfish allergy in 2 Asian populations. J Allergy Clin Immunol 2010;126(2):324–31, 331.e1–7.
81. Green TD, LaBelle VS, Steele PH, et al. Clinical characteristics of peanut-allergic children: recent changes. Pediatrics 2007;120(6):1304–10.
82. Vereda A, van Hage M, Ahlstedt S, et al. Peanut allergy: clinical and immunologic differences among patients from 3 different geographic regions. J Allergy Clin Immunol 2011;127(3):603–7.
83. Savage JH, Limb SL, Brereton NH, et al. The natural history of peanut allergy: extending our knowledge beyond childhood. J Allergy Clin Immunol 2007; 120(3):717–9.
84. Bock SA, Atkins FM. The natural history of peanut allergy. J Allergy Clin Immunol 1989;83(5):900–4.
85. Skolnick HS, Conover-Walker MK, Koerner CB, et al. The natural history of peanut allergy. J Allergy Clin Immunol 2001;107(2):367–74.
86. Fleischer DM, Conover-Walker MK, Christie L, et al. The natural progression of peanut allergy: resolution and the possibility of recurrence. J Allergy Clin Immunol 2003;112(1):183–9.
87. Fleischer DM, Conover-Walker MK, Christie L, et al. Peanut allergy: recurrence and its management. J Allergy Clin Immunol 2004;114(5):1195–201.
88. Fleischer DM, Conover-Walker MK, Matsui EC, et al. The natural history of tree nut allergy. J Allergy Clin Immunol 2005;116(5):1087–93.
89. Sicherer SH, Sampson HA. 9. Food allergy. J Allergy Clin Immunol 2006;117(2 Suppl Mini-Primer):S470–5.
90. Sampson HA, McCaskill CM. Food hypersensitivity in atopic dermatitis: evaluation of 113 patients. J Pediatr 1985;107(5):669–75.
91. Savage JH, Kaeding A, Matsui E, et al. The natural history of soy allergy. J Allergy Clin Immunol 2010;125(3):683–6.
92. BallmerWeber BK, Vieths S. Soy allergy in perspective. Curr Opin Allergy Clin Immunol 2008;8(3):270–5.
93. Kotaniemi-Syrjanen A, Palosuo K, Jartti T, et al. The prognosis of wheat hypersensitivity in children. Pediatr Allergy Immunol 2010;21(2 Pt 2):e421–8.
94. Keet C, Matsui E, Dhillon G, et al. The natural history of wheat allergy. Ann Allergy Asthma Immunol 2009;102(5):410.
95. Czaja-Bulsa GY, Bulsa M. The natural history of IgE mediated wheat allergy in children with dominant gastrointestinal symptoms. Allergy Asthma Clin Immunol 2014;10(1):12.
96. Cohen A, Goldberg M, Levy B, et al. Sesame food allergy and sensitization in children: the natural history and long-term follow-up. Pediatr Allergy Immunol 2007;18(3):217–23.
97. Aaronov D, Tasher D, Levine A, et al. Natural history of food allergy in infants and children in Israel. Ann Allergy Asthma Immunol 2008;101(6):637–40.
98. Sicherer SH, Munoz-Furlong A, Sampson HA. Prevalence of seafood allergy in the United States determined by a random telephone survey. J Allergy Clin Immunol 2004;114(1):159–65.

99. Commins SP, Satinover SM, Hosen J, et al. Delayed anaphylaxis, angioedema, or urticaria after consumption of red meat in patients with IgE antibodies specific for galactose-alpha-1,3-galactose. J Allergy Clin Immunol 2009;123(2):426–33.
100. Perry TT, Matsui EC, Kay Conover-Walker M, et al. The relationship of allergen-specific IgE levels and oral food challenge outcome. J Allergy Clin Immunol 2004;114(1):144–9.
101. Komata T, Soderstrom L, Borres M, et al. Usefulness of wheat and soybean specific IgE Antibody titers for the diagnosis of food allergy. Allergol Int 2009;58(4): 599–603.
102. Neuman-Sunshine DL, Eckman JA, Keet CA, et al. The natural history of persistent peanut allergy. Ann Allergy Asthma Immunol 2012;108(5):326–31.e3.
103. Wood RA. The likelihood of remission of food allergy in children: when is the optimal time for challenge? Curr Allergy Asthma Rep 2012;12(1):42–7.
104. Fleischer DM, Spergel JM, Assa'ad AH, et al. Primary prevention of allergic disease through nutritional interventions. J Allergy Clin Immunol Pract 2013;1(1): 29–36.
105. Palmer DJ, Metcalfe J, Makrides M, et al. Early regular egg exposure in infants with eczema: a randomized controlled trial. J Allergy Clin Immunol 2013;132(2): 387–92.e1.
106. Jones SM, Pons L, Roberts JL, et al. Clinical efficacy and immune regulation with peanut oral immunotherapy. J Allergy Clin Immunol 2009;124(2): 292–300.e7.
107. Keet C, Frischmeyer-Guerrerio P, Thyagarajan A, et al. The safety and efficacy of sublingual and oral immunotherapy for milk allergy. J Allergy Clin Immunol 2012; 129(2):448–55.
108. Enrique E, Pineda F, Malek T, et al. Sublingual immunotherapy for hazelnut food allergy: a randomized, double-blind, placebo-controlled study with a standardized hazelnut extract. J Allergy Clin Immunol 2005;116(5):1073–9.
109. Buchanan AD, Green TD, Jones SM, et al. Egg oral immunotherapy in nonanaphylactic children with egg allergy. J Allergy Clin Immunol 2007;119(1):199–205.
110. Chatchatee P, Jarvinen KM, Bardina L, et al. Identification of IgE- and IgG-binding epitopes on alpha(s1)-casein: differences In patients with persistent and transient cow's milk allergy. J Allergy Clin Immunol 2001;107(2):379–83.
111. Shreffler WG. Microarrayed recombinant allergens for diagnostic testing. J Allergy Clin Immunol 2011;127(4):843–9 [quiz: 850–1].
112. Ford LS, Bloom KA, Nowak-Wegrzyn AH, et al. Basophil reactivity, wheal size, and immunoglobulin levels distinguish degrees of cow's milk tolerance. J Allergy Clin Immunol 2013;131(1):180–6.e3.

Optimizing the Diagnosis of Food Allergy

Jacob D. Kattan, MD*, Scott H. Sicherer, MD

KEYWORDS

- Diagnosis • Food allergy • Skin prick testing • Food-specific IgE
- Oral food challenge • Component-resolved diagnostics • Epitope
- Basophil activation

KEY POINTS

- Accurate diagnosis of food allergies is vital to identify patients who may have severe, life-threatening allergic reactions, and to exclude suspected allergies that could lead to unnecessary dietary restrictions.
- Traditional tests for food allergy have several limitations; skin prick testing and food-specific IgE levels are excellent tools for detecting sensitization to foods, but, often, positive tests are clinically irrelevant. Although oral food challenges are the gold standard for diagnosing food allergy, they are time-consuming and costly, and they may result in an allergic reaction.
- Recent studies have identified several testing modalities that may improve the ability to identify true clinical reactivity or severity, including component-resolved diagnostics, basophil activation studies, T-cell proliferative responses, and measurement of platelet-activating factor.

INTRODUCTION

An accurate diagnosis of food allergies is necessary to ensure that an individual is avoiding foods that could trigger severe allergic reactions or contribute to chronic symptoms. Importantly, misdiagnosis could also result in unnecessary dietary restrictions that carry social and nutritional consequences. In 2010, the National Institute of Allergy and Infectious Diseases sponsored an expert panel that published recommendations on the diagnosis of food allergy, endorsing use of the medical history and physical examination, elimination diets, skin prick testing (SPT), serum food-specific IgE (sIgE) levels, and oral food challenges (OFCs).[1] These key diagnostic tools, often used together, are essential for arriving at an accurate diagnosis. Unfortunately, they also carry various limitations. For example, SPTs and sIgE levels are sensitive tools for

Department of Pediatric Allergy and Immunology, Jaffe Food Allergy Institute, Icahn School of Medicine at Mount Sinai, 1 Gustave L. Levy Place, Box 1198, New York, NY 10029, USA
* Corresponding author.
E-mail address: jacob.kattan@mssm.edu

Immunol Allergy Clin N Am 35 (2015) 61–76
http://dx.doi.org/10.1016/j.iac.2014.09.009   immunology.theclinics.com

identifying the presence of food-sIgE antibodies (sensitization) that can be associated with acute allergic reactions, but sensitization often exists without clinical consequence. Additionally, there are circumstances when these tests are negative despite the presence of a true food allergy. The medically supervised OFC is a very specific diagnostic test, but the procedure is time consuming, costly, and may result in a severe allergic reaction. In recent years, several testing modalities have been investigated that may improve food allergy diagnostics, including component-resolved diagnostics (CRD), basophil activation studies, T-cell proliferation assays, and measurement of platelet-activating factor (PAF).

STANDARD DIAGNOSTIC TESTS

The typical diagnostic routine (**Fig. 1**) begins with a medical history to determine whether the symptoms are potentially related to ingestion of specific foods; whether adverse reactions are allergic in nature; and, if so, the likely pathophysiologic basis. Knowledge of the epidemiology of food allergy and details of the history may identify potential triggers to which simple tests, such as SPT and sIgE, can be applied and interpreted in the context of the history and a knowledge of test limitations. When the diagnosis is uncertain, an OFC can be used as the diagnostic gold standard.

The Medical History

The evaluation for a patient with a possible food allergy begins with a thorough history and physical examination. The history should focus on possible triggers of a reaction, the quantity ingested, the time course of the reaction, whether there were ancillary or facilitating factors around the time of the reaction that might have promoted reactivity (exercise, illness, medications such as aspirin), and the specific

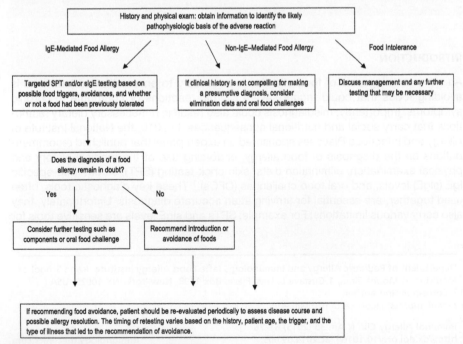

Fig. 1. Food allergy diagnostic algorithm.

symptoms that led to concern for an allergic reaction.[2] The history is important in determining the likely pathophysiologic basis of the reaction, specifically whether the food-induced allergic reaction is IgE-mediated. This is important because tests of food-sIgE would not be diagnostic for disorders that are cell-mediated or non-IgE mediated such as food protein–induced enterocolitis syndrome. Once a possible food trigger is identified, additional history can help decipher if that food is the likely culprit for the reaction. For example, a food that was not previously ingested or was ingested infrequently is more likely to have caused an acute reaction than one that had been regularly tolerated. Common (major) allergens such as milk, egg, wheat, soy, peanut, tree nuts, fish, and shellfish are more likely to be triggers than other foods. The history is, therefore, an important tool to guide allergy test selection and interpretation.

Skin Prick Testing

SPT is extremely sensitive and has a negative predictive value of greater than 90%.[3] This form of testing is often helpful to rapidly rule out an IgE-mediated food allergy. It can also help confirm a food allergy when positive in the setting of a recent clear history of an acute allergic reaction to the tested food (high-priority probability). Unfortunately, the specificity of skin testing is not 100%. Although a positive test, defined in most studies as a mean wheal diameter 3 mm larger than the saline control, is able to confirm sensitization to an allergen, it does not confirm a diagnosis of food allergy. However, evaluating the SPT test result according to wheal size, rather than solely as a positive response, can add to its diagnostic usefulness because studies suggest that the likelihood of a reaction to the tested food increases with increasing SPT wheal size.[2,4]

Researchers have attempted to identify wheal diameter sizes above which virtually no one would be able to tolerate a food, but these values exist for only a few foods and vary among populations. In one Australian study of children presenting to a tertiary allergy clinic, no child was able to pass an OFC if the skin test wheal diameter was above 8 mm for milk, 7 mm for egg, or 8 mm for peanut.[5] A similar study that evaluated a population-based Australian cohort of infants reported 95% predictive values for allergic reactions for egg (SPT wheal $\geq$4 mm), peanut (SPT wheal $\geq$8 mm), and sesame (SPT wheal $\geq$8 mm).[6] These cutoffs were not validated when researchers from Montreal, Canada, looked retrospectively at children evaluated for peanut allergy. Of 140 children examined, 64 had positive SPT responses, and 18 reacted during oral peanut challenge. Of 17 subjects who had an SPT wheal greater than or equal to 10 mm, only 8 had a positive peanut challenge.[7] Although not specific, the SPT testing was sensitive because all 18 subjects with a positive peanut challenge had a wheal diameter greater than or equal to 5 mm. These studies demonstrate that predictive values may vary according to different foods, ages, and populations, and that skin test results cannot be used as an isolated diagnostic tool without a thorough history and, possibly, other testing. Furthermore, commercial food extracts for skin testing have not been standardized, and may contain differing concentrations of relevant proteins, leading to variable results.[8,9] Commercial extracts are also not available for some food allergens. Finally, in some instances, testing may be more accurate using fresh foods (especially fruits and vegetables) by doing a prick-prick test rather than using commercial extracts because relevant labile proteins may not be present in the commercial extracts.[10,11] For ease of use in the clinical setting, fresh fruits can be frozen and used later for skin testing.[12] Skin tests provide quick results and are considered highly sensitive, but they require the patient to be off antihistamines and to have an area of skin free of rash for testing.

Serum IgE Testing

Serum immunoassays that measure food-sIgE antibodies are another common diagnostic tool used in the evaluation of IgE-mediated food allergy. Similar to SPT, in which larger wheal sizes correlate with increased risk of clinical allergy, higher concentrations of food-sIgE correlate with increased risk of true food allergy. As with skin testing, predictive values may differ among populations for various reasons.[13] Proposed cutoffs that predict 50% and 95% likelihood of a reaction to an OFC based on food-sIgE levels for egg, cow's milk, and peanut have been calculated based on several studies of referral populations (**Table 1**).[14] A recent study examining an Australian cohort of infants revealed different predictive levels for egg (95% positive: ≥1.7 kUA/L) and peanut (95% positive: ≥34 kUA/L), which highlights the variability among studies due to geographic differences, subject age, referral base, test characteristics, interpretation of the OFC outcomes, and other factors.[6]

It is also important to note that sIgE levels that have been reported in various studies may use different test systems and that the results between these systems are not directly comparable.[15] Another important limitation is that sIgE levels are not highly correlated with reaction severity.[16,17]

Limitations of skin prick testing and specific IgE

Neither SPT nor sIgE are sufficient to diagnose food allergy on their own.[1] These tests are not predictive of reaction severity. Importantly, there are situations in which clinical reactions occur despite negative tests either because the allergy is not IgE-mediated, for example with food protein-induced enterocolitis syndrome, or because the test does not detect the relevant antigen. These limitations underscore the importance of the medical history. If the suspicion is high, a negative test may not be sufficient to exclude a food allergy.[3,18] Cross-reactivity among foods is often not clinically relevant and this must also be considered in test interpretation. For example, 50% of persons with peanut allergy test positive to other legumes, but 95% tolerate these legumes.[19]

Oral Food Challenge

Given the limitations of current testing modalities, it is often necessary to perform an OFC to make the distinction between a patient who is simply sensitized to an allergen and a patient who is clinically reactive to it. OFCs are also helpful to determine if a child has outgrown their allergy. An OFC is a physician-supervised oral provocation procedure performed in a hospital or outpatient office in which a patient ingests gradually increasing amounts of a food under medical supervision until an age-appropriate serving is reached or the feeding is terminated because of symptoms. There are several factors that must be considered before performing an OFC, including the

Table 1			
Predictive specific IgE values for reactivity to egg, milk, and peanut			
Food	Mean Age 5 y, 50% React	Mean Age 5 y, ~95% React	Age <2 y, ~95% React
Egg (kUA/L)	2	7	2
Milk (kUA/L)	2	15	5
Peanut (kUA/L)	2 (with a clinical history) 5 (without a clinical history)	14	—

Data from Sicherer SH, Sampson HA. Food allergy: epidemiology, pathogenesis, diagnosis, and treatment. J Allergy Clin Immunol 2014;133:291–307.

patient's medical history, age, past adverse food reactions, SPT and serum food allergen–sIgE results, and the importance of the food to the patient, both socially and nutritionally. Indications for performing the OFC can be found in **Box 1**.[13] The OFC is usually performed when the patient's history and test results suggest that the allergy may not exist or may have resolved. The clinician can use the medical history and test results to estimate a probability of tolerance, and the odds can then be considered in the context of the patient's needs, weighing the risks and benefits.

The OFC can be performed as an open feeding or as a single-blind or double-blind placebo-controlled food challenge (DBPCFC). In an open challenge, the subject is aware that they are ingesting the potentially problematic food, which can lead to symptoms from anxiety, biasing the test. Although an open feeding is the most common approach used clinically for OFCs, this bias must be considered if the child fails the challenge. The DBPCFC is the most specific test for the diagnosis of a food allergy.[1] In this test, the food is masked in a carrier, and the food to be tested or placebo is randomly administered at different times. Although the DBPCFC is currently the gold standard test for diagnosing food allergy, due to the time and labor-intensive nature of this method, it is typically only performed in research studies and select cases in clinical practice.[20,21] A single-blind placebo-controlled OFC may be helpful if the subject is suspected of having a psychological response. The open challenge is a reasonable first choice when the need for OFC is established because less than one-third of suspected foods result in a positive challenge, and many of these positive OFCs will have objective symptoms.[18,20,22]

How a food is processed can affect the challenge outcome. Heating can change the protein conformation of certain foods and may result in a change in allergenicity.[23] This is seen with milk and egg, as well as with several fruits and vegetables implicated in pollen-food allergy syndrome.[24–27] Based on studies of peanut, patients may be at risk of their allergy recurring if they fail to incorporate the food into their diet on a regular basis after passing an OFC.[28,29]

When considering whether or not to perform an OFC in the office setting, safety is a concern, and patients should be made aware of the risks and benefits of the OFC. Lieberman and colleagues[30] reported the results of all OFCs performed between August 2008 and May 2010 at the Jaffe Food Allergy Institute, the authors' university-based, outpatient practice. This was a retrospective chart review that included all subjects referred by 9 allergists; subjects were typically challenged when the likelihood of a

---

Box 1
Indications for an oral food challenge

Identify foods causing acute reactions for initial diagnosis of food allergy and for monitoring resolution of food allergy.

Determine whether food allergens associated with chronic conditions such as atopic dermatitis or allergic eosinophilic esophagitis will cause immediate reactions.

Expand the diet in persons with multiple dietary restrictions, usually because of subjective complaints such as headaches or hyperactive behavior.

Assess the status of tolerance to cross-reactive foods.

Assess the effect of food processing on food tolerability, including fruits and vegetables that may be tolerated in cooked form in the pollen-food allergy syndrome.

From Nowak-Wegrzyn A, Assa'ad AH, Bahna SL, et al. Work Group report: oral food challenge testing. J Allergy Clin Immunol 2009;123:S366; with permission.

reaction was thought to be less than 50%, though no specific cutoffs for SPT size or sIgE precluded a challenge. There were 701 OFCs performed in 521 subjects who ranged in age from 8 months to 21.8 years. OFCs were performed to a wide variety of foods, most commonly milk, egg, peanut, tree nuts, soy, fish, shellfish, sesame, and wheat. Overall, 132 (18.8%) challenges elicited a reaction. Most of those reactions were cutaneous (56.8%), and 9.1% were treated with epinephrine, with one requiring 2 doses. Because, overall, only 1.7% of challenges required treatment with epinephrine, the investigators concluded that open OFCs are a safe and effective method of ascertaining tolerance in patients with potential food allergy.

The benefits of performing OFCs, in particular eliminating unnecessary dietary restrictions, have been demonstrated in several studies. Using OFCs, Nicolaou and colleagues[31] demonstrated the high rate of false-positive SPT and sIgE to peanut. In a population-based birth cohort from the United Kingdom of 933 children, 110 (11.8%) were peanut-sensitized at 8 years of age. OFCs were performed on those children without a convincing history of reaction and on those who had a peanut-sIgE less than or equal to 15 kUA/L, and peanut skin test wheal less than or equal to 8 mm. Based on OFC results, the estimated prevalence of clinical peanut allergy was only 22.4% among sensitized children. In a study from Denver of 125 children, primarily with atopic dermatitis, who were avoiding foods largely due to previous immunoassay and SPT results, 89% of 364 OFCs were passed, allowing significant dietary expansion.[32] The investigators concluded that, in the absence of anaphylaxis, the primary reliance on serum food-sIgE testing to make the diagnosis of food allergy, particularly in children with atopic dermatitis, is not sufficient.

EMERGING DIAGNOSTIC TESTS
Component-Resolved Diagnostics

Allergen CRDs have garnered a lot of attention in recent years, with the hope of offering a more accurate assessment of allergic status. Instead of using crude allergen extracts consisting of a mixture of components, CRD measures IgE to individual allergen proteins. In recent years, several studies on a variety of food allergens have demonstrated that CRD can improve the specificity of allergy testing.

The usefulness of CRD has been best demonstrated in studies on peanut allergy.[33] In 2004, Koppelman and colleagues[34] suggested the importance of the peanut component, Ara h 2, in predicting reactivity or tolerance to peanut. The level of IgE to Ara h 2, one of the major peanut allergens, was most important for predicting allergic status in their cohort of 32 subjects, with 26 out of 32 peanut-allergic subjects testing positive to this component. Similarly, Dang and colleagues[35] reported that Ara h 2 sIgE levels provide higher diagnostic accuracy than whole peanut-sIgE levels. In the Australian HealthNuts study,[36] 11- to 15-month-old infants underwent SPT to peanut, and if a positive wheal reaction was elicited, the infant was invited for a formal open OFC. Overall, 411 peanut-sensitized infants underwent a peanut OFC, 137 of which were positive. Nonsensitized subjects (n = 140) also underwent a peanut OFC as negative controls. Another 100 peanut-allergic subjects and 100 peanut-tolerant subjects were randomly selected for Ara h 2 testing, and whole peanut–IgE testing was also performed. Compared with currently used whole peanut–sIgE levels, Ara h 2 sIgE levels were more accurate in determining peanut allergy. An Ara h 2 sIgE level of 0.46 less than or equal to provided 95% specificity and 73% sensitivity, whereas a peanut-sIgE level of 6.2 kUA/L provided 95% specificity but only 44% sensitivity. In comparison, a peanut-sIgE level of 15 kUA/L provided a 95% PPV and 98% specificity but the sensitivity dropped to 26%. An Ara h 2 level of 1.19

kUA/L provided 98% specificity but offered sensitivity of 60%. Given the improved accuracy found in the Ara h 2 sIgE diagnostic testing, it was concluded that this test could become a preferred diagnostic tool for diagnosing peanut allergy. However, similar to the problems with food-sIgE testing, predictive cutoff levels for Ara h 2 have varied from study to study. Among children in a referral population in the United States, the positive predictive value was reported to be 75% at 2 kUA/L, and the negative predictive value was 91% at 0.23 kUA/L.[37] Researchers from the Netherlands examined Ara h 2 levels among children with suspected peanut allergy and reported that a cutoff of 5 kUA/L had the best overall predictive value, with a positive predictive value of 96% and a negative predictive value of 71%.[38] Although the studies all report benefits with the use of Ara h 2 in the diagnosis of peanut allergy, the differing cutoffs for predictive values likely reflect differences in sensitization among different geographic locations and populations, and demonstrate that there are subjects with positive test results to Ara h 2 who are still able to tolerate peanut. Ara h 2 levels also do not seem to clearly predict severity among subjects with peanut allergy.[39]

The peanut component Ara h 6 is structurally similar to Ara h 2 and has been reported to be a relevant allergen in peanut allergy, though it is unclear if assessment of IgE levels to this component would offer additional diagnostic value to that of Ara h 2 alone as part of CRD.[40] Asarnoj and colleagues[41] reported a case of a 15-year-old boy who was sensitized to Ara h 8 but not to Ara h 1, 2, or 3, who developed anaphylaxis, including vomiting, diarrhea, and lower respiratory obstruction, following peanut ingestion. He was found to have marked sensitization to Ara h 6 (24 kUA/L), whereas Ara h 2 remained below 0.35 kUA/L (0.12 kUA/L). A recent study by Klemans and colleagues[42] assessing the diagnostic value of sIgE to Ara h 6 in an adult population in the Netherlands with suspected peanut allergy, demonstrated that the discriminative ability of Ara h 6 was as good as sIgE to Ara h 2, though they did not demonstrate an added benefit to analyzing Ara h 6 instead of, or in addition to, the measurement of Ara h 2. Component testing to peanut is more likely to be informative if the patient has a history of no or mild reactions, a remote clinical reaction with development of birch tree pollen sensitization over time, a peanut-sIgE between 0.35 and 15 kUA/L, birch pollen sensitization, or if the patient is older.[33]

CRD has the potential to be a very useful tool in the diagnosis of hazelnut allergy as well. It is well known that cross-reactivity between proteins found in pollens and foods can account for positive test results to a variety of plant-derived foods. Hazelnut is one such food. Cor a 1 proteins cross-react with the birch pollen allergen, Bet v 1. In 2007, it was noted that many subjects had higher than expected serum hazelnut-sIgE levels.[43] At that time, the hazelnut extract in one manufacturer's test was supplemented with additional recombinant Cor a 1 to improve the test's sensitivity for birch-related reactions to hazelnut; however, this made it difficult to distinguish patients who had a serious allergy to hazelnut versus those who were sensitized to hazelnut only as a result of cross-reactivity from their birch pollen allergy. Phadia Immunology Reference Laboratory developed commercial IgE testing to the hazelnut components Cor a 1 and Cor a 8, and later added Cor a 9 and Cor a 14 to their hazelnut panel. In reports from the Mediterranean area, systemic reactions to hazelnut are generally mediated by IgE to Cor a 8, a lipid transfer protein.[44,45] In reports from the United States and Europe, sensitization to Cor a 9, an 11S globulin, and Cor a 14, a 2S albumin, have been associated with severe hazelnut allergy in children.[46–49] In a Dutch study by Masthoff and colleagues,[48] sensitization to Cor a 9 and Cor a 14 was highly specific for identifying subjects with objective symptoms to hazelnut. In this study, IgE levels of 1 kUA/L or greater to Cor a 9 or 5 kUA/L or greater to Cor a 14 in children, and 1 kUA/L or greater to Cor a 9 or 1 kUA/L or greater to Cor a 14 in adults, gave a specificity of greater than 90% for predicting true allergy to hazelnut. Similar findings were noted by the authors' group in a birch endemic area of the United States, where the specificity of hazelnut testing was greatly improved when using hazelnut components that included Cor a 9 and 14.[49] These components were both highly sensitive and specific, particularly when used in combination.

Although several studies have reported the usefulness of component testing for allergies to egg, milk, wheat, soy, and fruits, results from these studies have varied, likely reflecting different study populations and methods, manners of sensitization, environmental exposures, and degree of sensitization to various food components.[50–63] In studies on cow's milk, hen's egg, and shrimp component testing, CRD offered increased specificity but decreased sensitivity when compared with traditional SPT and serum-sIgE testing.[52,53,62] From a practical standpoint, this means that CRD for these foods could be used as an adjunct to currently used allergy tests to avoid performing some OFCs, but it is not ready to be used on its own in ruling out a food allergy.

The reported usefulness of component testing for diagnosing wheat allergy is also quite variable. Omega-5 gliadin has been identified as a major allergen in children for provoking wheat-dependent, exercise-induced anaphylaxis.[56] Studies from Finland and Japan have reported that omega-5 gliadin is a significant allergen in children with immediate reactions to wheat, and that this component can be used to predict the outcome of oral wheat challenges.[57,58] A collaborative study examining wheat allergy in both American and German children found no correlation between omega-5 gliadin levels and the outcomes of oral wheat challenges, and the investigators concluded that omega-5 gliadin–sIgE levels in wheat-sensitized subjects seem not to be helpful for diagnosis.[59] A recent European study reported that IgE to the wheat component rTri a 36 accurately identified more subjects with true wheat allergy than did IgE to omega-5 gliadin.[60] Although the different results reported from these studies could result from different sensitization patterns in different geographic locations, they also likely reflect different inclusion criteria and other differences in the populations tested.

FUTURE DIAGNOSTIC TESTS

Several tests are undergoing study and may have advantages compared with currently available tests for diagnosing food allergy (**Table 2**).

Epitope Binding

Just as immune responses against different proteins within a food may carry different clinical implications, the location (epitope) and strength of binding (affinity) of IgE antibodies within a protein may also have clinical ramifications. Having IgE antibodies directed to a greater number of epitopes, or to epitopes that are not easily destroyed by denaturation and digestion (eg, sequential or linear epitopes instead of those which depend on folding and conformation) may be associated with clinical allergy.[64] The role of sequential IgE-binding epitopes in subjects with persistent milk allergy has been reported in several studies.[65,66] A recent study from Finland, in which investigators compared IgE, IgG4, and IgA binding to cow's milk epitopes in subjects with early resolution versus persistent cow's milk allergy, demonstrated that cow's milk tolerance is associated with decreased IgE epitope binding and increased epitope binding by IgG4.[67] They compared results from serum samples obtained at the time of diagnosis, 1 year later, and at follow-up years later in 11 subjects with IgE-mediated cow's milk allergy that was persistent to age 8 to 9 years, and in 12 subjects who recovered

Table 2
Emerging and future diagnostic tests

Testing Modality	Potential Advantages	Pitfalls
CRDs	• Some components offer increased specificity compared with SPT and sIgE • Requires a small amount of patient serum	• Decreased sensitivity for a variety of food allergens • In studies for several foods, results vary, likely reflecting differences among study populations, manners of sensitization, and environmental exposures
Epitope Binding	• May be a marker of allergy persistence • More specific marker of clinical reactivity	• Yet to be studied for several common food allergens
T-Cell Responses	• Improved specificity over SPT and sIgE	• Difficult to measure, unlikely to become commercially available in the near future
Basophil Activation	• May better distinguish between milk allergic patients who can tolerate baked milk and those who cannot • A potential marker of allergy severity	• Requires the ability to perform flow cytometry • Not yet evaluated in several common food allergens
PAF and PAF Acetylhydrolase	• A potential marker of allergy severity and risk for anaphylaxis	• Clinical usefulness yet to be substantiated in multiple studies • Unclear if this can be used as a marker of allergy severity at baseline

by age 3 years. Although the IgE epitope-binding patterns were stable over time in the subjects whose allergy to cow's milk persisted, binding decreased in those subjects who recovered early.

Ayuso and colleagues[68] investigated whether the recognition of particular IgE epitopes of certain shrimp allergens are good biomarkers for clinical reactivity to shrimp. They performed DBPCFC on 37 consecutive subjects with clinical histories of shrimp allergy and analyzed their IgE binding to synthetic overlapping peptides representing the sequence of 4 allergens of the Pacific white shrimp, Lit v 1, 2, 3 and 4. The 17 subjects with a positive challenge to shrimp had more intense and diverse epitope recognition to all 4 shrimp allergens. They concluded that IgE antibodies to these epitopes could be used as biomarkers for predicting clinical reactivity in subjects sensitized to shrimp. Studies have also demonstrated potential benefits from analyzing IgE epitope binding in studies of egg and wheat allergy.[69,70] It may not be long before epitope binding assays make their way to the clinical arena.

T-Cell Responses

In recent years, researchers have examined T-cell responses to food allergens, and it has been reported that analysis of allergen-specific T-cell responses may be useful for distinguishing sensitization from clinical reactivity.[71,72] Flinterman and colleagues[73] examined T-cell responses to the major peanut allergens Ara h 1, 2, 3, and 6 in peanut-allergic children, nonallergic peanut-sensitized children, and nonatopic adults. The peanut-allergic children were the only subjects who demonstrated increased IL-13 production in response to Ara h 1, 3 and 6. Further studies will be necessary to confirm the usefulness of T-cell proliferative responses in the diagnosis of food allergy.

Basophil Activation

Several studies have reported that markers of basophil activation, specifically upregulation of cell-surface molecules such as CD63 and CD203c using flow cytometry, may be helpful in the diagnosis of food allergy. Sato and colleagues[74] reported their findings from a Japanese cohort examining the performance of basophil activation for predicting challenge outcomes to egg and milk. In a group of 71 children with egg or milk allergy previously diagnosed by challenge outcomes or convincing history, they found that assessment of food antigen–induced CD203c expression on basophils was useful in determining whether a child will outgrow a food allergy and in deciding whether or not to perform an OFC. In a study evaluating tolerance to baked milk among children with cow's milk allergy, Ford and colleagues[75] compared basophil reactivity among subjects with milk allergy who reacted to baked milk and those who could tolerate it. They reported that the median basophil reactivity to cow's milk, as well as spontaneous basophil activation, were significantly higher among subjects who reacted to baked milk versus those who were able to tolerate milk in a baked form. Furthermore, they reported that spontaneous basophil activation was greater among subjects with more severe clinical milk reactivity. This discovery lends hope to clinicians looking for a potential test to predict the severity of a patient's food allergy. Further studies are necessary to elucidate the usefulness of basophil activation for use in clinical practice.

Platelet-Activating Factor and Platelet-Activating Factor Acetylhydrolase

There are currently no means to accurately predict the severity of an allergic reaction. Researchers have examined serum PAF and PAF acetylhydrolase (PAF-AH) levels as potential markers of allergy severity. PAF is a proinflammatory phospholipid synthesized and secreted by mast cells, basophils, monocytes, and macrophages. It has various biological activities, including platelet activation, airway constriction, hypotension, and vascular permeation.[76–78] Circulating levels of PAF are, in part, controlled by the activity of PAF-AH, an enzyme that controls activity by cleaving PAF, rendering it inactive. It has been demonstrated that anaphylactic symptoms can be mimicked by PAF injection in animals.[78,79] PAF-receptor antagonists protect against anaphylaxis in mice, rabbits, and rats.[80] PAF-receptor knockout mice are protected from fatal anaphylaxis in contrast to wild-type mice with intact PAF receptors.[81]

Vadas and colleagues[82] measured serum PAF levels and PAF-AH activity in 41 subjects with anaphylaxis and 23 control subjects. PAF-AH activity was also compared in 9 subjects who had fatal anaphylaxis with those in nonallergic control subjects, children with mild peanut allergy, and subjects with nonfatal anaphylaxis. Serum PAF levels were directly correlated and serum PAF-AH activity was inversely correlated with the severity of anaphylaxis. Further studies are necessary to establish the role of PAF and its related catabolic enzymes in the prediction and confirmation of anaphylaxis.

CONTROVERSIAL AND UNPROVEN TESTS

There are several tests that have been examined that are not recommended for the diagnosis of food allergy. Intradermal testing should not be used. Not only is intradermal injection of allergens overly sensitive, but it also carries a higher risk of adverse reactions than SPT.[1,83] The National Institute of Allergy and Infectious Diseases expert guidelines published in 2010 also suggest that atopy patch testing (APT) should not be used in the routine evaluation of noncontact food allergy. Although some studies have suggested that APT may be useful in the evaluation of food allergy in subjects with eosinophilic esophagitis or atopic dermatitis, the sensitivity and specificity is variable among different studies, and there is no consensus on the appropriate reagents or methods to use, or on how to interpret these tests.[1,84–87] Measuring the total serum IgE level is not recommended for routine use in making a diagnosis of food allergy.[1] When researchers have examined the predictive value of the ratio of sIgE to total IgE for the diagnosis of food allergy compared with the DBPCFC, it was concluded that the ratio did not offer an advantage over sIgE alone,[88] although emerging studies may suggest otherwise.[89] Finally, other nonstandardized tests that are not recommended for the routine evaluation of IgE-mediated food allergy include facial thermography, gastric juice analysis, applied kinesiology, allergen-sIgG₄ levels, hair analysis, and electrodermal testing.[1]

FUTURE CONSIDERATIONS AND SUMMARY

The work-up of a potential food allergy can be a complex assessment involving the clinical history, SPT, and sIgE levels, although ultimately these diagnostic tools may be inadequate to definitively diagnose a food allergy. Currently, OFCs remain the most definitive test in the diagnosis of food allergy, but they are time consuming, costly, and have the potential to elicit a severe allergic reaction. In recent years, several different testing modalities, including CRD, basophil activation studies, T-cell proliferation assays, and measurement of PAF have demonstrated potential to aid the allergist in better identifying a patient with true clinical reactivity to an allergen. Although CRD is currently used clinically, the remaining tests are promising but require further evaluation before they are ready for implementation in clinical practice.

REFERENCES

1. Boyce JA, Assa'ad A, Burks AW, et al. Guidelines for the diagnosis and management of food allergy in the United States: report of the NIAD-sponsored expert panel. J Allergy Clin Immunol 2010;126:S1–58.
2. American College of Allergy, Asthma, & Immunology. Food allergy: a practice parameter. Ann Allergy Asthma Immunol 2006;9:S1–68.
3. Sicherer SH, Sampson HA. Food allergy. J Allergy Clin Immunol 2010;125:S116–25.
4. Knight AK, Shreffler WG, Sampson HA, et al. Skin prick test to egg white provides additional diagnostic utility to serum egg white-specific IgE antibody concentration in children. J Allergy Clin Immunol 2006;117:842–7.
5. Sporik R, Hill DJ, Hosking CS. Specificity of allergen skin testing in predicting positive open food challenges to milk, egg, and peanut in children. Clin Exp Allergy 2000;30:1541–6.
6. Peters RL, Allen KJ, Dharmage SC, et al. Skin prick test responses and allergen-specific IgE levels as predictors of peanut, egg, and sesame allergy in infants. J Allergy Clin Immunol 2013;132:874–80.
7. Pucar F, Kagan R, Lim H, et al. Peanut challenge: a retrospective study of 140 patients. Clin Exp Allergy 2001;31:40–6.
8. Sampson HA. Comparative study of commercial food antigen extracts for the diagnosis of food hypersensitivity. J Allergy Clin Immunol 1988;82:718–26.
9. Hefle SL, Helm RN, Burks AW, et al. Comparison of commercial peanut skin test extracts. J Allergy Clin Immunol 1995;95:837–42.

10. Rancé F, Juchet A, Brémont F, et al. Correlations between skin prick tests using commercial extracts and fresh foods, specific IgE, and food challenges. Allergy 1997;52:1031–5.
11. Vertege A, Mehl A, Rolinck-Werninghaus C. The predictive value of skin prick test wheal size for the outcome of oral food challenges. Clin Exp Allergy 2005;35: 1220–6.
12. Begin P, Des RA, Nguyen M, et al. Freezing does not alter antigenic properties of fresh fruits for skin testing in patients with birch tree pollen-induced oral allergy syndrome. J Allergy Clin Immunol 2011;127:1624–6.
13. Nowak-Wegrzyn A, Assa'ad AH, Bahna SL, et al. Work group report: oral food challenge testing. J Allergy Clin Immunol 2009;123:S365–83.
14. Sicherer SH, Sampson HA. Food allergy: epidemiology, pathogenesis, diagnosis, and treatment. J Allergy Clin Immunol 2014;133:291–307.
15. Wang J, Godbold JH, Sampson HA. Correlation of serum allergy (IgE) tests performed by different assay systems. J Allergy Clin Immunol 2008;121:1219–24.
16. Perry TT, Matsui EC, Kay Conover-Walker M, et al. The relationship of allergen-specific IgE levels and oral food challenge outcome. J Allergy Clin Immunol 2004;114:144–9.
17. Sicherer SH, Morrow EH, Sampson HA. Dose-response in double-blind, placebo-controlled oral food challenges in children with atopic dermatitis. J Allergy Clin Immunol 2000;105:582–6.
18. Sicherer SH, Wood RA. Allergy testing in childhood: using allergen-specific IgE tests. Pediatrics 2012;129:193–7.
19. Sicherer SH. Clinical implications of cross-reactive food allergens. J Allergy Clin Immunol 2001;108:881–90.
20. Sampson HA, Gerth van Wijk R, Bindslev-Jensen C, et al. Standardizing double-blind, placebo-controlled oral food challenges: American Academy of Allergy, Asthma & Immunology-European Academy of Allergy and Clinical Immunology PRACTALL consensus report. J Allergy Clin Immunol 2012;130:1260–74.
21. Bindslev-Jensen C, Ballmer-Weber BK, Bengtsson U, et al. Standardization of food challenges in patients with immediate reactions to foods—position paper from the European Academy of Allergology and Clinical Immunology. Allergy 2004;59:690–7.
22. Bahna SL. Blind food challenge testing with wide-open eyes. Ann Allergy 1994; 72:235–8.
23. Thomas K, Herouet-Guicheney C, Ladics G, et al. Evaluating the effect of food processing on the potential human allergenicity of novel proteins: international workshop report. Food Chem Toxicol 2007;45:1116–22.
24. Eigenmann PA. Anaphylactic reactions to raw eggs after negative challenges with cooked egg. J Allergy Clin Immunol 2000;105:587–8.
25. Beyer K, Morrow E, Li XM, et al. Effects of cooking methods on peanut allergenicity. J Allergy Clin Immunol 2001;107:1077–81.
26. Nowak-Wegrzyn A, Bloom KA, Sicherer SH, et al. Tolerance to extensively heated milk in children with cow's milk allergy. J Allergy Clin Immunol 2008;122:342–7.
27. Lemon-Mule H, Sampson HA, Sicherer SH, et al. Immunologic changes in children with egg allergy ingesting extensively heated egg. J Allergy Clin Immunol 2008;122:977–83.
28. Busse PJ, Nowak-Wegrzyn AH, Noone SA, et al. Recurrent peanut allergy. N Engl J Med 2002;347:1535–6.
29. Fleischer DM, Conover-Walker MK, Christie L, et al. Peanut allergy: recurrence and its management. J Allergy Clin Immunol 2004;114:1195–201.

30. Lieberman JA, Cox AL, Vitale M, et al. Outcomes of office-based, open food challenges in the management of food allergy. J Allergy Clin Immunol 2011;128(5): 1120–2.
31. Nicolaou N, Poorafshar M, Murray C, et al. Allergy or tolerance in children sensitized to peanut: prevalence and differentiation using component-resolved diagnostics. J Allergy Clin Immunol 2010;125:191–7.
32. Fleischer DM, Bock SA, Spears GC, et al. Oral food challenges in children with a diagnosis of food allery. J Pediatr 2011;158:578–83.
33. Sicherer SH, Wood RA. Advances in diagnosing peanut allergy. J Allergy Clin Immunol Pract 2013;1:1–13.
34. Koppelman SJ, Wensing M, Ertmann M, et al. Relevance of Ara h1, Ara h2 and Ara h3 in peanut-allergic patients, as determined by immunoglobulin E Western blotting, basophil-histamine release and intracutaneous testing: Ara h2 is the most important peanut allergen. Clin Exp Allergy 2004;34:583–90.
35. Dang TD, Tang M, Choo S, et al. Increasing the accuracy of peanut allergy diagnosis by using Ara h 2. J Allergy Clin Immunol 2012;129:1056–63.
36. Osborne NJ, Koplin JJ, Martin PE, et al. The HealthNuts population-based study of paediatric food allergy: validity, safety and acceptability. Clin Exp Allergy 2010; 40:1516–22.
37. Keet CA, Johnson K, Savage JH, et al. Evaluation of Ara h 2 IgE thresholds in the diagnosis of peanut allergy in a clinical population. J Allergy Clin Immunol Pract 2013;1:101–3.
38. Lopes de Oliveira LC, Aderhold M, Brill M, et al. The value of specific IgE to peanut and its component Ara-h 2 in the diagnosis of peanut allergy. J Allergy Clin Immunol Pract 2013;1:394–8.
39. Klemans RJ, Otte D, Knol M, et al. The diagnostic value of specific IgE to Ara h 2 to predict peanut allergy in children is comparable to a validated and updated diagnostic prediction model. J Allergy Clin Immunol 2013;131:157–63.
40. Koppelman SJ, de Jong GA, Laaper-Ertmann M, et al. Purification and immunoglobulin E-binding properties of peanut allergen Ara h 6: evidence for cross-reactivity with Ara h 2. Clin Exp Allergy 2005;35:490–7.
41. Asarnoj A, Glaumann S, Elfström L, et al. Anaphylaxis to peanut in a patient predominantly sensitized to Ara h 6. Int Arch Allergy Immunol 2012;159:209–12.
42. Klemans RJ, Knol EF, Bruijnzeel-Koomen CA, et al. The diagnostic accuracy of specific IgE to Ara h 6 in adults is as good as Ara h 2. Allergy 2014;69(8):112–4.
43. Sicherer SH, Dhillon G, Laughery KA, et al. Caution: the Phadia hazelnut ImmunoCAP (f17) has been supplemented with recombinant Cor a 1 and now detects Bet v 1-specific IgE, which leads to elevated values for persons with birch pollen allergy. J Allergy Clin Immunol 2008;122:413–4.
44. Ortolani C, Ballmer-Weber BK, Hansen KS, et al. Hazelnut allergy: a double-blind, placebo-controlled food challenge multicenter study. J Allergy Clin Immunol 2000;105:577–81.
45. Flinterman AE, Akkerdaas JH, den Hartog Jager CF, et al. Lipid transfer protein-linked hazelnut allergy in children from a non-Mediterranean birch-endemic area. J Allergy Clin Immunol 2008;121:423–8.
46. Beyer K, Grishina G, Bardina L, et al. Identification of an 11S globulin as a major hazelnut food allergen in hazelnut-induced systemic reactions. J Allergy Clin Immunol 2002;110:517–23.
47. De Knop KJ, Verweij MM, Grimmelikhuijsen M, et al. Age-related sensitization profiles for hazelnut (Corylus avellana) in a birch-endemic region. Pediatr Allergy Immunol 2011;22:e139–49.

48. Masthoff LJ, Mattsson L, Zuidmeer-Jongejan L, et al. Sensitization to Cor a 9 and Cor a 14 is highly specific for a hazelnut allergy with objective symptoms in Dutch children and adults. J Allergy Clin Immunol 2013;132:393–9.
49. Kattan JD, Sicherer SH, Sampson HA. Clinical reactivity to hazelnut may be better identified by component testing than traditional testing methods. J Allergy Clin Immunol Pract 2014;2(5):633–4.e1.
50. Bartnikas LM, Sheehan WJ, Larabee KS, et al. Ovomucoid is not superior to egg white testing in predicting tolerance to baked egg. J Allergy Clin Immunol Pract 2013;1:354–60.
51. Ott H, Baron JM, Heise R, et al. Clinical usefulness of microarray-based IgE detection in children with suspected food allergy. Allergy 2008;63:1521–8.
52. D'Urbano LE, Pellegrino K, Artesani MC, et al. Performance of a component-based allergen-microarray in the diagnosis of cow's milk and hen's egg allergy. Clin Exp Allergy 2010;40:1561–70.
53. Alessandri C, Zennaro D, Scala E, et al. Ovomucoid (Gal d 1) specific IgE detected by microarray system predict tolerability to boiled hen's egg and an increased risk to progress to multiple environmental allergen sensitisation. Clin Exp Allergy 2012;42:441–50.
54. Caubet JC, Bencharitiwong R, Moshier E, et al. Significance of ovomucoid- and ovalbumin-specific IgE/IgG(4) ratios in egg allergy. J Allergy Clin Immunol 2012; 129:739–47.
55. Caubet JC, Nowak-Wegrzyn A, Moshier E, et al. Utility of casein-specific IgE levels in predicting reactivity to baked milk. J Allergy Clin Immunol 2013;131: 222–4.
56. Matsuo H, Dahlstrom J, Tanaka A, et al. Sensitivity and specificity of recombinant omega-5 gliadin-specific IgE measurement for the diagnosis of wheat-dependent exercise-induced anaphylaxis. Allergy 2008;63:233–6.
57. Palosuo K, Varjonen E, Kekki OM, et al. Wheat omega-5 gliadin is a major allergen in children with immediate allergy to ingested wheat. J Allergy Clin Immunol 2001;108:634–8.
58. Shibata R, Nishima S, Tanaka A, et al. Usefulness of specific IgE antibodies to ω-5 gliadin in the diagnosis and follow-up of Japanese children with wheat allergy. Ann Allergy Asthma Immunol 2011;107:337–43.
59. Beyer K, Chung D, Schulz G, et al. The role of wheat omega-5 gliadin IgE antibodies as a diagnostic tool for wheat allergy in childhood. J Allergy Clin Immunol 2008;122:419–21.
60. Baar A, Pahr S, Constantin C, et al. Specific IgE reactivity to Tri a 36 in children with wheat food allergy. J Allergy Clin Immunol 2014;133:585–7.
61. Gómez-Casado C, Garrido-Arandia M, Pereira C, et al. Component-resolved diagnosis of wheat flour allergy in baker's asthma. J Allergy Clin Immunol 2014; 134(2):480–3.
62. Gámez C, Sánchez-García S, Ibáñez MD, et al. Tropomyosin IgE-positive results are a good predictor of shrimp allergy. Allergy 2011;66:1375–83.
63. Ebisawa M, Brostedt P, Sjolander S, et al. Gly m 2S albumin is a major allergen with a high diagnostic value in soybean-allergic children. J Allergy Clin Immunol 2013;132:976–8.
64. Sampson HA. Improving in-vitro tests for the diagnosis of food hypersensitivity. Curr Opin Allergy Clin Immunol 2002;2:257–61.
65. Chatchatee P, Jarvinen KM, Bardina L, et al. Identification of IgE- and IgG-binding epitopes on alpha(s1)-casein: differences in patients with persistent and transient cow's milk allergy. J Allergy Clin Immunol 2001;107:379–83.

66. Chatchatee P, Järvinen KM, Bardina L, et al. Identification of IgE and IgG binding epitopes on beta- and kappa-casein in cow's milk allergic patients. Clin Exp Allergy 2001;31:1256–62.
67. Savilahti EM, Rantanen V, Lin JS, et al. Early recovery from cow's milk allergy is associated with decreasing IgE and increasing IgG4 binding to cow's milk epitopes. J Allergy Clin Immunol 2010;125:1315–21.
68. Ayuso R, Sanchez-Garcia S, Pascal M, et al. Is epitope recognition of shrimp allergens useful to predict clinical reactivity? Clin Exp Allergy 2012;42:293–304.
69. Cooke SK, Sampson HA. Allergenic properties of ovomucoid in man. J Immunol 1997;159:2026–32.
70. Battais F, Mothes T, Moneret-Vautrin DA, et al. Identification of IgE-binding epitopes on gliadins for patients with food allergy to wheat. Allergy 2005;60: 815–21.
71. Hoffman KM, Ho DG, Sampson HA. Evaluation of the usefulness of lymphocyte proliferation assays in the diagnosis of allergy to cow's milk. J Allergy Clin Immunol 1997;99:360–6.
72. Thottingal TB, Stefura BP, Simons FE, et al. Human subjects without peanut allergy demonstrate T cell-dependent, TH2-biased, peanut-specific cytokine and chemokine responses independent of TH1 expression. J Allergy Clin Immunol 2006;118:905–14.
73. Flinterman AE, Pasmans SG, den Hartog Jager CF, et al. T cell responses to major peanut allergens in children with and without peanut allergy. Clin Exp Allergy 2010;40:590–7.
74. Sato S, Tachimoto H, Shukuya A, et al. Basophil activation marker CD203c is useful in the diagnosis of hen's egg and cow's milk allergies in children. Int Arch Allergy Immunol 2010;152:54–61.
75. Ford LS, Bloom KA, Nowak-Wegrzyn A, et al. Basophil reactivity, wheal size, and immunoglobulin levels distinguish degrees of cow's milk tolerance. J Allergy Clin Immunol 2013;131:180–6.
76. Hanahan DJ. Platelet activating factor: a biologically active phosphoglyceride. Annu Rev Biochem 1986;55:483–509.
77. Prescott SM, Zimmerman GA, McIntyre TM. Platelet-activating factor. J Biol Chem 1990;265:17381–4.
78. Imaizumi TA, Stafforini DM, Yamada Y, et al. Platelet-activating factor: a mediator for clinicians. J Intern Med 1995;238:5 20.
79. Izumi T, Shimizu T. Platelet-activating factor receptor: gene expression and signal transduction. Biochim Biophys Acta 1995;1259:317–33.
80. Finkelman FD, Rothenberg ME, Brandt EB, et al. Molecular mechanisms of anaphylaxis: lessons from studies with murine models. J Allergy Clin Immunol 2005;115:449–57.
81. Ishii S, Kuwaki T, Nagase T, et al. Impaired anaphylactic responses with intact sensitivity to endotoxin in mice lacking a platelet-activating factor receptor. J Exp Med 1998;187:1779–88.
82. Vadas P, Gold M, Perelman B, et al. Platelet-activating factor, PAF acetylhydrolase, and severe anaphylaxis. N Engl J Med 2008;358:28–35.
83. Bock SA, Buckley J, Holst A, et al. Proper use of skin tests with food extracts in diagnosis of hypersensitivity to food in children. Clin Allergy 1977;7: 375–83.
84. Mehl A, Rolinck-Werninghaus C, Staden U, et al. The atopy patch test in the diagnostic workup of suspected food-related symptoms in children. J Allergy Clin Immunol 2006;118:923–9.

85. Keskin O, Tuncer A, Adalioglu G, et al. Evaluation of the utility of atopy patch testing, skin prick testing, and total and specific IgE assays in the diagnosis of cow's milk allergy. Ann Allergy Asthma Immunol 2005;94:553–60.
86. Spergel JM, Beausoleil JL, Mascarenhas M, et al. The use of skin prick tests and patch tests to identify causative foods in eosinophilic esophagitis. J Allergy Clin Immunol 2002;109:363–8.
87. Isolauri E, Turjanmaa K. Combined skin prick and patch testing enhances identification of food allergy in infants with atopic dermatitis. J Allergy Clin Immunol 1996;97:9–15.
88. Mehl A, Verstege A, Staden U, et al. Utility of the ratio of food-specific IgE/total IgE in predicting symptomatic food allergy in children. Allergy 2005;60:1034–9.
89. Gupta RS, Lau CH, Hamilton RG, et al. Predicting outcomes of oral food challenges by using the allergen-specific IgE-total IgE ratio. J Allergy Clin Immunol Pract 2014;2:300–5.

Potential Treatments for Food Allergy

Stephanie Albin, MD[a], Anna Nowak-Węgrzyn, MD[b],*

KEYWORDS

- Food allergy • Food immunotherapy • Desensitization • Tolerance • Omalizumab

KEY POINTS

- There is currently no cure for food allergy, and standard of care remains strict avoidance of foods to which a patient is allergic.
- Immunotherapy is based on established protocols for desensitization, and it involves administering increasing doses of an allergenic food over a period of several months to increase tolerance. Goals of ongoing immunotherapy trials are to achieve sustained unresponsiveness and permanent tolerance, although this has not yet been consistently established.
- The oral route appears to be the preferred method of food allergen delivery, but immunotherapy is also being studied through sublingual and epicutaneous routes.
- Improvements in immunotherapy safety and outcomes may come with anti-immunoglobulin E monoclonal antibody adjuncts, modified food antigens, and recombinant vaccines.
- Allergen nonspecific treatments could potentially be used to treat various and multiple food allergies.

INTRODUCTION

Food allergy has been a subject of increasing research interest in the past decade. Data from multiple centers and various study designs indicate that there is a potential to effectively treat food allergy with immunomodulating therapies in both allergen-specific and nonspecific ways. This review serves to highlight the major therapeutics under investigation for food allergy, and the treatments discussed herein are summarized in **Fig. 1**.

Funding Sources: No funding for this article.
Conflict of Interest: No conflicts of interest for this article.
[a] Division of Allergy and Immunology, Department of Pediatrics, Icahn School of Medicine at Mount Sinai, One Gustave L. Levy Place, Box 1198, New York, NY 10029, USA; [b] Division of Allergy and Immunology, Department of Pediatrics, Kravis Children's Hospital, Jaffe Food Allergy Institute, Icahn School of Medicine at Mount Sinai, One Gustave L. Levy Place, Box 1198, New York, NY 10029, USA
* Corresponding author.
E-mail address: anna.nowak-wegrzyn@mssm.edu

Immunol Allergy Clin N Am 35 (2015) 77–100
http://dx.doi.org/10.1016/j.iac.2014.09.011
0889-8561/15/$ – see front matter
immunology.theclinics.com

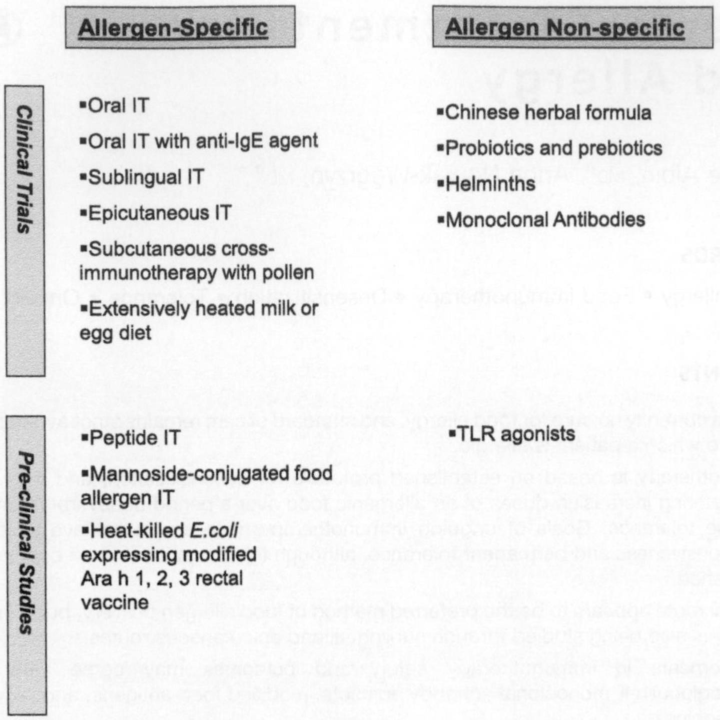

Allergen-Specific	Allergen Non-specific
Clinical Trials	
▪Oral IT	▪Chinese herbal formula
▪Oral IT with anti-IgE agent	▪Probiotics and prebiotics
▪Sublingual IT	▪Helminths
▪Epicutaneous IT	▪Monoclonal Antibodies
▪Subcutaneous cross-immunotherapy with pollen	
▪Extensively heated milk or egg diet	
Pre-clinical Studies	
▪Peptide IT	▪TLR agonists
▪Mannoside-conjugated food allergen IT	
▪Heat-killed *E.coli* expressing modified Ara h 1, 2, 3 rectal vaccine	

Fig. 1. Food allergy therapy. IT, immunotherapy.

Current Standard of Care for Food Allergy

Currently, there is no cure for food allergy, and standard of care hinges on strict avoidance of those foods to which a patient is allergic. The National Institute of Allergy and Infectious Diseases has put forth guidelines for the management of food allergy in the United States, which emphasizes the importance of food avoidance and label-reading, nutritional guidance and growth monitoring, and regular follow-up with an allergist.[1] An international consensus document endorses similar strategies, but concedes that no randomized clinical studies have proven the superiority of allergen avoidance or whether food allergen avoidance diminishes nutritional status.[2]

Avoidance is difficult in many situations, and as such, management always also necessitates education on timely and appropriate treatment of accidental exposures.[3] In the registry of fatal food-induced anaphylaxis, most fatal reactions were reported in the subjects who unknowingly ingested an offending food, thus highlighting the need for a more definitive approach to food allergy management.[4]

POTENTIAL ALLERGEN-SPECIFIC TREATMENTS FOR FOOD ALLERGY
Concept of Immunotherapy

Given that there is currently no cure for food allergy, there is great interest in researching methods of tolerance induction, particularly food-specific immunotherapy. Food immunotherapy is based on established protocols for drug desensitization and aeroallergen/venom immunotherapy, and it involves administering increasing doses of an allergenic food over a period of several months.[5] For example, in oral immunotherapy (OIT), typically there is an initial rapid dose escalation, followed by further dose escalation on a biweekly schedule in a controlled clinical setting until maintenance dose is achieved. Daily ingestion of tolerated doses during the build-up and maintenance phases occurs at home. The oral route appears to be the preferred method of food allergen delivery, but immunotherapy is also being studied through sublingual and epicutaneous routes. Of note, subcutaneous immunotherapy for food allergy was abandoned following early pilot studies, demonstrating serious side effects during all phases of treatment.[6,7]

Mechanism of Oral Immunotherapy

The exact mechanism of desensitization in food immunotherapy is not known, but associated immunologic changes include decreased reactivity of mast cells and basophils, increased food-specific serum immunoglobulin (Ig) G_4 antibodies, and initially increased but eventually decreased serum food-specific IgE antibodies.[8] Specific regulatory T cells (Tregs) increase and peak at around 12 months, with a subsequent decrease over time.[9] Increased antigen-induced Treg function is associated with hypomethylation of forkhead box protein 3.[10]

Desensitization Versus Sustained Unresponsiveness

Early clinical trials in immunotherapy aimed to safely desensitize subjects to a maintenance dose equivalent to a small serving of allergenic food, to protect allergic subjects from accidental exposures.[11–15] Current, more rigorous clinical trials are aiming for a sustained protective effect (sustained unresponsiveness), whereby subjects have a prolonged ability to ingest large amounts of allergenic food without the continuation of scheduled immunotherapy. Although consistent methods and mechanisms for induction of permanent tolerance have not yet been demonstrated, clinical trials have shown that OIT can "successfully desensitize a large number of individuals without major morbidity or mortality; at the end of the all of the studies, the greater part of patients can tolerate more of the food than at the start."[16]

Two studies provide insight into sustained unresponsiveness following peanut OIT. In a study by Vickery and colleagues,[17] 24 subjects were treated up to 5 years with peanut OIT, with a maintenance daily dose of 4000 mg peanut protein and a mean duration of 3.98 years (SD, 1.8 years). Twelve (50%) of 24 passed a peanut challenge to 5000 mg of peanut protein 1 month after stopping OIT, were considered to have achieved sustained unresponsiveness, and added unrestricted peanut to their diet. At baseline and at the time of the final peanut challenge, subjects who achieved sustained unresponsiveness had smaller skin test results, lower serum peanut-specific IgE antibody levels for peanut, Ara h 1, Ara h 2, and lower ratios of peanut-specific IgE/total IgE compared with subjects who did not achieve achieved sustained unresponsiveness.

Syed and colleagues[10] showed that with a shorter duration of peanut OIT (24 months of daily dosing with 4000 mg of peanut protein), 20 of 24 (83%) treated subjects became desensitized, as determined by a peanut challenge while on OIT. However, after 3 months of strict peanut elimination, only 7 of 24 (29%) subjects passed the peanut challenge with 4000 mg of peanut protein. Following an additional 3 months of peanut avoidance (a total of 6 months after discontinuation of peanut OIT), 3 of those 7 subjects (12.5% of original treatment group) remained tolerant to peanut during a final peanut challenge. These observations suggest that sustained responsiveness to peanut following peanut OIT is likely dose-dependent and duration-dependent.

Effect of Oral Immunotherapy on Quality of Life

Studies looking at quality of life in the setting of food immunotherapy have identified improvement in domains, including dietary and social limitations, risk of accidental exposure, and anxiety after immunotherapy.[18,19]

Oral Immunotherapy

Clinical trials have been undertaken to study the effect of OIT in the context of peanut, milk, and egg allergy.[20]

Peanut oral immunotherapy

In 2010, Blumchen and colleagues[21] investigated the efficacy and safety of OIT in patients with peanut allergy. Of 22 subjects who completed a rush protocol followed by 8 weeks of OIT, only 14 (64%) reached a goal maintenance dose of 500 mg of peanut. At the final double-blind, placebo-controlled food challenge (DBPCFC) however, subjects tolerated a median of 1000 mg (range, 250–4000 mg) in comparison with 190 mg peanut at the DBPCFC before OIT. The authors concluded that peanut OIT appeared to be safe and of some benefit in patients with peanut allergy, as the intervention increased threshold levels of ingestion. In 2011, Varshney and colleagues[9] reported the results of the first randomized, double-blind, placebo-controlled trial evaluating peanut OIT that proved effective desensitization. After 1 year of treatment, those who completed a peanut OIT protocol ingested the maximum cumulative dose of 5000 mg of peanuts, whereas placebo subjects ingested a median cumulative dose of 280 mg (range, 0–1900 mg). In 2013, Vickery and colleagues[17] went on to demonstrate sustained unresponsiveness after stopping peanut OIT. Of 24 subjects who completed up to 5 years of peanut OIT, 12 (50%) successfully passed a 5000-mg challenge 1 month after stopping OIT and introduced peanut into their diet. Most recently, in 2014, Anagnostou and colleagues[22] published a randomized controlled trial showing an estimate of the effect size, benefits, and risks of desensitization with peanut OIT. In this study group, desensitization (defined as passing a 1400 mg [roughly 10 peanuts] DBPCFC) was achieved for 24 of 49 (62%) subjects receiving peanut OIT for 6 months, and for none of the control group abiding by strict peanut avoidance. There was an increase in median peanut threshold after OIT to 1345 mg (range, 45–1400 mg). Quality-of-life scores improved in the group receiving OIT, and side effects were mild in most participants.

Although these studies are promising, a meta-analysis of published peanut OIT trials concluded that only one small randomized controlled trial demonstrated that peanut OIT can result in desensitization with immune modulation.[23] They went on to point out that this study (as with most OIT studies) was associated with a substantial risk of adverse events, although most were mild. The meta-analysis, as well as other expert opinion, supports that peanut OIT cannot be currently recommended as a treatment for management of IgE-mediated peanut allergy, and larger randomized control trials are needed.[24]

Milk/egg oral immunotherapy

In 2007, Staden and colleagues[25] sought to examine the efficacy of milk and egg OIT as compared with strict avoidance. Subjects had immunotherapy maintenance doses increased (according to individual tolerance) to a maximum dose of 8250 mg of cow's milk or 2800 mg hen's egg protein, with a minimum dose of 3300 mg cow's milk or 1600 mg hen's egg protein. Of the 25 subjects randomized to OIT, 16 (64%) were able to integrate the food allergen into their diet in some form: 9 subjects (36%) receiving OIT showed sustained unresponsiveness after a secondary 2-month elimination diet; 3 subjects (12%) showed tolerance with regular intake; and 4 subjects (16%) were partial responders who did not meet the planned, full maintenance dose. In contrast, only 7 of 20 control subjects (35%) developed natural tolerance during the elimination diet, as evidenced by passing a DBPCFC (cumulative goal dose of cow's milk protein 4770 mg, cumulative goal dose of hen's egg protein 6200 mg) after a median interval of 21 months.

Skripak and colleagues[26] went on to publish the first randomized, double-blind, placebo-controlled study of milk OIT in 2008, showing efficacy in the treatment group with an increase in the median threshold of ingested milk protein from 40 mg to 5140 mg (without a change in the placebo group). A follow-up, open-label study in 2009 showed that after 13 to 75 weeks of open-label dosing (median dose 7000 mg), 6 of 13 subjects (46%) tolerated 16,000 mg milk protein without reaction and 7 subjects reacted at doses 3000 to 16,000 mg.[27] Most recently, the clinical status of 32 subjects from 2 of this group's study protocols[26,28] evaluated the long-term outcomes of milk immunotherapy.[29] Sixteen subjects were followed up after a median of 4.5 years (range, 1.3–5.3 years)[26] and 16 were followed up after a median of 3.2 years (range, 2.6–3.4 years)[28] from the end of dose escalation. Twenty-five of 32 subjects (78%) were ingesting some amount of uncooked milk, although only 6 (19%) reported unlimited milk consumption. Two subjects (6%) were ingesting trace or baked milk products, and 5 subjects (16%) reported no milk consumption. Most worrisome, the authors reported that some subjects who initially did well and passed interim oral food challenges (OFCs) subsequently had increased symptoms (including severe symptoms), which led to the restriction of cow's milk.

Other studies have focused on dosing schedules of milk OIT in consideration of feasibility and compliance. Pajno and colleagues[30] found that after achieving desensitization to cow's milk with OIT, a maintenance regimen with milk given twice weekly was as effective as daily maintenance. However, in terms of "clinical readiness," a systematic review of randomized controlled trials for milk OIT concluded the overall low quality of evidence "leaves important uncertainty about anticipated effects of immunotherapy due to very serious imprecision of the estimates of effects and the likelihood of publication bias for some of the critical outcomes…[there were] frequent and sometimes serious adverse effects…and additional, larger [trials] measuring all patient-important outcomes are still needed."[31]

There have been relatively fewer trials for egg immunotherapy. Small pilot and proof-of-concept studies have shown feasibility and safety of egg OIT,[11–13,32,33] and, in 2012, Burks and colleagues[34] published the first randomized, double-blind, placebo-controlled trial for egg OIT. Forty subjects received egg OIT with a goal maintenance dose of 2000 mg egg protein daily, and 15 subjects received placebo. At a 10-month desensitization challenge, 22 of 40 OIT subjects (55%) tolerated 5000 mg of egg protein, as compared with none of the placebo group. At a 22-month desensitization challenge, 30 of 40 OIT subjects (75%) tolerated 5000 mg of egg protein. However, at a 24-month tolerance challenge after 6 to 8 weeks off of OIT, only 11 of 29 subjects (28%) tolerated 5000 mg of egg protein, raising concerns about the long-term protection afforded by the protocol. In keeping with meta-analyses of specific food OIT, a meta-analysis of general food OIT concluded that it cannot yet be recommended in routine practice as a means to induce tolerance in children with IgE-mediated food allergy.[35]

Safety of Oral Immunotherapy

OIT is associated with adverse effects in virtually all published trials, although side effects are often mild and localized to the oropharynx. A study looking at safety in the different phases of OIT showed that reactions were most frequent during the initial escalation day when subjects underwent oral desensitization, and doses were better tolerated during the buildup phase and home dosing.[36] Factors such as febrile illness, exercise, and menstruation can reduce tolerated threshold doses.[37] The predominance of gastrointestinal symptoms merits a thoughtful consideration regarding eosinophilic esophagitis (EoE), as the risk is estimated to be about 10% to 20% in those treated with OIT.[38,39]

Oral Immunotherapy with Anti-Immunoglobulin E

An anti-IgE agent, omalizumab, is currently approved for moderate-to-severe allergic asthma. It functions by depleting free IgE and downregulating FcεRI on effector cells, such as mast cells and basophils, and on antigen-presenting cells, such as dendritic cells and B cells.[40] Omalizumab may also have a role to play in food allergy immunotherapy, as it minimizes IgE-mediated side effects and may contribute to mechanisms of tolerance. Pretreatment with omalizumab for 9 to 12 weeks before starting OIT and combined treatment during the build-up phase of OIT appears to reduce side effects and accelerate buildup dosing. Preliminary studies evaluating safety of omalizumab in combination with milk, peanut, and multifood OIT have been published (**Table 1**).[41–43]

Sublingual and Epicutaneous Immunotherapy

In sublingual immunotherapy (SLIT), a food allergen extract is kept in the mouth for 2 to 3 minutes and then spit out or swallowed. It is generally better tolerated and uses significantly lower doses than OIT, but appears to have inferior clinical effects of desensitization.[44] Clinical trials of food SLIT have been reported for milk, peanut, hazelnut, and peach extracts (**Table 2**).[28,44–50]

Epicutaneous immunotherapy (EPIT) uses a skin patch containing soluble allergen that is absorbed into intact stratum corneum. It is an attractive approach to noninvasive immunotherapy with minimal side effects, and studies have demonstrated that EPIT commonly causes local reactions but almost never induces serious systemic adverse events.[51] Pilot trials are currently underway for milk and peanut (see **Table 2**).[51,52]

Role for Aeroallergen Immunotherapy for Pollen Cross-Reactive Foods

Pollen immunotherapy has typically been considered a therapeutic option for patients with allergic rhinitis and asthma, but studies have also shown an effect on symptoms of pollen food syndrome (PFS). In PFS, cross-reactive IgE antibodies recognize homologous allergens in pollen and raw fruits, vegetables, and nuts. These allergens are typically broken down during the process of digestion, but patients with pollen allergies can develop oropharyngeal symptoms (commonly pruritus or swelling of the mouth, face, lip, tongue, and throat) with ingestion of various plant-based foods. Multiple studies have successfully used subcutaneous birch pollen immunotherapy to treat apple allergy in this context.[53–57] Birch-pollen immunotherapy has been demonstrated to decrease skin prick test (SPT) reactivity for recombinant Bet v 1 (major birch allergen) and recombinant Mal d 1 (major apple allergen), induce IgG_4 antibodies against Bet v 1 (which display cross-reactivity to Mal d 1), and increase the amount of fresh apple ingested at a DBPCFC after 1 year.[56] In addition, the beneficial effects of immunotherapy on PFS appear to be long lasting after treatment, despite a propensity for apple resensitization over time.[54]

Immunotherapy with Modified Food Antigens

Recently, there has been a movement toward modifying food antigens to create more effective and safe immunotherapeutic materials. One of the most commonly used approaches to immunomodulation with modified food antigens is the incorporation of extensively heated egg and milk products into the diet of selected allergic patients. Certain egg and milk conformational epitopes are destroyed by high temperatures, making it possible for some allergic patients to consume small amounts of these foods in the baked form.[58] Most patients with cow's milk and egg allergy tolerate extensively heated products, and the addition of baked milk and baked egg to the diet of children tolerating such foods appears to accelerate the development of unheated milk and egg tolerance compared with strict avoidance.[59,60] Immunologic changes induced by a diet containing baked milk and egg are similar to changes that have been observed during OIT trials, although individuals who are tolerant to heated milk products may represent a milder milk allergy phenotype with evidence of greater immune regulation, such as lower specific IgE, higher specific IgG_4, lower basophil reactivity to milk proteins, and a higher frequency of milk-specific Tregs.[61-63]

Additional immunotherapy with modified food antigens includes peptide immunotherapy and mannose-conjugated food allergen immunotherapy, which are both currently under investigation in preclinical studies (**Table 3**).[64-68]

Immunotherapy with Recombinant Peanut Rectal Vaccine

In another model of modification, Bannon and colleagues[69] have successfully developed and characterized cDNA clones for 3 major peanut allergens, Ara h 1, Ara h 2, and Ara h 3. The group substituted amino acids through site-directed mutagenesis of the cDNA clones and performed recombinant production of the modified allergens. In a murine model of peanut allergy using the heat-killed *Escherichia coli* producing mutated Ara h 1, 2, and 3 (HKE-MP123), mice had reduced symptom scores on challenge, lower IgE levels, and decreased Th2 cytokines/increased Th1 cytokines from peanut-stimulated splenocytes in vitro.[70] Most recently, a phase I safety study was undertaken, giving 5 healthy adult controls and 10 peanut-allergic adult subjects weekly dose escalations of EMP-123, a rectally administered suspension of recombinant Ara h 1, Ara h 2, and Ara h 3.[71] There were no significant effects on the healthy controls, but there were severe allergic reactions in 20% of the peanut-allergic subjects, and the authors concluded that "future studies with this product, if any, will require alterations in the dosing scheme and/or route of delivery."[71]

POTENTIAL ALLERGEN NON-SPECIFIC TREATMENTS FOR FOOD ALLERGY

Although significant resources are being put toward allergen-specific immunotherapy, there is a parallel effort toward developing nonspecific treatments that could potentially be used to treat various and multiple food allergies. One promising example of this is Chinese herbal formulas, and others include probiotics/prebiotics, helminths, monoclonal antibodies, and toll-like receptor (TLR) agonists.

Chinese Herbal Formulas

Chinese herbal medicine studies in the setting of food allergy were initially done using food allergy herbal formula-1 (FAHF-1), an 11-herb formula containing the classical Wu-Mei Wan (a combination of 10 herbs previously used for intestinal parasitic infection, gastroenteritis, and asthma) and Ling Shi (an additional herb with purported anti-inflammatory properties).[72] The herbs Xi-Xin and Zhi-Fu-Zi were removed from the formula for safety concerns, and the resultant 9-herb formula, FAHF-2, has been used in both murine research and early clinical trials (**Table 4**).[73-76] These herbal formulas are thought to have synergistic anti-inflammatory effects, with reduced side effects in formulation as compared with individual herbs.[72] In general, results from

Table 1
Oral immunotherapy and anti-IgE safety studies

Study/Subjects	Success Rate	Immunologic Changes	Side Effects/Comments
Nadeau et al,[41] 2011 n = 11; age 7–17 y Pilot phase I study using omalizumab in combination with oral milk desensitization (desensitization performed 9 wk after start of omalizumab treatment) Goal maintenance dose: 2000 mg milk protein/d	The mean frequency for total reactions reported by week 24 was 1.6% (32 reactions of 2199 doses total for all 11 subjects). All subjects experienced some adverse events, though most reactions were defined as mild and needed no treatment. One dose of epinephrine was given during rush desensitization, and 2 subjects received epinephrine at home during the maintenance phase. Nine of the 11 subjects tolerated desensitization to a dose of 2000 mg milk within a period of 7–11 wk.	Within a week of treatment, the CD4+ T-cell response to milk was nearly eliminated. Over the following 3 mo, the CD4+ T-cell response returned, characterized by a shift from IL-4 to IFN-γ. Milk-IgE decreased, and milk-IgG$_4$ increased 15-fold.	This was a phase I study, and the primary objectives were to examine the safety of this approach and to determine whether subjects could be dosed up to 2000 mg milk within 7–11 wk of initiating desensitization.
Schneider et al,[42] 2013 n = 13; age 8–16 y Pilot study using omalizumab in combination with oral peanut desensitization (desensitization performed 12 wk after start of omalizumab treatment) Goal maintenance dose: 4000 mg peanut protein/d	All 13 subjects (100%) reached the 500 mg peanut desensitization dose on the first day (cumulative dose, 992 mg), which was the primary outcome of the study, with minimal or no symptoms. Twelve of the 13 subjects (92%) reached the 4000 mg maintenance dose, which was a secondary outcome of the study, requiring median time of 8 wk. Twelve weeks after stopping omalizumab (week 32), 12 subjects underwent a DBPCFC (cumulative dose, 8000 mg peanut). Eleven of the subjects (85%) tolerated this challenge, and the twelfth subject later passed an open challenge of 8000 mg peanut. Therefore, 12 of the 13 subjects (92%) tolerated an 8000-mg dose of peanut.	Not reported	There were a total of 72 reactions during the study (2% of the 3502 total peanut doses ingested). During the study, 6 of the 13 subjects experienced mild or no allergic reactions; 5 subjects had grade 2 reactions, and 2 subjects had grade 3 reactions, all of which responded rapidly to treatment.

Bégin et al,[43] 2014 n = 25; age 4–15 y Phase I study using up to 5 different food allergens rush OIT simultaneously with omalizumab (omalizumab was administered for 8 wk before and 8 wk following the initiation of rush OIT) Goal maintenance dose: 4000 mg protein per allergen	The median time to reach maintenance dose (4000 mg per allergen) was 18 wk (range, 7–36 wk) with all subjects able to reach this dose by 9 mo. All subjects had reached a dose equivalent to a 10-fold increase of all their allergens by 2 mo of therapy. Over the study period, there were 3 withdrawals because of noncompliance with study medication.	Peanut-specific IgG_4 levels increased and peanut SPT decreased. Peanut-specific IgE did not change significantly.	This was a proof of concept study and evaluated subjects for desensitization. Thirteen subjects (52%) experienced some symptoms on their initial dose escalation day. With home dosing, 401 of the 7530 doses (5.3%) triggered reactions, and most home reactions occurred in the first months of therapy. Most (94%) allergic reactions were mild. One severe reaction requiring epinephrine occurred shortly after a subject reached maintenance phase (16,000 mg).

Table 2
Selected sublingual and epicutaneous immunotherapy studies

Study/Subjects	Success Rate	Immunologic Changes	Side Effects/Comments
SLIT			
Milk Keet et al,[28] 2012 n = 30; age 6–17 y Randomized clinical trial comparing milk OIT and SLIT with challenge performed after 12 and 60 wk Goal maintenance dose: SLIT: 7 mg daily Low-dose OIT: 1000 mg High-dose OIT: 2000 mg	One of 10 subjects in the SLIT group, 6 of 10 subjects in the SLIT/low-dose OIT group, and 8 of 10 subjects in the SLIT/high-dose OIT group passed the 8 g milk protein challenge ($P = .002$, SLIT vs OIT). After avoidance, 6 of 15 subjects (3 subjects in each OIT group) regained reactivity, 2 after only 1 wk off therapy.	Titrated milk SPT wheal diameter and basophil activity decreased in all groups. Milk-specific IgG_4 increased in all groups. Milk-specific IgE and spontaneous histamine release decreased in only the OIT group.	OIT was more efficacious for desensitization than SLIT alone, but was accompanied by more systemic side effects. There were symptoms with 1802 (29%) of 6246 SLIT doses and 2402 (23%) of 10,645 OIT doses. However, OIT had significantly more multisystem, upper respiratory tract, gastrointestinal, and lower respiratory tract symptoms than SLIT.
Peanut Fleischer et al,[50] 2013 n = 40; age 12–37 y Randomized, double-blind, placebo-controlled multicenter trial comparing peanut SLIT and placebo after 44 wk; placebo-treated patients were unblinded, then crossed over into a higher dose peanut SLIT for 44 wk Goal maintenance dose: minimum dose of 165 µg and maximum dose of 1386 µg daily Crossover group: maximum maintenance dose of 3696 µg daily	After 44 wk of SLIT, 14 of 20 subjects receiving peanut SLIT passed a 5 g peanut powder challenge (or ingested at least 10-fold more peanut powder than the baseline OFC), compared with 3 of 20 subjects receiving placebo ($P<.001$). Seven of 16 crossover subjects passed a 5 g peanut powder challenge (or ingested at least 10-fold more peanut powder than the baseline OFC) after 44 wk. Median successfully consumed doses of peanut powder increased with duration of SLIT.	Peanut-specific IgE levels increased in SLIT group between baseline and week 44, but not in the placebo or crossover group. Peanut-specific IgG_4 increased in SLIT and crossover group between baseline and week 44, but not in placebo group. Basophil activity decreased in SLIT group.	Of 10,855 peanut doses through the week 44 OFCs, 63.1% were symptom-free; excluding oral-pharyngeal symptoms, 95.2% were symptom-free.

Hazelnut Enrique et al,[46] 2005 n = 23; age 19–53 y Randomized, double-blind, placebo-controlled trial comparing hazelnut SLIT (with standardized hazelnut extract) and placebo after 8–12 wk Goal maintenance dose: 22 mg daily	Twenty-two subjects reached their planned maximum dose after 4 d. Mean hazelnut quantity provoking objective symptoms increased from 2.29 g to 11.56 g in the treated group ($P = .02$) vs 3.49 g–4.14 g in the placebo group (not significant). Almost 50% of subjects who underwent treatment reached the highest dose of hazelnut (20 g) during the DBPCFC, as compared with 9% of placebo subjects.	IgG_4 and IL-10 levels increased after immunotherapy in only the active group.	A total of 1466 doses were administered: 309 during the build-up phase and 1157 during maintenance. Systemic reactions were observed in only 0.2% of the total doses administered, and they appeared only in the buildup phase. A follow-up study showed that beneficial effect increases with a long-lasting period of hazelnut SLIT, and even after treatment interruptions, the beneficial effects seem to persist.[47]
Peach Fernandez-Rivas,[48] 2009 n = 49; age 18–65 y Randomized, double-blind, placebo-controlled trial comparing peach SLIT (with standardized peach extract) and placebo after 6 mo Goal maintenance dose: 10 µg of Pru p 3 three times a week	All 33 subjects in the SLIT group tolerated at least 3 times (3–9 times) more peach in the DBPCFC after 6 mo of SLIT.	Pru p 3–specific IgE and IgG_4 increased in the SLIT group. The SLIT group had a decrease in SPT.	No serious adverse events were reported. Systemic reactions were mild and observed with a similar frequency in both groups. Local reactions were significantly more frequent in the active group (3 times), and 95% of them were restricted to the oral cavity.
EPIT			
Milk Dupont et al,[51] 2010 n = 19; age 10 mo–7 y Double-blind, placebo-controlled 2 center trial comparing milk EPIT (patch with milk powder) and placebo after 3 mo	After 90 d, EPIT treatment tended to increase the cumulative tolerated dose, from a mean ± SD of 1.77 ± 2.98 mL at day 0 to 23.61 ± 28.61 mL at day 90 ($P = .18$). Mean cumulative tolerated dose did not vary in the placebo group (4.36 ± 5.87 mL at day 0 vs 5.44 ± 5.88 mL	Milk-specific IgE did not increase in the EPIT group.	Typically, local erythema occurred at the site of patch application and remained visible for 4–14 d. Local adverse events were reported for 4 subjects in the active group and 2 in the placebo group. Among the intention-to-treat population, 24 systemic adverse

(continued on next page)

Table 2
(continued)

Study/Subjects	Success Rate	Immunologic Changes	Side Effects/Comments
Goal maintenance dose: 1 mg 3 times a week	at day 90). The mean cumulative tolerated dose increment was 12-fold in the active group vs 8% in placebo group ($P = .13$).		events occurred in the active group and 8 in the placebo group, with no anaphylaxis. The estimated risk of local eczema was higher in the active group than in the placebo group.
Peanut Dupont et al,[52] 2014 n = 54; age 5–17 y Multicenter study evaluating 18 mo of daily peanut EPIT (patch with peanut protein), as well as a second regimen of placebo for 6 mo followed by 12 mo of daily peanut EPIT Goal maintenance dose: 100 µg peanut protein daily	Twenty-five subjects receiving 18-mo EPIT showed a treatment response of 40% overall. The subgroup of 15 subjects aged 5–11 y receiving 18-mo EPIT showed a 67% response rate. Cumulative reactive dose for this group increased constantly over time; at baseline, it was 24.27 ± 29.98 mg peanut protein and by 18 mo it was 357.7 ± 542.9 mg peanut protein ($P<.001$ between serial values).	In the 5–11 y age group receiving 18-mo EPIT, a progressive IgG$_4$ was seen over time.	Abstract; study not yet published.

Table 3
Selected studies of modified food antigen immunotherapy

Modified Food Antigen Immunotherapy	Rationale	Study Design	Results
Peanut peptide Prickett et al,[65] 2013	Immunotherapy with intact peanut protein can induce life-threatening, IgE-mediated adverse events. Degradation of whole protein into smaller immunoregulatory peptides with decreased IgE reactivity could allow for larger doses to be given, thereby stimulating more significant T-cell responses.	Ara h 1–specific CD4+ T-cell lines were generated from PBMCs of peanut-allergic subjects, and T-cell epitopes were identified using CFSE and thymidine-based proliferation assays. Epitope HLA-restriction was also investigated. Peanut-specific IgE reactivity to peptides was assessed by functional basophil activation assay.	Seven non-basophil-reactive peptides encompassing all core epitopes were designed and validated in peanut-allergic donor PBMC T-cell assays.
Peanut peptide Pascal et al,[68] 2013	See above.	In silico predictive algorithms were used to identify candidate peptides for an Ara h 2 peptide-based vaccine using peanut-allergic subjects' PBMCs in vitro.	Four dominant regions in Ara h 2 were identified that could be potential candidates for future peanut peptide vaccine.
Man(51)-BSA Zhou et al,[66] 2010	Targeting intestinal DCs with sugar-modified antigen mimics highly mannosylated pathogens, which could lead to the induction of oral tolerance via CLRs.	A mouse model was used to investigate whether mannoside-conjugated BSA (as compared with unconjugated BSA) mediated a differential immune response in vivo.	Oral delivery of Man(51)-BSA substantially reduced the BSA-induced anaphylactic response. It selectively targeted LPDCs through SIGNR1 and induced the expression of IL-10, likely leading to the induction of tolerance.
Glycated OVA Rupa et al,[67] 2014	See above, although authors also state that "detailed molecular mechanisms on what causes the mannose form to attenuate allergic response remains to be elucidated."	A mouse model was used to investigate whether various forms of glycated OVA (in previously sensitized mice) affected outcomes in an oral challenge.	Clinical signs and specific IgE were decreased and Treg percentage was increased in the mannose- and glucomannan-treated groups. The OVA-mannose group also had reduced maturation and uptake by DCs, less histamine, MMCP-1, specific IgG, IL-4, and IL-17, and more IL-12p70.

Abbreviations: CFSE, carboxyfluorescein succinimidyl ester; CLR, C-type lectin receptors; DC, dendritic cell; LPDC, lamina propria dendritic cells; Man(51)-BSA, bovine serum albumin bearing 51 molecules of mannoside; MMCP-1, mouse mast cell protease 1; OVA, ovalbumin; PBMC, peripheral blood mononuclear cells; SIGNR1, a C-type lectin receptor.

Table 4
Selected studies of Chinese herbal formula and food allergy

Study/Subjects	Study Design	Results	Safety Profile
FAHF-2 and peanut allergy/murine model Srivastava et al,[73] 2005	Mice allergic to peanut were treated with FAHF-2 for 7 wk and then were challenged with peanut at 1, 3, or 5 wk after therapy.	During peanut challenges, there were no signs of anaphylactic reactions or elevation of plasma histamine levels in FAHF-2-treated mice (while all controls developed anaphylaxis). In FAHF-2-treated mice, IgE levels were significantly reduced. Peanut-stimulated splenocytes showed significantly reduced IL-4, IL-5, and IL-13, and enhanced IFN-γ.	In a preliminary assessment of safety, FAHF-2 was tested for lethality (LD50 test). No mouse died within 1 wk after feeding 12 times the effective mouse daily dose of FAHF-2, nor did any die within 2 wk after feeding 24 times the effective mouse daily dose of FAHF-2 (n = 10). Mice had normal CBC, BUN, and ALT after being given FAHF-2. All of the major organs analyzed appeared normal.
FAHF-2 and peanut allergy/murine model Qu et al,[74] 2007	Mice allergic to peanut were treated with FAHF-2 for 7 wk and then were challenged with peanut at 1 d and 4 wk after therapy.	During peanut challenges, there were no signs of anaphylactic reactions or elevation of plasma histamine levels in FAHF-2-treated mice (while all controls developed anaphylaxis). In FAHF-2-treated mice, peanut-specific IgE levels were reduced and IgG2a levels were increased. MLN cells showed significantly reduced IL-4 and IL-5, and enhanced IFN-γ with increased numbers of IFN-γ-producing CD8+ cells.	No additional safety studies done.

FAHF-2 and food allergy (peanut, tree nut, fish, or shellfish)/ clinical trial Wang et al,[75] 2010	n = 19; ages 12–45 y of age Randomized, double-blind, placebo-controlled phase 1 trial Subjects received 1 of 3 doses of FAHF-2 or placebo: 2.2 g (4 tablets), 3.3 g (6 tablets), or 6.6 g (12 tablets) 3 times a day for 7 d. Of 19 subjects enrolled, 18 completed the study: 4 active and 2 placebo patients were treated at each dose level.	No significant differences were found in vital signs, physical examination, pulmonary function tests, and electrocardiogram data obtained before and after treatment visits. No significant changes were found in allergen-specific IgE or SPT results before or after 7 d of treatment. No significant changes were found in serum cytokine levels before and after treatment. Significantly decreased IL-5 levels were found in the active treatment group after 7 d. In vitro studies of peripheral blood mononuclear cells cultured with FAHF-2 also demonstrated a significant decrease in IL-5 and an increase in culture supernatant IFN-γ and IL-10 levels.	No patients had grade 3 adverse events. Two patients (1 in the FAHF-2 group and 1 in the placebo group) reported mild gastrointestinal symptoms. One patient withdrew from the study after the second day (sixth dose) because of an allergic reaction that was unlikely related to the study medication.
FAHF-2 and food allergy (peanut, tree nut, fish, or shellfish)/ clinical trial Patil et al,[76] 2011	n = 18; ages 12–45 y of age Extended phase 1 clinical trial (open-label) Subjects received 3.3 g (6 tablets) of FAHF-2 three times a day for 6 mo. Of 18 subjects enrolled, 14 completed the study.	No significant drug-associated differences were found in laboratory parameters, pulmonary function study results, or electrocardiographic findings before and after treatment. There were no changes in SPT results after treatment. There was a significant reduction in basophil CD63 expression in response to ex vivo stimulation at 6 mo. There was also a trend toward a reduction in eosinophil and basophil numbers after treatment.	One patient had a history of EoE (not active or requiring treatment at time of study); after 5½ wk on FAHF-2 treatment, she reported a recurrence of her EoE. She was seen by a gastroenterologist and started on medication for active disease. She was restarted on FAHF-2 two months later and completed the study with no other abdominal complaints.

Abbreviations: ALT, alanine aminotransferase; BUN, blood urea nitrogen; CBC, complete blood count; MLN, mesenteric lymph node.

studies suggest that Chinese herbal formulas may be a safe and effective way to treat food allergies, and a phase II trial is underway.

Probiotics and Prebiotics

A probiotic is a consumable micro-organism with potential health benefit, and a prebiotic is a nondigestable food ingredient that can stimulate the growth and activity of beneficial bacteria in the gut. With recent emphasis on the microbiome's role in immune development, it is not surprising that work has been done to elucidate whether probiotics and prebiotics may have a role in the prevention and treatment of atopic disease. Children with allergy have been shown to have different gut microflora than healthy controls (ie, higher levels of clostridia and lower levels of bifidobacteria),[77] and some hypothesize that beneficial microbes support immunoregulation by inducing the development of Treg.[78] There are conflicting results from clinical trials in allergic rhinitis, atopic dermatitis, and asthma, and the routine use of therapeutic probiotics in patients with these diseases has not yet been recommended.[79–83]

In food allergy, a mouse model has shown that treatment with a probiotic mixture was effective in protection against anaphylaxis as well as redirection of allergen-specific Th2-polarized immune responses toward Th1-T regulatory responses.[84] Although the first randomized, controlled trial of probiotic supplementation (*Lactobacillus casei* CRL431 and *Bifidobacterium lactis* Bb-12) in the setting of cow's milk allergy did not demonstrate accelerated tolerance in infants,[85] a recent trial demonstrated that supplementation of an extensively hydrolyzed casein formula with a different probiotic (*Lactobacillus* GG) accelerated the development of tolerance to milk in infants with milk allergy as confirmed by DBPCFC (age, 1–12 months).[86] After 6 months of treatment, 22 of 28 subjects (79%) receiving formula alone compared with 11 of 27 subjects (41%) receiving formula with probiotic supplementation had a positive DBPCFC. Subjects with persistent cow's milk allergy were challenged again after 12 months of treatment, and 13 of 22 subjects (60%) receiving formula alone compared with 5 of 11 subjects (45%) receiving formula with probiotic supplementation had a positive DBPCFC. Although the rate of tolerance acquisition was higher in infants treated with probiotic supplementation, it should be noted that there is a natural tendency to outgrow milk allergy over time, particularly in non-IgE-mediated milk allergy, which comprised a majority of subjects in each treatment arm.

Helminth Treatment

Helminths are parasitic worms with life cycles involving residency in various host tissues, and observational and experimental studies have investigated their benefit in immune-mediated diseases, most notably inflammatory bowel disease.[87] It is postulated that therapeutic helminths release helminth-derived immunomodulatory molecules that activate several distinct regulatory pathways involving both the innate and the adaptive immune system to mitigate inflammation.[88]

Outside of inflammatory bowel disease, helminthic therapy is also actively being investigated in atopic disorders. Recent population studies have shown that early, heavy helminthic infection can be inversely associated with allergic disorders and decrease the odds of SPT reactivity.[89] With such epidemiologic data in mind, peanut-allergic mouse models have shown that enteric helminth infection downregulates peanut-specific IgE, reduces anaphylactic symptoms, and protects against the development of food allergy.[90] Helminths (particularly *Trichuris suis* ova, the eggs of pig whipworm) have been used in a clinical trial for allergic rhinitis and a case report of pecan allergy,[91,92] although there are currently no definitive, beneficial results to recommend incorporation of helminths into clinical practice.

Monoclonal Antibodies

Production of monoclonal antibodies involving human-mouse hybrid cells was first described in the 1970s,[93,94] but these biologics are now commonly used for a variety of diseases including cancers, autoimmune diseases, and allergic disorders. Two major monoclonal antibodies, omalizumab (anti-IgE) and mepolizumab (anti-interleukin-5 [IL5]), are being studied in the context of food allergy.

As described above, omalizumab has been used successfully in conjunction with food immunotherapy, but monoclonal anti-IgE antibodies have also been investigated as monotherapies.[95,96] Leung and colleagues[95] conducted a double-blind, randomized, dose-ranging trial of TNX-901, a humanized IgG$_1$ monoclonal antibody, in children and adults with peanut allergy. Subjects were randomly assigned to receive either TNX-901 (150, 300, or 450 mg) or placebo subcutaneously, and they underwent a final OFC 2 to 4 weeks after 4 treatment doses. The study showed that the 450-mg dosing of TNX-901 significantly increased the threshold of sensitivity to peanut on OFC from a level equal to approximately half a peanut (178 mg) to a level equal to approximately 8 peanuts (2805 mg). As a next step, Sampson and colleagues[96] conducted a phase II randomized, double-blind, placebo-controlled trial of omalizumab in children with peanut allergy, although it was terminated early because of the safety concerns regarding the baseline pretreatment oral peanut challenges. Limited data from this trial suggested an increase in tolerability to peanut flour in the omalizumab-treated versus placebo-treated subjects: 4 (44.4%) omalizumab-treated subjects versus 1 (20%) placebo-treated subject could tolerate 1000 mg peanut flour or more during an OFC after 24 weeks of treatment.

Mepolizumab antagonizes IL-5 (and subsequent downstream stimulation of eosinophils), and as such, has been used mostly in food allergy models of EoE. In a randomized, double-blind, placebo-controlled trial of 11 adults with active EoE, subjects were randomized to 2 to 4 doses of mepolizumab, and the effect of treatment was assessed clinically, endoscopically, and histologically.[97] Mepolizumab significantly reduced eosinophil numbers in esophageal biopsies but had limited effect on improving clinical symptoms. A randomized, double-blind, multicenter trial of mepolizumab in 59 children with active EoE also showed reduced esophageal eosinophilic inflammation.[98] Follow-up research in this pediatric cohort showed biopsies of mepolizumab-treated subjects had significantly fewer mast cells, IL-9+ cells, and mast cell-eosinophil couplets in the esophageal epithelium.[99]

Toll-like Receptor Agonists

Systemic TLR stimulation may be able to protect against the development of allergic conditions when it is implemented early enough in the natural history of the disease.[100] This finding has been related back to the hygiene hypothesis, whereby infections early in life may protect against atopy by engaging with TLR receptors and an overall skewing of the immune system toward a Th1 (rather than Th2) responses.

Early murine models investigated the effects of different TLR agonists on Th2-mediated responses in the airway, and results have shown that therapeutics such as TLR7 and TLR9 may have the potential to treat allergic disorders in human trials.[101] There have been promising clinical trials looking at the efficacy, safety, and tolerability of QbG10 (recombinant viral protein shell filled with DNA and a ligand for TLR9) in the setting of allergic asthma, and a clinical trial has also been done to look at the safety, tolerability, and pharmacodynamics of GSK2245035 (a highly selective TLR7 agonist) in allergic rhinitis.[102,103]

In the preventative murine model of peanut allergy, mice treated with a combination of an oral synthetic TLR9 agonist and peanut had decreased specific peanut IgE and increased IgG2a levels, inhibition of IL-5 and IL-13 production in stimulated splenocytes, and increased production of interferon (IFN)-γ in stimulated splenocytes as compared with mice sensitized with peanut alone.[104] Findings were similar in the treatment model, and the authors concluded that TLR9 agonists might be suitable candidates for the management of peanut-induced allergy. More recent work has shown promise in treating mouse models of food allergy with *Listeria monocytogenes–*derived flagellin A (a TLR5 agonist),[105] and the accumulation of data on TLR agonists supports that they may be important for future therapeutics in patients with IgE-mediated allergy.

SUMMARY

Among the potential treatments for food allergy discussed in this review, there is no doubt that food immunotherapy has the greatest share of research interest and activity. OIT with multiple foods and triple therapy, combining OIT, anti-IgE, and Chinese herbal formula, are being actively investigated. However, although current food immunotherapy studies are encouraging, relatively high rates of adverse reactions and the lack of evidence for long-term tolerance are problematic. The future holds promise in terms of identifying patients who are most likely to benefit from food immunotherapy, as well as modifying treatment protocols to be more safe and effective. Diagnostic tests including peptide microarrays and component profiles may be able to help identify those phenotypes best positioned to benefit from immunotherapy. Bacterial adjuvants, such as heat-killed *L monocytogenes* or probiotic bacteria, may be useful because they can enhance IFN-γ (Th1) and inhibit IL-4 (Th2) immune responses in the setting of immunotherapy.[106,107] Antigen delivery vehicles, such as nanoparticles, can assist in the preferential uptake of food antigens to be more efficiently delivered to gut-associated lymphoid tissue in the setting of immunotherapy.[108] Continuing to pursue trials with more potent anti-IgE antibodies (as they become available) represents another future direction, and as with all potential improvements, it is hoped to bring us closer to a cure for food allergy.

REFERENCES

1. Boyce JA, Assa'ad A, Burks AW, et al. Guidelines for the diagnosis and management of food allergy in the United States: report of the NIAID-sponsored expert panel. J Allergy Clin Immunol 2010;126:S1–58.
2. Burks AW, Tang M, Sicherer S, et al. ICON: food allergy. J Allergy Clin Immunol 2012;129:906–20.
3. Sicherer SH, Sampson HA. Food allergy: epidemiology, pathogenesis, diagnosis, and treatment. J Allergy Clin Immunol 2014;133:291–307.e5.
4. Bock SA, Munoz-Furlong A, Sampson HA. Fatalities due to anaphylactic reactions to foods. J Allergy Clin Immunol 2001;107:191–3.
5. Kulis M, Vickery BP, Burks AW. Pioneering immunotherapy for food allergy: clinical outcomes and modulation of the immune response. Immunol Res 2011;49:216–26.
6. Oppenheimer JJ, Nelson HS, Bock SA, et al. Treatment of peanut allergy with rush immunotherapy. J Allergy Clin Immunol 1992;90:256–62.
7. Nelson HS, Lahr J, Rule R, et al. Treatment of anaphylactic sensitivity to peanuts by immunotherapy with injections of aqueous peanut extract. J Allergy Clin Immunol 1997;99:744–51.

8. Thyagarajan A, Burks AW. Food allergy: present and future management. World Allergy Organ J 2009;2:282–8.
9. Varshney P, Jones SM, Scurlock AM, et al. A randomized controlled study of peanut oral immunotherapy: clinical desensitization and modulation of the allergic response. J Allergy Clin Immunol 2011;127:654–60.
10. Syed A, Garcia MA, Lyu SC, et al. Peanut oral immunotherapy results in increased antigen-induced regulatory T-cell function and hypomethylation of forkhead box protein 3 (FOXP3). J Allergy Clin Immunol 2014;133:500–10.e511.
11. Patriarca G, Nucera E, Pollastrini E, et al. Oral specific desensitization in food-allergic children. Dig Dis Sci 2007;52:1662–72.
12. Patriarca G, Nucera E, Roncallo C, et al. Oral desensitizing treatment in food allergy: clinical and immunological results. Aliment Pharmacol Ther 2003;17:459–65.
13. Morisset M, Moneret-Vautrin DA, Guenard L, et al. Oral desensitization in children with milk and egg allergies obtains recovery in a significant proportion of cases. A randomized study in 60 children with cow's milk allergy and 90 children with egg allergy. Eur Ann Allergy Clin Immunol 2007;39:12–9.
14. Meglio P, Bartone E, Plantamura M, et al. A protocol for oral desensitization in children with IgE-mediated cow's milk allergy. Allergy 2004;59:980–7.
15. Longo G, Barbi E, Berti I, et al. Specific oral tolerance induction in children with very severe cow's milk-induced reactions. J Allergy Clin Immunol 2008;121:343–7.
16. Pajno GB, Caminiti L, Crisafulli G, et al. Recent advances in immunotherapy: the active treatment of food allergy on the horizon. Expert Rev Clin Immunol 2013;9:891–3.
17. Vickery BP, Scurlock AM, Kulis M, et al. Sustained unresponsiveness to peanut in subjects who have completed peanut oral immunotherapy. J Allergy Clin Immunol 2014;133:468–75.e6.
18. Factor JM, Mendelson L, Lee J, et al. Effect of oral immunotherapy to peanut on food-specific quality of life. Ann Allergy Asthma Immunol 2012;109:348–52.e342.
19. Carraro S, Frigo AC, Perin M, et al. Impact of oral immunotherapy on quality of life in children with cow milk allergy: a pilot study. Int J Immunopathol Pharmacol 2012;25:793–8.
20. Nowak-Wegrzyn A, Sampson HA. Future therapies for food allergies. J Allergy Clin Immunol 2011;127:558–73.
21. Blumchen K, Ulbricht H, Staden U, et al. Oral peanut immunotherapy in children with peanut anaphylaxis. J Allergy Clin Immunol 2010;126:83–91.e81.
22. Anagnostou K, Islam S, King Y, et al. Assessing the efficacy of oral immunotherapy for the desensitisation of peanut allergy in children (STOP II): a phase 2 randomised controlled trial. Lancet 2014;383:1297–304.
23. Nurmatov U, Venderbosch I, Devereux G, et al. Allergen-specific oral immunotherapy for peanut allergy [Systematic reviews and meta-analyses]. Cochrane Database Syst Rev 2012;(9):CD009014.
24. Sampson HA. Peanut oral immunotherapy: is it ready for clinical practice? J Allergy Clin Immunol Pract 2013;1:15–21.
25. Staden U, Rolinck-Werninghaus C, Brewe F, et al. Specific oral tolerance induction in food allergy in children: efficacy and clinical patterns of reaction. Allergy 2007;62:1261–9.
26. Skripak JM, Nash SD, Rowley H, et al. A randomized, double-blind, placebo-controlled study of milk oral immunotherapy for cow's milk allergy. J Allergy Clin Immunol 2008;122:1154–60.

27. Narisety SD, Skripak JM, Steele P, et al. Open-label maintenance after milk oral immunotherapy for IgE-mediated cow's milk allergy. J Allergy Clin Immunol 2009;124:610–2.
28. Keet CA, Frischmeyer-Guerrerio PA, Thyagarajan A, et al. The safety and efficacy of sublingual and oral immunotherapy for milk allergy. J Allergy Clin Immunol 2012;129:448–55, 455.e1–5.
29. Keet CA, Seopaul S, Knorr S, et al. Long-term follow-up of oral immunotherapy for cow's milk allergy. J Allergy Clin Immunol 2013;132:737–9.e6.
30. Pajno GB, Caminiti L, Salzano G, et al. Comparison between two maintenance feeding regimens after successful cow's milk oral desensitization. Pediatr Allergy Immunol 2013;24:376–81.
31. Brozek JL, Terracciano L, Hsu J, et al. Oral immunotherapy for IgE-mediated cow's milk allergy: a systematic review and meta-analysis [Systematic reviews and meta-analyses]. Clin Exp Allergy 2012;42:363–74.
32. Buchanan AD, Green TD, Jones SM, et al. Egg oral immunotherapy in non-anaphylactic children with egg allergy. J Allergy Clin Immunol 2007;119: 199–205.
33. Vickery BP, Pons L, Kulis M, et al. Individualized IgE-based dosing of egg oral immunotherapy and the development of tolerance. Ann Allergy Asthma Immunol 2010;105:444–50.
34. Burks AW, Jones SM, Wood RA, et al. Oral immunotherapy for treatment of egg allergy in children. N Engl J Med 2012;367:233–43.
35. Fisher HR, du Toit G, Lack G. Specific oral tolerance induction in food allergic children: is oral desensitisation more effective than allergen avoidance?: a meta-analysis of published RCTs [Systematic reviews and meta-analyses]. Arch Dis Child 2011;96:259–64.
36. Hofmann AM, Scurlock AM, Jones SM, et al. Safety of a peanut oral immuno-therapy protocol in children with peanut allergy. J Allergy Clin Immunol 2009; 124:286–91, 291.e1–6.
37. Varshney P, Steele PH, Vickery BP, et al. Adverse reactions during peanut oral immunotherapy home dosing. J Allergy Clin Immunol 2009;124:1351–2.
38. Sanchez-Garcia S, Rodriguez Del Rio P, Escudero C, et al. Possible eosinophilic esophagitis induced by milk oral immunotherapy. J Allergy Clin Immunol 2012; 129:1155–7.
39. Ridolo E, De Angelis GL, Dall'aglio P. Eosinophilic esophagitis after specific oral tolerance induction for egg protein. Ann Allergy Asthma Immunol 2011; 106:73–4.
40. Shankar T, Petrov AA. Omalizumab and hypersensitivity reactions. Curr Opin Allergy Clin Immunol 2013;13:19–24.
41. Nadeau KC, Schneider LC, Hoyte L, et al. Rapid oral desensitization in combi-nation with omalizumab therapy in patients with cow's milk allergy. J Allergy Clin Immunol 2011;127:1622–4.
42. Schneider LC, Rachid R, LeBovidge J, et al. A pilot study of omalizumab to facil-itate rapid oral desensitization in high-risk peanut-allergic patients. J Allergy Clin Immunol 2013;132:1368–74.
43. Bégin P, Dominguez T, Wilson SP, et al. Phase 1 results of safety and tolerability in a rush oral immunotherapy protocol to multiple foods using Omalizumab. Allergy Asthma Clin Immunol 2014;10:7.
44. Chin SJ, Vickery BP, Kulis MD, et al. Sublingual versus oral immunotherapy for peanut-allergic children: a retrospective comparison. J Allergy Clin Immunol 2013;132:476–8.e2.

45. de Boissieu D, Dupont C. Sublingual immunotherapy for cow's milk protein allergy: a preliminary report. Allergy 2006;61:1238–9.
46. Enrique E, Pineda F, Malek T, et al. Sublingual immunotherapy for hazelnut food allergy: a randomized, double-blind, placebo-controlled study with a standardized hazelnut extract. J Allergy Clin Immunol 2005;116:1073–9.
47. Enrique E, Malek T, Pineda F, et al. Sublingual immunotherapy for hazelnut food allergy: a follow-up study. Ann Allergy Asthma Immunol 2008;100:283–4.
48. Fernandez-Rivas M, Garrido Fernandez S, Nadal JA, et al. Randomized double-blind, placebo-controlled trial of sublingual immunotherapy with a Pru p 3 quantified peach extract. Allergy 2009;64:876–83.
49. Kim EH, Bird JA, Kulis M, et al. Sublingual immunotherapy for peanut allergy: clinical and immunologic evidence of desensitization. J Allergy Clin Immunol 2011;127:640–6.e1.
50. Fleischer DM, Burks AW, Vickery BP, et al. Sublingual immunotherapy for peanut allergy: a randomized, double-blind, placebo-controlled multicenter trial. J Allergy Clin Immunol 2013;131:119, 127.e1–7.
51. Dupont C, Kalach N, Soulaines P, et al. Cow's milk epicutaneous immunotherapy in children: a pilot trial of safety, acceptability, and impact on allergic reactivity. J Allergy Clin Immunol 2010;125:1165–7.
52. Dupont C, de Blay F, Guenard-Bilbault L, et al. Peanut epicutaneous immunotherapy (EPIT) in peanut-allergic children: 18 months treatment in the Arachild Study. J Allergy Clin Immunol 2014;133:AB102.
53. Asero R. Effects of birch pollen-specific immunotherapy on apple allergy in birch pollen-hypersensitive patients. Clin Exp Allergy 1998;28:1368–73.
54. Asero R. How long does the effect of birch pollen injection SIT on apple allergy last? Allergy 2003;58:435–8.
55. Asero R. Effects of birch pollen SIT on apple allergy: a matter of dosage? Allergy 2004;59:1269–71.
56. Bolhaar ST, Tiemessen MM, Zuidmeer L, et al. Efficacy of birch-pollen immunotherapy on cross-reactive food allergy confirmed by skin tests and double-blind food challenges. Clin Exp Allergy 2004;34:761–9.
57. Bucher X, Pichler WJ, Dahinden CA, et al. Effect of tree pollen specific, subcutaneous immunotherapy on the oral allergy syndrome to apple and hazelnut. Allergy 2004;59:1272–6.
58. Konstantinou GN, Giavi S, Kalobatsou A, et al. Consumption of heat-treated egg by children allergic or sensitized to egg can affect the natural course of egg allergy: hypothesis-generating observations. J Allergy Clin Immunol 2008;122:414–5.
59. Kim JS, Nowak-Wegrzyn A, Sicherer SH, et al. Dietary baked milk accelerates the resolution of cow's milk allergy in children. J Allergy Clin Immunol 2011;128:125–31.e2.
60. Leonard SA, Sampson HA, Sicherer SH, et al. Dietary baked egg accelerates resolution of egg allergy in children. J Allergy Clin Immunol 2012;130:473–80.e1.
61. Huang F, Nowak-Wegrzyn A. Extensively heated milk and egg as oral immunotherapy. Curr Opin Allergy Clin Immunol 2012;12:283–92.
62. Shreffler WG, Wanich N, Moloney M, et al. Association of allergen-specific regulatory T cells with the onset of clinical tolerance to milk protein. J Allergy Clin Immunol 2009;123:43–52.e7.
63. Ford LS, Bloom KA, Nowak-Wegrzyn AH, et al. Basophil reactivity, wheal size, and immunoglobulin levels distinguish degrees of cow's milk tolerance. J Allergy Clin Immunol 2013;131:180–6.e1–3.

64. Hong SJ, Michael JG, Fehringer A, et al. Pepsin-digested peanut contains T-cell epitopes but no IgE epitopes. J Allergy Clin Immunol 1999;104:473–8.
65. Prickett SR, Voskamp AL, Phan T, et al. Ara h 1 CD4+ T cell epitope-based peptides: candidates for a peanut allergy therapeutic. Clin Exp Allergy 2013; 43:684–97.
66. Zhou Y, Kawasaki H, Hsu SC, et al. Oral tolerance to food-induced systemic anaphylaxis mediated by the C-type lectin SIGNR1. Nat Med 2010;16:1128–33.
67. Rupa P, Nakamura S, Katayama S, et al. Effects of ovalbumin glycoconjugates on alleviation of orally induced egg allergy in mice via dendritic-cell maturation and T-cell activation. Mol Nutr Food Res 2014;58:405–17.
68. Pascal M, Konstantinou GN, Masilamani M, et al. In silico prediction of Ara h 2 T cell epitopes in peanut-allergic children. Clin Exp Allergy 2013;43:116–27.
69. Bannon GA, Cockrell G, Connaughton C, et al. Engineering, characterization and in vitro efficacy of the major peanut allergens for use in immunotherapy. Int Arch Allergy Immunol 2001;124:70–2.
70. Li XM, Srivastava K, Grishin A, et al. Persistent protective effect of heat-killed Escherichia coli producing "engineered," recombinant peanut proteins in a murine model of peanut allergy. J Allergy Clin Immunol 2003;112:159–67.
71. Wood RA, Sicherer SH, Burks AW, et al. A phase 1 study of heat/phenol-killed, E. coli-encapsulated, recombinant modified peanut proteins Ara h 1, Ara h 2, and Ara h 3 (EMP-123) for the treatment of peanut allergy. Allergy 2013;68:803–8.
72. Wang J. Treatment of food anaphylaxis with traditional Chinese herbal remedies: from mouse model to human clinical trials. Curr Opin Allergy Clin Immunol 2013; 13:386–91.
73. Srivastava KD, Kattan JD, Zou ZM, et al. The Chinese herbal medicine formula FAHF-2 completely blocks anaphylactic reactions in a murine model of peanut allergy. J Allergy Clin Immunol 2005;115:171–8.
74. Qu C, Srivastava K, Ko J, et al. Induction of tolerance after establishment of peanut allergy by the food allergy herbal formula-2 is associated with up-regulation of interferon-gamma. Clin Exp Allergy 2007;37:846–55.
75. Wang J, Patil SP, Yang N, et al. Safety, tolerability, and immunologic effects of a food allergy herbal formula in food allergic individuals: a randomized, double-blinded, placebo-controlled, dose escalation, phase 1 study. Ann Allergy Asthma Immunol 2010;105:75–84.
76. Patil SP, Wang J, Song Y, et al. Clinical safety of Food Allergy Herbal Formula-2 (FAHF-2) and inhibitory effect on basophils from patients with food allergy: extended phase I study. J Allergy Clin Immunol 2011;128:1259–65.e2.
77. Kalliomaki M, Kirjavainen P, Eerola E, et al. Distinct patterns of neonatal gut microflora in infants in whom atopy was and was not developing. J Allergy Clin Immunol 2001;107:129–34.
78. Vitaliti G, Pavone P, Guglielmo F, et al. The immunomodulatory effect of probiotics beyond atopy: an update [Systematic reviews and meta-analyses]. J Asthma 2014;51:320–32.
79. Gore C, Custovic A, Tannock GW, et al. Treatment and secondary prevention effects of the probiotics Lactobacillus paracasei or Bifidobacterium lactis on early infant eczema: randomized controlled trial with follow-up until age 3 years. Clin Exp Allergy 2012;42:112–22.
80. Perrin Y, Nutten S, Audran R, et al. Comparison of two oral probiotic preparations in a randomized crossover trial highlights a potentially beneficial effect of Lactobacillus paracasei NCC2461 in patients with allergic rhinitis. Clin Transl Allergy 2014;4:1.

81. Cabana MD. No consistent evidence to date that prenatal or postnatal probiotic supplementation prevents childhood asthma and wheeze [Systematic reviews and meta-analyses]. Evid Based Med 2014;19:144.
82. Silverberg JI. Atopic dermatitis: an evidence-based treatment update [Systematic reviews and meta-analyses]. Am J Clin Dermatol 2014;15:149–64.
83. Foolad N, Armstrong AW. Prebiotics and probiotics: the prevention and reduction in severity of atopic dermatitis in children [Systematic reviews and meta-analyses]. Benef Microbes 2014;5:151–60.
84. Schiavi E, Barletta B, Butteroni C, et al. Oral therapeutic administration of a probiotic mixture suppresses established Th2 responses and systemic anaphylaxis in a murine model of food allergy. Allergy 2011;66:499–508.
85. Hol J, van Leer EH, Elink Schuurman BE, et al. The acquisition of tolerance toward cow's milk through probiotic supplementation: a randomized, controlled trial. J Allergy Clin Immunol 2008;121:1448–54.
86. Berni Canani R, Nocerino R, Terrin G, et al. Effect of Lactobacillus GG on tolerance acquisition in infants with cow's milk allergy: a randomized trial. J Allergy Clin Immunol 2012;129:580–2, 582.e1–5.
87. Garg SK, Croft AM, Bager P. Helminth therapy (worms) for induction of remission in inflammatory bowel disease [Systematic reviews and meta-analyses]. Cochrane Database Syst Rev 2014;(1):CD009400.
88. Heylen M, Ruyssers NE, Gielis EM, et al. Of worms, mice and man: an overview of experimental and clinical helminth-based therapy for inflammatory bowel disease. Pharmacol Ther 2014;143:153–67.
89. Amoah AS, Boakye DA, van Ree R, et al. Parasitic worms and allergies in childhood: insights from population studies 2008-2013. Pediatr Allergy Immunol 2014;25:208–17.
90. Nagler-Anderson C. Helminth-induced immunoregulation of an allergic response to food. Chem Immunol Allergy 2006;90:1–13.
91. Bager P, Arnved J, Ronborg S, et al. Trichuris suis ova therapy for allergic rhinitis: a randomized, double-blind, placebo-controlled clinical trial. J Allergy Clin Immunol 2010;125:123–30.e1–3.
92. Jouvin MH, Kinet JP. Trichuris suis ova: testing a helminth-based therapy as an extension of the hygiene hypothesis. J Allergy Clin Immunol 2012;130:3–10 [quiz: 11–2].
93. Schwaber J, Cohen EP. Human x mouse somatic cell hybrid clone secreting immunoglobulins of both parental types. Nature 1973;244:444–7.
94. Kohler G, Milstein C. Continuous cultures of fused cells secreting antibody of predefined specificity. Nature 1975;256:495–7.
95. Leung DY, Sampson HA, Yunginger JW, et al. Effect of anti-IgE therapy in patients with peanut allergy. N Engl J Med 2003;348:986–93.
96. Sampson HA, Leung DY, Burks AW, et al. A phase II, randomized, double-blind, parallel-group, placebo-controlled oral food challenge trial of Xolair (omalizumab) in peanut allergy. J Allergy Clin Immunol 2011;127:1309–10.e1.
97. Straumann A, Conus S, Grzonka P, et al. Anti-interleukin-5 antibody treatment (mepolizumab) in active eosinophilic oesophagitis: a randomised, placebo-controlled, double-blind trial. Gut 2010;59:21–30.
98. Assa'ad AH, Gupta SK, Collins MH, et al. An antibody against IL-5 reduces numbers of esophageal intraepithelial eosinophils in children with eosinophilic esophagitis. Gastroenterology 2011;141:1593–604.
99. Otani IM, Anilkumar AA, Newbury RO, et al. Anti-IL-5 therapy reduces mast cell and IL-9 cell numbers in pediatric patients with eosinophilic esophagitis. J Allergy Clin Immunol 2013;131:1576–82.

100. Aumeunier A, Grela F, Ramadan A, et al. Systemic Toll-like receptor stimulation suppresses experimental allergic asthma and autoimmune diabetes in NOD mice. PLoS One 2010;5:e11484.
101. Duechs MJ, Hahn C, Benediktus E, et al. TLR agonist mediated suppression of allergic responses is associated with increased innate inflammation in the airways. Pulm Pharmacol Ther 2011;24:203–14.
102. Beeh KM, Kanniess F, Wagner F, et al. The novel TLR-9 agonist QbG10 shows clinical efficacy in persistent allergic asthma. J Allergy Clin Immunol 2013;131: 866–74.
103. ClinicalTrials.gov [Internet]. Bethesda (MD): National Library of Medicine (US). 2012 March 8-Identifier NCT01480271, An investigation of the safety, tolerability, pharmacokinetics and pharmacodynamics of GSK2245035 in healthy volunteers and allergic rhinitics. Available at: http://clinicaltrials.gov/ct/show/NCT00287391?order=1. Accessed April 28, 2014.
104. Zhu FG, Kandimalla ER, Yu D, et al. Oral administration of a synthetic agonist of Toll-like receptor 9 potently modulates peanut-induced allergy in mice. J Allergy Clin Immunol 2007;120:631–7.
105. Schulke S, Burggraf M, Waibler Z, et al. A fusion protein of flagellin and ovalbumin suppresses the TH2 response and prevents murine intestinal allergy. J Allergy Clin Immunol 2011;128:1340–8.e12.
106. Li XM, Srivastava K, Huleatt JW, et al. Engineered recombinant peanut protein and heat-killed Listeria monocytogenes coadministration protects against peanut-induced anaphylaxis in a murine model. J Immunol 2003; 170:3289–95.
107. Frossard CP, Steidler L, Eigenmann PA. Oral administration of an IL-10-secreting Lactococcus lactis strain prevents food-induced IgE sensitization. J Allergy Clin Immunol 2007;119:952–9.
108. Roy K, Mao HQ, Huang SK, et al. Oral gene delivery with chitosan–DNA nanoparticles generates immunologic protection in a murine model of peanut allergy. Nat Med 1999;5:387–91.

Inner City Asthma

Peter J. Gergen, MD, MPH*, Alkis Togias, MD

KEYWORDS

- Asthma • Inner city • Severity • Poverty • Disparities • Intervention

KEY POINTS

- Inner cities are areas of high asthma morbidity and mortality.
- Many asthma risk factors present; no single one predominates.
- Structure and function of medical care contribute to the problem.
- Social inequities contribute to the problem.
- Successful interventions exist.

SCOPE OF THE PROBLEM
Prevalence

In the United States, asthma prevalence increased at a rate of 1.4% per year between 2001 to 2010 in children and adolescents 17 years and younger, so that by 2008 to 2010, the prevalence reached 9.5%.[1] Asthma prevalence varies among racial/ethnic groups; African American children have 1.6 times the level of current asthma than white children.[2] Asthma prevalence varies greatly in the Hispanic groups in the United States. Puerto Rican children have among the highest prevalence, approximately 2.4 times that of white children, whereas Mexican American children have levels lower than white children.[2,3] Differences in prevalence can represent true differences in disease or differences in diagnosis. An analyses of children aged 3 to 17 years with reported wheezing in the past year from the 1999 National Health Interview Study (NHIS) found that compared with non-Hispanic white children, the adjusted relative risk for reporting a diagnosis of asthma was increased for Puerto Rican (1.43), non-Hispanic black (1.22), and Mexican American children (1.19),[4] suggesting that part of the reported differences in prevalence can be explained by differential rates of diagnosis.

In addition to varying in different racial/ethnic groups, asthma prevalence can vary both across and within neighborhoods. Neighborhoods with the highest asthma prevalence tend to have high minority concentration and low income levels. In Chicago, the neighborhood prevalence of asthma ranges from 0% to 44%, with the highest levels

Allergy, Asthma, Airway Biology Branch (AAABB), MD, USA
* Corresponding author. NIH/DAIT/AAABB, 5601 Fishers Lane, Room 6B58, Rockville, MD 20892.
E-mail address: pgergen@niaid.nih.gov

Immunol Allergy Clin N Am 35 (2015) 101–114
http://dx.doi.org/10.1016/j.iac.2014.09.006
0889-8561/15/$ – see front matter Published by Elsevier Inc.

seen in African American and Hispanic neighborhoods.[5] Within a single neighborhood in New York City, asthma prevalence has been reported at 5.3% for Dominicans and other Latinos versus 13.2% for Puerto Ricans.[6]

The factors contributing to the high prevalence of asthma in Puerto Rican children are not clear. Despite having higher socioeconomic status (SES), lower rates of prematurity, and less exposure to prenatal smoke exposure, the prevalence of asthma is higher in Puerto Rican children living in Puerto Rico compared with Puerto Rican children living in the south Bronx.[7] Differences in prevalence between island resident Puerto Rican children and those living in the US mainland are not caused by increased severity when Global Initiative for Asthma severity criteria and pulmonary function are considered, but island Puerto Rican children have a higher rate of emergency room visits and lowest use of inhaled steroids.[8] Differences in perception of disease may contribute to the differences noted in Puerto Rican children. Comparison of subjective estimates of peak expiratory flow rates (PEFR) compared with measurement of PEFR over a 5-week period in 512 children aged 7 to 16 years living in Puerto Rico and Rhode Island found that island Puerto Ricans had the lowest accuracy of estimating their PEFR, with Rhode Island Latinos better. However, both groups were significantly worse than non-Hispanic white children. The investigators also reported that self-reported asthma morbidity increased as ability to estimate the pulmonary function decreased.[9]

Morbidity and Mortality

Data from a national database report in 2006 indicated that asthma was the reason for 3.4 million visits to physician offices, 500,000 visits to hospital outpatient departments, 593,000 emergency visits, and 155,000 hospitalizations. In 2005, there were 167 deaths from asthma in children and adolescents (most asthma deaths occur in the elderly). African American children and adolescents had a 7.6 times higher death rate, 2.6 times higher emergency department (ED) visits, 3 times higher hospitalization, but 20% lower nonemergency asthma ambulatory care than whites. Data on Hispanics at the national level are more limited, but ED usage by this ethnic group is approximately double that of whites, although there is a similar asthma death rate. The magnitude of the disparity between white and African American children is confounded by the approach taken in analyzing the data. Asthma morbidity and mortality data for children 0 to 17 years of age collected by the National Center for Health Statistics found between 2001 and 2010 show that racial disparities have remained unchanged if the rates are based on the total population. If, however, rates are calculated based on the number of children with asthma within each racial group, a disparity for asthma attack prevalence is no longer evident and the level of disparity for ED visits and hospitalization is decreased. However, the disparity in asthma mortality remains.[10]

CONTRIBUTING FACTORS
Disease Severity

Reduced responsiveness to therapy for intrinsic or extrinsic reasons has been considered as a possible explanation for the higher rates of morbidity and mortality found in poor and minority children and adolescents. However, several studies such as the Inner City Asthma Consortium ACE (Asthma Control Evaluation) study[11] and the BreathMobile[12] found that, after providing high-quality, comprehensive asthma care and the ability to obtain the needed medication, most poor and minority children and adolescents with asthma can be well controlled.

Although proportionally more ED visits occur in children who live in low-income, urban environments, the severity of asthma exacerbations does not seem to differ between children of varying socioeconomic strata. As part of the Multicenter Airway Research Collaboration,[13] 40 EDs across the United States evaluated 1095 children and adolescents 2 to 17 years of age presenting with an attack of asthma. In multivariate analyses, after controlling for socioeconomic factors, race/ethnicity was not related to respiratory distress at presentation or outcomes as measured by a pulmonary index score, which included severity of wheeze, respiratory rate and accessory muscle use, ED management, hospitalization for asthma, or outcome 2 weeks after discharge from the ED.

One explanation for the increased burden of asthma in low-income, urban, minority children and adolescents may lie in the role of physician's and patient's perception of severity and need for treatment. In 3494 adult asthmatics in 15 managed care organizations in the United States, the severity of asthma estimated from patient-reported symptoms was compared with physician estimates of severity. Physicians were more likely to estimate the severity of asthma lower than the patient's perception of severity in blacks compared with whites patients (odds ratio [OR] = 1.39, 95% CI 1.08–1.79). This underestimation was associated with undertreatment with inhaled corticosteroid.[14]

Poverty

To better understand the differences in morbidity and mortality, the social environment in which these children and adolescents live must be considered.

In 2012, the percentage of African American (36.7%) and Hispanic (33.8%) children living in poverty was almost 3 times that of white children (12.3%). This disparity in poverty in children has not decreased since 2000.[15] However, the relation between asthma prevalence and income is complex. Analyses of the 1997 NHIS for children and adolescents younger than 18 years found that, after controlling for relevant confounders, only in families living on income less than half the federal poverty level was asthma prevalence increased in African American compared with white children.[16] Using a composite socioeconomic index in 8-year-old to 21-year-old participants in the Genes-Environment and Admixture in Latino Americans (GALA II) and Study of African Americans, Asthma, Genes and Environments (SAGE II) studies (large asthma genetic studies focusing on African American and Latinos), the investigators found that, in African American children, asthma prevalence increased, whereas the index decreased. In contrast, Mexican American children showed a decrease in asthma prevalence as the socioeconomic index decreased. These findings did not change when acculturation was taken into account.[17]

Comparisons based solely on income do not adequately explain the disparities between the racial/ethnic groups in the United States. Controlling for income, African American and Puerto Rican populations, compared with whites, live in neighborhoods with poorer quality of life as a result of less economic investment, lower-quality schools, and less access to medical services.[18] Although racial segregation has declined in the United States, African Americans as a group continue to experience the highest level of housing segregation.[19] Worse community functioning as measured by increased crime, incarceration rate, or exposure to violence has been associated with higher asthma prevalence,[20] lower adherence to inhaled corticosteroids,[21] and more asthma symptoms.[22]

A more complete understanding of the role of SES in health disparities is hindered by the conceptualization of SES. Many studies operationalize SES with 2 variables: family income, with or without adjustment for family size; and education level. Other important individual factors, such as wealth, and nonindividual factors, such as the social and physical environment, which includes residence in a poor neighborhood, are not taken into account. A study of asthma readmission rates in 1-year-old to 16-year-old children in the Cincinnati, OH area, where African American children had approximately twice the readmission rate of white children, used 2 approaches to understand the reasons for this racial difference. Conventional SES variables (income, education) explained approximately 8% of the difference, whereas the addition of variables such as car or house ownership, marriage status, looking for work, and source from which to borrow money increased the ability to explain the difference to almost 41%.[23] A neighborhood analysis of childhood (1–16 years of age) asthma admission rates from Hamilton County, OH found that neighborhood-level education, car access, and population density explained most ($R^2 = 0.55$) of the neighborhood variation in asthma admissions.[24] Simply placing many variables in a statistical model is not an optimal methodology compared with using more advanced statistical approaches such as propensity scores to better account for SES differences between racial/ethnic groups.

Quality of Care

Uncontrolled asthma results in higher health care use. In a study by Guilbert and colleagues,[25] children with uncontrolled asthma (Asthma Control Test score $\leq$19) had an OR of 4.6 for an asthma-related doctor's visit and OR of 1.7 for an ED visit compared with children with well-controlled asthma, over a 9-month period. Access to quality care is an important factor in how asthma is controlled. In a study of asthma hospital readmissions in 1-year-old to 16-year-old children in Ohio, the readmission rate was lowest in children with private insurance and good access to care.[26]

Disparities exist in how poor and minority children are treated. Minority children frequently have lower use of controller medication and higher use of reliever medication to control their asthma.[27] In children 1 to 6 years of age who were hospitalized for asthma, minority children were less likely to be prescribed a nebulizer on discharge than white children.[28] Hispanic children with asthma received fewer inhaled steroid prescriptions regardless whether they received their care at a private practice or a clinic.[29] Even within a system with equal access, military dependents covered by Tricare Prime, African American, and Hispanic children had higher rates of ED visits and hospitalizations, although they were less likely to receive care from an asthma specialist.[30]

In addition to being prescribed proper treatment of asthma, it is important that children use the treatment. Lack of adherence to inhaled corticosteroids has been associated with exacerbations; for example, with every 25% increase in adherence to inhaled corticosteroids, there was a decrease of 11% in asthma exacerbations in adults.[31] Factors found to be associated with adherence include the family's belief about the need for the medication, the parental expectation about asthma control, non-English speaking, and family organization/functioning.[32,33] Neighborhood factors such as crime level have also been related to adherence.[21] Of course, increasing adherence may have relatively little impact if the child is prescribed inadequate dose of a controller medication: a community study of 5-year-olds to 12-year-olds found that, although 76% reported to be using daily controller medication, 74% were on an inadequate controller dose.[34] Prescribing an inadequate dose can also lead to worse adherence, because patients or their families may question the benefit when efficacy is low.

Although guidelines exist as to how to manage asthma, care must be taken to ensure that the method or tool used is appropriate for the population. For example, written action plans are often used as a measure of good quality of care. However, when the impact of action plans is evaluated, they are not always found to be effective.[35] An evaluation of 30 asthma action plans used by 27 state Departments of Health determined that readability was at seventh grade level instead of the third to fifth level that is recommended for low literate populations. Based on ease of use and readability, more than 40% of these action plans were considered unsuitable.[36]

Allergens/Sensitization

Exposure and sensitization to allergens play an important role in asthma morbidity. Increased exposure to certain allergens such as mite or cockroach is associated with increased rate of sensitization,[37,38] and sensitization and exposure to allergens such as those deriving from cockroaches,[39] mice,[40] rats,[41] or molds are associated with increased asthma symptoms and health care use.

Exposure to indoor allergens varies widely based on many factors, several of which are linked to poverty. Older homes, poor condition of the house (eg, cracks in the wall, water leaks), and low family income are associated with increased levels of cockroach, mite, and mouse allergens.[42-44] Urban areas and high-rise apartment buildings are specifically linked to increased cockroach allergen.[43] Single-family homes and high bedroom humidity are associated with mite allergen.[42] Pet (cat or dog) ownership is the most important marker of pet allergens.[45] Because pet ownership increases with increasing income, these allergens are relatively less common in poor urban areas.[45] Exposure in the bedroom seems to be the most important in regards to developing sensitization.[38] Much effort has been directed at lowering allergen exposure in the home, specifically the bedroom, but that high levels of allergen and mold exposure can occur at school or daycare.[46,47]

Data from the US population collected in the National Health and Nutrition Examination Survey (NHANES) show that non-Hispanic African Americans and Mexican Americans have higher rates of allergen sensitization than non-Hispanic whites.[48] African American and Mexican American children, 6 to 16 years of age, have higher rates of sensitization to allergens associated with asthma morbidity, such as cockroach and dust mite.[49] It is not known if these differences are solely caused by differential exposure to allergens or if genetic differences play a role.

Housing

Housing quality in poor neighborhoods plays an important role in exposing the child or adolescent to a variety of asthma triggers. Public housing has been associated with some of the highest prevalence of asthma.[50] Data from the Puerto Rican Asthma Project in New York City[51] found that buildings with serious or medium level housing code violations had higher home allergen levels after adjustment for other neighborhood characteristics. A New York City study[52] of 7-year-old to 8-year-old children living in high asthma prevalence area found higher levels of cockroach, cat, and mouse allergens in their homes compared with children living in low asthma prevalence areas.

Conflicting data exist as to whether or not the homes of children with asthma differ from those without asthma within the same community. In a study conducted in Baltimore, MD, no difference in the levels of indoor pollutants ($PM_{2.5}$, PM_{10}, NO_2, O_3) and allergens (cat, dust mite, cockroach, dog, and mouse) was found when the homes of children 2 to 6 years of age with and without asthma were compared.[53] In contrast, a multicity study across the United States using the Environmental Relative Moldiness Index, which was developed by the Environmental Protection Agency (EPA) and the US Department of Housing and Urban Development to quantify mold contamination in housing, found that within the same geographic area, homes of people with asthma had higher relative burden of mold compared with the homes of people without asthma.[54]

Environmental Tobacco Smoke

Exposure to environmental tobacco smoke (ETS) is associated with increased asthma prevalence, symptoms, asthma-related school absenteeism, asthma exacerbations, and decreased pulmonary function in children and adolescents.[55,56] The highest rates of active cigarette smoking are in the poor and those with low education.[57] Analysis of NHANES data from 2005 to 2010 showed that 53.2% of the children and adolescents with asthma who did not use tobacco products were exposed to ETS based on increased serum cotinine levels. This figure increased to 70.1% in low-income children and adolescents. The level of exposure to ETS has been decreasing since 1988, but the rate of decrease has slowed considerably since 2004.[58] The factors most strongly associated with ETS exposure in inner city children are the number of smokers in the house and younger age.[59]

Nitrogen Dioxide

Nitrogen dioxide (NO_2) is a common respiratory irritant in inner city homes. This situation is mostly caused by the high use of gas stoves. High levels of NO_2 have been associated with an increase in asthma symptoms.[60,61] The National Cooperative Inner City Asthma Study (NCICAS) reported the effect of NO_2 on children who were not allergen skin test positive. The investigators speculated that the sensitized children were not immune to the effects of NO_2, but rather the prevalent allergen exposure in the children's homes was causing the sensitized children to have such a high level of symptoms that the effect of NO_2 was not seen.[61]

Outdoor Pollution

Air pollution has repeatedly been shown to play an important role in asthma. Five of the 6 criteria pollutants (nitrogen oxides, particulate matter, ozone, sulfur dioxide, carbon monoxide) monitored by the EPA have been associated with increased asthma prevalence or morbidity.[62–64] Studies have also found that the closer a child lives to a source of outdoor pollutants such as a major highway or bus route, the more problems with asthma symptoms and exacerbations they experience.[65,66] A Rochester, MN study[67] found that after matching for other asthma risk factors using propensity scores to equalize asthma risk, children living in census tracks close to a major highway or railroad had a higher risk of asthma. Pollutant and interaction with allergens may play a role in the increased sensitization seen in inner city communities: in 5-year-olds to 7 year-olds in New York City, higher levels of polycyclic aromatic hydrocarbons were associated with increased levels of cockroach sensitization. This increased risk was highest in the children with a null genotype for GSTM1.[68]

Lower-income, minority communities have higher exposures to environmental pollutants because of the disproportionately higher numbers of toxic waste dumps, major highways, bus terminals, industry, and so forth located nearby.[69,70] The US Centers for Disease Control and Prevention reported that in 2010 approximately 4% of the US population lived within 150 m of a major highway. Being a member of a racial/ethnic minority group (non-Hispanic black 4.4%, Hispanic 5%, non-Hispanic white 3.1%), being foreign born (5.1% vs 3.5% native born), and speaking a language other than English at home (Spanish 5.1% vs English 3.3%) increases the probability of living close to a major highway.[71]

Studies that focus on immigrants give us a better understanding of the influence of the local environment on asthma. Data from the NHIS 2001 to 2009[72] found higher prevalence of asthma in all ages in individuals born in the United States compared with foreign-born individuals. These differences were present in all racial/ethnic groups. In the foreign born, time living in the United States seems to be important. After 10 years or more living in the United States, foreign-born individuals had higher rates of asthma compared with more recent arrivals.

Obesity

Obesity is a major problem in poor and minority communities. In children and adolescents in the United States during 2009 to 2010, 39.4% of Mexican Americans, 39.1% of non-Hispanic blacks, and 27.9% of non-Hispanic whites were overweight (body mass index [BMI], calculated as weight in kilograms divided by the square of height in meters, $\geq 85\%$). Greater differences existed when obesity (BMI$\geq$95%) was considered: 21.2% in Mexican Americans, 24.3% in non-Hispanic blacks, and 14% in non-Hispanic whites. Overweight/obesity has been shown to be associated with increased asthma prevalence, symptoms, and exacerbations. This difference was not related to differences in allergic sensitization.[73,74] A randomized control trail reported that weight loss in obese asthmatics resulted in improvement in static lung function and asthma control without changes in inflammation.[75]

Prematurity

Higher rates of asthma in children and adolescents have been found to be associated with certain birth characteristics, such as low birth weight or premature birth.[76,77] In a study of middle-class, racially diverse children, 6 to 8 years of age, living in the suburbs of Detroit, MI, approximately one-third of the black-white differences in physician-diagnosed asthma was accounted for by the difference in low birth weight.[78] Extreme prematurity (gestation 23–27 weeks) seems to be the period when the highest risk for developing asthma exists.[79] Natality data from the United States in 2012 show that non-Hispanic African American mothers experience up to twice the rate of premature or low-birth-weight births. This finding is true for births of less than 37 weeks' and 32 weeks' gestation and for birth weights less than 2500 g or 1500 g. The prematurity and low birth rates for Hispanics are either equal or slightly higher than non-Hispanic whites.[80]

Psychosocial Factors

Psychological factors play an important role in inner city asthma. Maternal mental health problems are associated with increased hospitalizations for childhood asthma,[81] maternal depression is associated with increased asthma ED visits,[82] and maternal stress levels with increased infant wheezing.[83] The child's psychological status is also important, because childhood behavioral problems are associated with wheezing and poorer functioning.[81]

INTERVENTIONS

Interventions in the inner city are challenging given the many factors contributing to the high burden of asthma in poor and minority children. Several interventions have been focused on the quality care received. One aspect of the problem of obtaining quality care in the inner city is the family's ability to successfully deal with the medical care system because of lack of knowledge/skills and other, competing major socioeconomic problems. The National Institute of Allergy and Infectious Diseases (NIAID)-

funded NCICAS[84] found that a tailored family-based intervention performed by an asthma counselor (an asthma-trained social worker) was effective in helping the families obtain better care and reduce the morbidity of their child's illness. Other successful interventions to improve medical care use have focused on the children or adolescents with asthma and have been school based either by providing asthma education to the students during the school day[85] or by direct observation of the use of asthma controller medications.[86] Lack of family participation limits the effectiveness of a program, as reported in an intervention using a trained parent mentor to help families with asthma.[87]

As discussed earlier, environmental triggers of asthma are highly prevalent in the living environment of poor and minority children. Concern has been raised as to the ability to decrease allergen levels and the impact on disease. For example, using an exterminator service only temporarily reduces the level of cockroach allergen.[88] The NIAID-funded Inner City Asthma Study (ICAS) completed a clinical trial evaluating the effect of a comprehensive environmental cleanup focused on home allergens and exposure to tobacco smoke. The intervention resulted in a decrease in the level of home allergens and a concomitant decrease in asthma symptoms, thus showing the feasibility of lower allergen levels but also the large effort required to accomplish this goal.[89] The effect of this approach appeared to be long lasting, because it remained present for at least 1 year after the intervention of the ICAS was completed.

Other interventions have focused on improving housing conditions. A program to weatherize homes resulted in decreased mold and moisture exposure and improvement in asthma control compared with a historical control group.[90] Taking advantage of a Seattle, WA public housing redevelopment project, investigators found that moving families of children and adolescents with asthma into asthma-friendly homes improved symptoms and asthma-related quality of life and reduced ED visits, compared with controls who received asthma education from a nurse at a primary care setting.[91]

Several factors influence whether or not an intervention is successful in the inner city. Interventions that are too narrowly focused, such as emphasizing nebulizer use[92] or using a high-efficiency particulate air filter alone,[93] tend to have limited to no effect. Although the targets of these interventions are important, the effects are overwhelmed by other factors that are left untreated. Lack of active participation and interest by the subjects of an asthma intervention is of importance and can lie in the design of the program itself or in the attitude and beliefs of the participants or their families. An evaluation of nonresponders in the PUFF City intervention (a computer-tailored intervention designed to aid urban African American adolescents gain better control of their asthma) found that several factors such as the Asthma Self-Regulation Interview (which measures acceptability of the chronic nature of the disease, perceived vulnerability, and ability to control it), rebelliousness, religiosity, and perceived emotional support from family and friends had varying impact on adherence to controller medication, availability of rescue medication, and smoking cessation.[94]

With the proper treatment, inner city asthma can be well controlled. With the provision of guidelines-driven care and assured access to the appropriate controller medication, the NIAID-fund ACE study reduced asthma symptoms to a low level.[11] The NIAID-funded ICATA study reported that asthma exacerbations could be decreased significantly with similar high-quality care. In addition, ICATA found that the addition of a biologic (omalizumab) could further reduce symptoms and exacerbations.[95] Although biologics are too expensive to be used widely, they show that future advances in therapies will allow inner city asthma to be even better controlled.

SUMMARY

Inner city asthma is a complex problem. Improving the efficacy of drugs to treat asthma or identifying a new environmental or genetic risk factor contributing to morbidity will add to our existing armamentarium but will have limited impact on reducing disparities. A multifaceted approach must be used that targets a broader spectrum of risk factors. Environmental interventions should not be limited to home allergens or indoor pollution but must be expanded to include housing quality and even outdoor sources of pollution, such as highways or dump sites in the neighborhood. Although guidelines-based management and new therapies targeting phenotype-specific pathways need to be implemented, it may not be sufficient for the inner city child and adolescent with asthma to receive the right drugs. The structure of the medical care system must change to allow the needed access to the required follow-ups and medications, education about asthma self-management, and appropriate environmental intervention. Physicians taking care of these patients need to consider the environmental and social factors which impact on asthma management. In addition, other factors such as instability of housing, access to transportation, or family function should be addressed to ensure that pediatric patients and their families are not otherwise overburdened to manage asthma. Only with expanded creative solutions can the disparities found in the inner city be decreased.

REFERENCES

1. Moorman JE, Akinbami LJ, Bailey CM, et al. National surveillance of asthma: United States, 2001-2010. Vital Health Stat 3 2012;1–67.
2. Akinbami LJ, Moorman JE, Garbe PL, et al. Status of childhood asthma in the United States, 1980-2007. Pediatrics 2009;123(Suppl 3):S131–45.
3. Carter-Pokras OD, Gergen PJ. Reported asthma among Puerto Rican, Mexican-American, and Cuban children, 1982 through 1984. Am J Public Health 1993;83: 580–2.
4. Akinbami LJ, Rhodes JC, Lara M. Racial and ethnic differences in asthma diagnosis among children who wheeze. Pediatrics 2005;115:1254–60.
5. Gupta RS, Zhang X, Sharp LK, et al. Geographic variability in childhood asthma prevalence in Chicago. J Allergy Clin Immunol 2008;121:639–45.e1.
6. Ledogar RJ, Penchaszadeh A, Garden CC, et al. Asthma and Latino cultures: different prevalence reported among groups sharing the same environment. Am J Public Health 2000;90:929–35.
7. Cohen RT, Canino GJ, Bird HR, et al. Area of residence, birthplace, and asthma in Puerto Rican children. Chest 2007;131:1331–8.
8. Esteban CA, Klein RB, McQuaid EL, et al. Conundrums in childhood asthma severity, control, and health care use: Puerto Rico versus Rhode Island. J Allergy Clin Immunol 2009;124:238–44, 244.e1–5.
9. Fritz GK, McQuaid EL, Kopel SJ, et al. Ethnic differences in perception of lung function: a factor in pediatric asthma disparities? Am J Respir Crit Care Med 2010;182:12–8.
10. Akinbami LJ, Moorman JE, Simon AE, et al. Trends in racial disparities for asthma outcomes among children 0 to 17 years, 2001-201. J Allergy Clin Immunol 2014; 134:547–53.
11. Szefler SJ, Mitchell H, Sorkness CA, et al. Management of asthma based on exhaled nitric oxide in addition to guideline-based treatment for inner-city adolescents and young adults: a randomised controlled trial. Lancet 2008;372:1065–72.

12. Kwong KY, Morphew T, Scott L, et al. Asthma control and future asthma-related morbidity in inner-city asthmatic children. Ann Allergy Asthma Immunol 2008; 101:144–52.
13. Boudreaux ED, Emond SD, Clark S, et al. Race/ethnicity and asthma among children presenting to the emergency department: differences in disease severity and management. Pediatrics 2003;111:e615–21.
14. Okelo SO, Wu AW, Merriman B, et al. Are physician estimates of asthma severity less accurate in black than in white patients? J Gen Intern Med 2007;22:976–81.
15. Information on poverty and income statistics: a summary of 2013 current population survey data. ASPE Issue Brief: Department of Health and Human Services, Office of the Assistant Secretary for Planning and Evaluation; 2013. Available at: aspe.hhs.gov/hsp/13/PovertyandIncomeEst/ib_poverty2013.pdf. Accessed January 29, 2014.
16. Smith LA, Hatcher-Ross JL, Wertheimer R, et al. Rethinking race/ethnicity, income, and childhood asthma: racial/ethnic disparities concentrated among the very poor. Public Health Rep 2005;120:109–16.
17. Thakur N, Oh SS, Nguyen EA, et al. Socioeconomic status and childhood asthma in urban minority youths. The GALA II and SAGE II studies. Am J Respir Crit Care Med 2013;188:1202–9.
18. Williams DR, Sternthal M, Wright RJ. Social determinants: taking the social context of asthma seriously. Pediatrics 2009;123(Suppl 3):S174–84.
19. Williams DR, Collins C. Racial residential segregation: a fundamental cause of racial disparities in health. Public Health Rep 2001;116(5):404–16.
20. Sternthal MJ, Jun HJ, Earls F, et al. Community violence and urban childhood asthma: a multilevel analysis. Eur Respir J 2010;36(6):1400–9.
21. Williams LK, Joseph CL, Peterson EL, et al. Race-ethnicity, crime, and other factors associated with adherence to inhaled corticosteroids. J Allergy Clin Immunol 2007;119:168–75.
22. Wright RJ, Mitchell H, Visness CM, et al. Community violence and asthma morbidity: the Inner-City Asthma Study. Am J Public Health 2004;94:625–32.
23. Beck AF, Huang B, Simmons JM, et al. Role of financial and social hardships in asthma racial disparities. Pediatrics 2014;133:1–9.
24. Beck AF, Moncrief T, Huang B, et al. Inequalities in neighborhood child asthma admission rates and underlying community characteristics in one US county. J Pediatr 2013;163:574–80.
25. Guilbert TW, Garris C, Jhingran P, et al. Asthma that is not well-controlled is associated with increased healthcare utilization and decreased quality of life. J Asthma 2011;48:126–32.
26. Auger KA, Kahn RS, Davis MM, et al. Medical home quality and readmission risk for children hospitalized with asthma exacerbations. Pediatrics 2013;131:64–70.
27. Crocker D, Brown C, Moolenaar R, et al. Racial and ethnic disparities in asthma medication usage and health-care utilization: data from the National Asthma Survey. Chest 2009;136:1063–71.
28. Finkelstein JA, Brown RW, Schneider LC, et al. Quality of care for preschool children with asthma: the role of social factors and practice setting. Pediatrics 1995; 95:389–94.
29. Ortega AN, Gergen PJ, Paltiel AD, et al. Impact of site of care, race, and Hispanic ethnicity on medication use for childhood asthma. Pediatrics 2002;109:E1.
30. Stewart KA, Higgins PC, McLaughlin CG, et al. Differences in prevalence, treatment, and outcomes of asthma among a diverse population of children with equal

access to care: findings from a study in the military health system. Arch Pediatr Adolesc Med 2010;164:720–6.

31. Williams LK, Peterson EL, Wells K, et al. Quantifying the proportion of severe asthma exacerbations attributable to inhaled corticosteroid nonadherence. J Allergy Clin Immunol 2011;128:1185–91.

32. McQuaid EL, Everhart RS, Seifer R, et al. Medication adherence among Latino and non-Latino white children with asthma. Pediatrics 2012;129:e1404–10.

33. Smith LA, Bokhour B, Hohman KH, et al. Modifiable risk factors for suboptimal control and controller medication underuse among children with asthma. Pediatrics 2008;122:760–9.

34. Bloomberg GR, Banister C, Sterkel R, et al. Socioeconomic, family, and pediatric practice factors that affect level of asthma control. Pediatrics 2009;123: 829–35.

35. Sunshine J, Song L, Krieger J. Written action plan use in inner-city children: is it independently associated with improved asthma outcomes? Ann Allergy Asthma Immunol 2011;107:207–13.

36. Yin HS, Gupta RS, Tomopoulos S, et al. Readability, suitability, and characteristics of asthma action plans: examination of factors that may impair understanding. Pediatrics 2013;131:e116–26.

37. Gruchalla RS, Pongracic J, Plaut M, et al. Inner City Asthma Study: relationships among sensitivity, allergen exposure, and asthma morbidity. J Allergy Clin Immunol 2005;115:478–85.

38. Eggleston PA, Rosenstreich D, Lynn H, et al. Relationship of indoor allergen exposure to skin test sensitivity in inner-city children with asthma. J Allergy Clin Immunol 1998;102:563–70.

39. Rosenstreich DL, Eggleston P, Kattan M, et al. The role of cockroach allergy and exposure to cockroach allergen in causing morbidity among inner-city children with asthma. N Engl J Med 1997;336:1356–63.

40. Phipatanakul W, Eggleston PA, Wright EC, et al. Mouse allergen. II. The relationship of mouse allergen exposure to mouse sensitization and asthma morbidity in inner-city children with asthma. J Allergy Clin Immunol 2000;106:1075–80.

41. Perry T, Matsui E, Merriman B, et al. The prevalence of rat allergen in inner-city homes and its relationship to sensitization and asthma morbidity. J Allergy Clin Immunol 2003;112:346–52.

42. Arbes SJ Jr, Cohn RD, Yin M, et al. House dust mite allergen in US beds: results from the First National Survey of Lead and Allergens in Housing. J Allergy Clin Immunol 2003;111:408–14.

43. Cohn RD, Arbes SJ Jr, Jaramillo R, et al. National prevalence and exposure risk for cockroach allergen in US households. Environ Health Perspect 2006;114:522–6.

44. Wilson J, Dixon SL, Breysse P, et al. Housing and allergens: a pooled analysis of nine US studies. Environ Res 2010;110:189–98.

45. Arbes SJ Jr, Cohn RD, Yin M, et al. Dog allergen (Can f 1) and cat allergen (Fel d 1) in US homes: results from the National Survey of Lead and Allergens in Housing. J Allergy Clin Immunol 2004;114:111–7.

46. Baxi SN, Muilenberg ML, Rogers CA, et al. Exposures to molds in school classrooms of children with asthma. Pediatr Allergy Immunol 2013;24:697–703.

47. Salo PM, Sever ML, Zeldin DC. Indoor allergens in school and day care environments. J Allergy Clin Immunol 2009;124:185–92.

48. Arbes SJ Jr, Gergen PJ, Elliott L, et al. Prevalences of positive skin test responses to 10 common allergens in the US population: results from the third National Health and Nutrition Examination Survey. J Allergy Clin Immunol 2005;116:377–83.

49. Stevenson LA, Gergen PJ, Hoover DR, et al. Sociodemographic correlates of indoor allergen sensitivity among United States children. J Allergy Clin Immunol 2001;108:747–52.
50. Northridge J, Ramirez OF, Stingone JA, et al. The role of housing type and housing quality in urban children with asthma. J Urban Health 2010;87:211–24.
51. Rosenfeld L, Rudd R, Chew GL, et al. Are neighborhood-level characteristics associated with indoor allergens in the household? J Asthma 2010;47:66–75.
52. Olmedo O, Goldstein IF, Acosta L, et al. Neighborhood differences in exposure and sensitization to cockroach, mouse, dust mite, cat, and dog allergens in New York City. J Allergy Clin Immunol 2011;128:284–92.
53. Diette GB, Hansel NN, Buckley TJ, et al. Home indoor pollutant exposures among inner-city children with and without asthma. Environ Health Perspect 2007;115: 1665–9.
54. Vesper S, Barnes C, Ciaccio CE, et al. Higher environmental relative moldiness index (ERMI) values measured in homes of asthmatic children in Boston, Kansas City, and San Diego. J Asthma 2013;50:155–61.
55. Akinbami LJ, Kit BK, Simon AE. Impact of environmental tobacco smoke on children with asthma, United States, 2003-2010. Acad Pediatr 2013;13:508–16.
56. Chilmonczyk BA, Salmun LM, Megathlin KN, et al. Association between exposure to environmental tobacco smoke and exacerbations of asthma in children. N Engl J Med 1993;328:1665–9.
57. National Center for Health Statistics. Health, United States, 2012: with special feature on emergency care. Hyattsville (MD): 2013.
58. Kit BK, Simon AE, Brody DJ, et al. US prevalence and trends in tobacco smoke exposure among children and adolescents with asthma. Pediatrics 2013;131:407–14.
59. Butz AM, Halterman JS, Bellin M, et al. Factors associated with second-hand smoke exposure in young inner-city children with asthma. J Asthma 2011;48: 449–57.
60. Belanger K, Gent JF, Triche EW, et al. Association of indoor nitrogen dioxide exposure with respiratory symptoms in children with asthma. Am J Respir Crit Care Med 2006;173:297–303.
61. Kattan M, Gergen PJ, Eggleston P, et al. Health effects of indoor nitrogen dioxide and passive smoking on urban asthmatic children. J Allergy Clin Immunol 2007; 120:618–24.
62. Akinbami LJ, Lynch CD, Parker JD, et al. The association between childhood asthma prevalence and monitored air pollutants in metropolitan areas, United States, 2001-2004. Environ Res 2010;110:294–301.
63. Gasana J, Dillikar D, Mendy A, et al. Motor vehicle air pollution and asthma in children: a meta-analysis. Environ Res 2012;117:36–45.
64. Nishimura KK, Galanter JM, Roth LA, et al. Early-life air pollution and asthma risk in minority children. The GALA II and SAGE II studies. Am J Respir Crit Care Med 2013;188:309–18.
65. Li S, Batterman S, Wasilevich E, et al. Asthma exacerbation and proximity of residence to major roads: a population-based matched case-control study among the pediatric Medicaid population in Detroit, Michigan. Environ Health 2011;10:34.
66. Patel MM, Quinn JW, Jung KH, et al. Traffic density and stationary sources of air pollution associated with wheeze, asthma, and immunoglobulin E from birth to age 5 years among New York City children. Environ Res 2011;111:1222–9.
67. Juhn YJ, Qin R, Urm S, et al. The influence of neighborhood environment on the incidence of childhood asthma: a propensity score approach. J Allergy Clin Immunol 2010;125:838–43.

68. Perzanowski MS, Chew GL, Divjan A, et al. Early-life cockroach allergen and polycyclic aromatic hydrocarbon exposures predict cockroach sensitization among inner-city children. J Allergy Clin Immunol 2013;131:886–93.
69. Ruffin J. A renewed commitment to environmental justice in health disparities research. Am J Public Health 2011;101(Suppl 1):S12–4.
70. Cureton S. Environmental victims: environmental injustice issues that threaten the health of children living in poverty. Rev Environ Health 2011;26:141–7.
71. Boehmer TK, Foster SL, Henry JR, et al. Residential proximity to major highways–United States, 2010. MMWR Surveill Summ 2013;62(Suppl 3):46–50.
72. Iqbal S, Oraka E, Chew GL, et al. Association between birthplace and current asthma: the role of environment and acculturation. Am J Public Health 2014;104(Suppl 1):S175–82.
73. Belamarich PF, Luder E, Kattan M, et al. Do obese inner-city children with asthma have more symptoms than nonobese children with asthma? Pediatrics 2000;106:1436–41.
74. Kattan M, Kumar R, Bloomberg GR, et al. Asthma control, adiposity, and adipokines among inner-city adolescents. J Allergy Clin Immunol 2010;125:584–92.
75. Jensen ME, Gibson PG, Collins CE, et al. Diet-induced weight loss in obese children with asthma: a randomized controlled trial. Clin Exp Allergy 2013;43:775–84.
76. Gessner BD, Chimonas MA. Asthma is associated with preterm birth but not with small for gestational age status among a population-based cohort of Medicaid-enrolled children <10 years of age. Thorax 2007;62:231–6.
77. Svanes C, Omenaas E, Heuch JM, et al. Birth characteristics and asthma symptoms in young adults: results from a population-based cohort study in Norway. Eur Respir J 1998;12:1366–70.
78. Joseph CL, Ownby DR, Peterson EL, et al. Does low birth weight help to explain the increased prevalence of asthma among African-Americans? Ann Allergy Asthma Immunol 2002;88:507–12.
79. Crump C, Winkleby MA, Sundquist J, et al. Risk of asthma in young adults who were born preterm: a Swedish National Cohort Study. Pediatrics 2011;127:e913–20.
80. Martin JA, Hamilton BE, Osterman MJ, et al. Births: final data for 2012. Natl Vital Stat Rep 2013;62(9):1–87.
81. Weil CM, Wade SL, Bauman LJ, et al. The relationship between psychosocial factors and asthma morbidity in inner-city children with asthma. Pediatrics 1999;104:1274–80.
82. Bartlett SJ, Kolodner K, Butz AM, et al. Maternal depressive symptoms and emergency department use among inner-city children with asthma. Arch Pediatr Adolesc Med 2001;155:347–53.
83. Wood RA, Bloomberg GR, Kattan M, et al. Relationships among environmental exposures, cord blood cytokine responses, allergy, and wheeze at 1 year of age in an inner-city birth cohort (Urban Environment and Childhood Asthma study). J Allergy Clin Immunol 2011;127:913–9.
84. Evans R 3rd, Gergen PJ, Mitchell H, et al. A randomized clinical trial to reduce asthma morbidity among inner-city children: results of the National Cooperative Inner-City Asthma Study. J Pediatr 1999;135:332–8.
85. Bruzzese JM, Sheares BJ, Vincent EJ, et al. Effects of a school-based intervention for urban adolescents with asthma. A controlled trial. Am J Respir Crit Care Med 2011;183:998–1006.
86. Halterman JS, Szilagyi PG, Fisher SG, et al. Randomized controlled trial to improve care for urban children with asthma: results of the School-Based Asthma Therapy trial. Arch Pediatr Adolesc Med 2011;165:262–8.

87. Flores G, Bridon C, Torres S, et al. Improving asthma outcomes in minority children: a randomized, controlled trial of parent mentors. Pediatrics 2009;124:1522–32.
88. Gergen PJ, Mortimer KM, Eggleston PA, et al. Results of the National Cooperative Inner-City Asthma Study (NCICAS) environmental intervention to reduce cockroach allergen exposure in inner-city homes. J Allergy Clin Immunol 1999;103: 501–6.
89. Morgan WJ, Crain EF, Gruchalla RS, et al. Results of a home-based environmental intervention among urban children with asthma. N Engl J Med 2004; 351:1068–80.
90. Breysse J, Dixon S, Gregory J, et al. Effect of weatherization combined with community health worker in-home education on asthma control. Am J Public Health 2014;104:e57–64.
91. Takaro TK, Krieger J, Song L, et al. The breathe-easy home: the impact of asthma-friendly home construction on clinical outcomes and trigger exposure. Am J Public Health 2011;101:55–62.
92. Butz AM, Tsoukleris MG, Donithan M, et al. Effectiveness of nebulizer use-targeted asthma education on underserved children with asthma. Arch Pediatr Adolesc Med 2006;160:622–8.
93. Lanphear BP, Hornung RW, Khoury J, et al. Effects of HEPA air cleaners on unscheduled asthma visits and asthma symptoms for children exposed to secondhand tobacco smoke. Pediatrics 2011;127:93–101.
94. Joseph CL, Havstad SL, Johnson D, et al. Factors associated with nonresponse to a computer-tailored asthma management program for urban adolescents with asthma. J Asthma 2010;47:667–73.
95. Busse WW, Morgan WJ, Gergen PJ, et al. Randomized trial of omalizumab (anti-IgE) for asthma in inner-city children. N Engl J Med 2011;364:1005–15.

Asthma
The Interplay Between Viral Infections and Allergic Diseases

Regina K. Rowe, MD, PhD[a], Michelle A. Gill, MD, PhD[b,c],*

KEYWORDS

- Asthma • Viral infection • Rhinovirus • Atopy • Allergy • Immunoglobulin E
- Type I interferon • Dendritic cells

KEY POINTS

- Respiratory viruses, especially rhinoviruses, are associated with both the development and exacerbation of asthma.
- Allergic sensitization increases the risk of virus-induced asthma exacerbation.
- Immunoglobulin E–mediated pathways block critical type I interferon responses after viral infection, representing one mechanism whereby viruses and allergens cooperatively induce asthmatic disease.
- Cytokine and chemokine responses between the epithelium, innate immune cells, and adaptive immune responses are regulated by both allergens and virus infection, and contribute to the synergistic effects of these factors on asthma pathogenesis.
- Therapeutic strategies targeting both viral and allergic inflammation may provide clinical benefit in asthma.

INTRODUCTION

The interaction between viral respiratory infections and allergic diseases, especially asthma, has long been appreciated. Much has been learned through both clinical and basic science studies on the synergy between these pathologic processes. This review discusses the clinical and molecular findings relevant to this intersection of viral

Disclosure Statement: The authors have no financial conflicts of interest to disclose.
[a] Pediatric Infectious Diseases Fellowship Program, Department of Pediatrics, UT Southwestern Medical Center, 5323 Harry Hines Boulevard, Dallas, TX 75390-9063, USA; [b] Department of Pediatrics, Division of Infectious Diseases and Division of Pulmonary Vascular Biology, UT Southwestern Medical Center, 5323 Harry Hines Boulevard, Dallas, TX 75390-9063, USA; [c] Department of Immunology, UT Southwestern Medical Center, 5323 Harry Hines Boulevard, Dallas, TX 75390-9063, USA
* Corresponding author. Department of Pediatrics and Immunology, Divisions of Infectious Diseases and Pulmonary Vascular Biology, UT Southwestern Medical Center, 5323 Harry Hines Boulevard, Dallas, TX 75390-9063.
E-mail address: michelle.gill@utsouthwestern.edu

Immunol Allergy Clin N Am 35 (2015) 115–127
http://dx.doi.org/10.1016/j.iac.2014.09.012
0889-8561/15/$ – see front matter © 2015 Elsevier Inc. All rights reserved.

and allergic diseases. The article focuses on recent studies investigating how these 2 disparate disease processes cooperatively affect asthma pathogenesis.

VIRAL INFECTIONS AND ASTHMA: CLINICAL ASSOCIATIONS
Viruses, Genetics, and Asthma Development

Multiple studies demonstrate strong correlations between early viral respiratory illness in childhood and the development of asthma.[1–3] Results of prospective birth cohort studies[4–7] have established correlations between the age at initial wheezing onset, severity of respiratory viral infection, and persistence of wheezing episodes with an increased risk of asthma at school age. Genetic predisposition (ie, family history of atopic disease) and concurrent atopy represented additional critical contributors to asthma pathogenesis,[4,8,9] suggesting a synergistic relationship between viral infections and allergic diseases.

The Childhood Origins of ASThma study (COAST) specifically targeted a high-risk cohort of children based on a parental history of atopy.[5] Whereas early respiratory syncytial virus (RSV) infection increased asthma risk at age 6 years by 3-fold, early-life human rhinovirus (RV) infection increased the risk by almost 10-fold in COAST participants,[10] suggesting a stronger link between early rhinovirus infection and asthma development in children genetically at risk.

Details regarding such genetic factors are beginning to emerge. Recent genomic analyses targeted the 17q21 chromosomal locus. A meta-analysis from 2 cohorts, the COAST and Copenhagen Studies on Asthma in Childhood (COPSAC), indicated a link between certain 17q21 genotypes and RV-related wheezing and asthma development.[11] Two genetic loci in this region, the ORMDL3 and GSDMB genes, were significantly upregulated in peripheral blood mononuclear cells (PBMCs) after in vitro RV exposure. Furthermore, COAST cohort participants homozygous for a specific single-nucleotide polymorphism (SNP) in the GSDMB gene had a 26-fold increased risk of developing asthma when combined with a history of prior rhinovirus infection. More studies are needed to define the exact functions of these genes and the specific host-virus interactions relevant to individuals with asthma.

Similarly, a second study linked SNPs in innate immunity genes to the development of asthma and atopy. Specifically, SNPs in the interleukin (IL)-1 receptor 2 and toll-like receptor (TLR)-1 genes linked picornavirus and RSV infections with airway hyperreactivity.[12] Although others have reported SNP associations with asthma and atopy,[13–15] these studies connect specific genotypes to asthma and virus-induced wheezing episodes, suggesting genetic interactions between viruses and atopy. However, not every child with risk factors develops asthma. Instead, a complex interplay of multiple risk factors, including genetic phenotypes prone to allergen sensitization, respiratory virus susceptibility, and atopic disease, all intersect, increasing an individual's risk for asthma development.

As described by the "2-hit hypothesis" of asthma development, genetic predisposition to atopy (the first hit) combined with a second environmental insult, specifically early respiratory viral infection (the second hit), may lead to asthma.[16] This hypothesis highlights the collaborative roles of genetics, viruses, and allergens in promoting asthma.

Viruses: Role in Asthma Exacerbations

In addition to their role in asthma development, respiratory viruses also contribute to ongoing disease as major causes of asthma exacerbations. The seasonality of RV-associated asthma exacerbations has been well described,[17] and multiple studies have shown a close temporal relationship between respiratory viral infection and disease exacerbation.[18–21] Rhinoviruses are most commonly isolated during asthma exacerbations, but other viruses, including human metapneumovirus[22] and influenza,[18,21] represent important contributors. During the 2009 influenza pandemic, an increase in disease severity and exacerbations was noted in pediatric asthmatic patients, with a disproportionate number requiring intensive care.[23]

Many studies point to diminished antiviral responses (**Box 1**) as one potential mechanism underlying viral-induced asthma exacerbations. For example, interferon (IFN)-γ production by viral or mitogen-stimulated cord blood monocytes inversely correlated with the number of wheezing episodes and respiratory viral infections during infancy.[24,25] Thus, one proposed mechanism of viral-induced wheezing and asthma development is increased susceptibility to respiratory viral infections secondary to diminished antiviral response. In addition, airway epithelial cells and immune cells recovered from asthmatic patients had diminished type I, II, and III IFN responses after rhinovirus exposure,[26–28] resulting in decreased release of IFN-dependent cytokines such as IL-15.[29] Deficient IFN-α secretion on in vitro exposure to viruses including influenza and RV has also been demonstrated in PBMCs and purified plasmacytoid dendritic cells (pDCs).[30,31] Furthermore, in vivo experimental RV inoculation of volunteers revealed more severe symptoms in asthmatics than in controls.[32] However, the inefficient innate immune response does not result in enhanced viral replication,[33] suggesting that a combination of factors including concomitant allergen exposure contributes to worsened viral disease. The remainder of this review focuses on clinical associations and potential mechanisms involved in the interplay between allergens and viral infection in asthma.

VIRUSES AND ALLERGENS: EVIDENCE OF SYNERGISM IN ASTHMA

Viral infections and allergic sensitization/allergen exposure together have been shown to synergistically increase the risk and severity of asthma exacerbations. The

---

Box 1
Virus-allergen synergism: potential mechanisms in asthma

- Genetic factors
- Deficient antiviral responses
- Immunoglobulin E–mediated effects
  - Inhibition of type I interferon responses
  - Impairment of monocyte function
  - Dendritic cell–driven induction of T-helper 2 (Th2) responses
- Other dendritic cell–mediated effects
- Enhanced Th2 responses
- Respiratory epithelial damage
- Respiratory epithelial mediators
  - Thymic stromal lymphopoietin
  - Interleukin-33
  - Interleukin-25
- Altered purinergic receptor activation
- Deficient interleukin-15 responses
- Altered T-regulatory and innate lymphocyte cell responses

mechanisms underlying this interplay between virus and atopy represent an area of intense investigation. Several recently published reviews detail these associations,[34–37] and a summary and relevant updates are discussed herein.

Clinical Associations

As previously mentioned, early-life respiratory viral infections, most notably rhinovirus and RSV, have been associated with subsequent development of allergic sensitization and asthma in children.[1,10,38] The synergism between atopy and rhinovirus infections persists throughout childhood; exacerbation rates are increased by the presence of allergic sensitization and exposure to aeroallergens including cockroach, dust mite, and cat allergens.[8,39,40] In a prospective study to determine relationships between rhinovirus infection and illness severity, Olenec and colleagues[41] collected weekly nasal lavage samples from asthmatic children during fall and spring months that corresponded with peak rhinovirus infection rates. Although the number of viral infections was not increased in the atopic group, the allergen-sensitized group experienced a 47% increase in viral respiratory tract illness and severity, including both cold and asthma symptoms, compared with the nonsensitized group. Other studies of asthma severity also highlight this virus-atopy collaboration in disease pathogenesis. The combination of virus detection, allergic sensitization, and allergen exposure were shown to significantly increase the risk of hospitalization in studies of both children and adults with asthma exacerbations.[42,43]

Viral-Atopy Associations in Experimental Rhinovirus Infections

Experimental rhinovirus infection directly affects components of the allergic response itself, resulting in increased histamine release and recruitment of eosinophils to the airway in adult allergic subjects,[44] suggesting that rhinovirus infection may induce an allergic state. Counter to this conclusion, however, are findings in prospective studies of children in the high-risk COAST birth cohort, which demonstrate that allergic sensitization actually precedes RV-induced wheezing.[8] Similarly, Zambrano and colleagues[45] demonstrated that the ability of experimental RV infection to induce asthma exacerbations correlated with sensitization to relevant aeroallergens; increased serum immunoglobulin E (IgE) concentrations were also associated with reduced lung function in response to RV infection. In another study, only the asthmatic subjects displayed increased eosinophilic airway inflammation, lower respiratory symptoms, lung function impairment, and enhanced T-helper 2 (Th2) cytokine release on RV infection; healthy control subjects did not exhibit these responses.[46] These studies confirm that atopy significantly affects the immune response to rhinovirus infection in individuals with allergic asthma, and suggest that allergic sensitization and exposure contribute to increased severity of lower respiratory tract infections and asthma exacerbations associated with RV infections.

MECHANISMS UNDERLYING VIRUS-ALLERGEN SYNERGISM IN ASTHMA

Multiple potential mechanisms underlying the interplay between viral infections and allergic sensitization in asthma have been postulated (see **Box 1**), as published in recent reviews.[34,47]

The Type I Interferon–Immunoglobulin E Axis: Evidence That Atopy Impairs Antiviral Responses

Type I IFN (IFN-α/β), a family of antiviral cytokines, is secreted in highest concentrations by pDCs, key antigen-presenting cells recruited to the airway during viral infections.[48] IFN-α/β is especially relevant to allergic disease in its ability to negatively regulate Th2 and Th17 lymphocyte responses.[49,50] IFN-α/β blocks Th2 effector cell secretion of IL-4, IL-5, and IL-13, and inhibits Th2 development in human CD4 T cells by suppressing GATA3, a major Th2 transcription factor.[49]

Counterregulation between antiviral responses and IgE-mediated pathways in pDCs represents a newly recognized mechanism by which allergens and viruses may cooperatively promote asthma exacerbations. Serum IgE and expression of its high-affinity receptor, FcϵRIα, are inversely correlated with IFN-α secretion from purified pDCs and PBMCs stimulated with viruses including influenza and rhinovirus in vitro.[30,31] In addition, IgE cross-linking significantly impairs viral and TLR-9 agonist-induced pDC IFN-α secretion, suggesting that allergen exposure in sensitized individuals may inhibit antiviral responses via in vivo cross-linking of allergen-specific IgE.[31,51] Exposure of pDCs from dust-mite allergic individuals to dust mite allergen (Der p 1) in vitro also significantly impaired pDC IFN-α responses to influenza.[31] Treatment of cat-allergic subjects with omalizumab, an anti-IgE monoclonal antibody that decreases both serum IgE and FcϵRI expression on innate immune cells, diminished the capacity of allergen-exposed DCs to drive Th2 inflammatory responses.[52]

Results of the recent National Institutes of Allergy and Infectious Diseases–sponsored Inner City Anti-IgE Therapy of Asthma trial provide further evidence of the relevance of this pathway; the group of children who received omalizumab experienced a near-complete elimination in the fall increase in asthma exacerbations, a seasonal increase known to be associated with the fall peak in rhinovirus infections.[53] Taken together, these studies suggest that pathways involving IgE, FcϵRI, allergens, and viral-induced IFN-α may play critical roles in the allergen-viral interplay in asthma pathogenesis. The role of dendritic cells and monocytes in this and other potential mechanisms underlying allergen and viral-associated exacerbation of asthma is illustrated in **Fig. 1** and has been reviewed elsewhere.[54]

IgE-mediated effects on monocytes and antigen-presenting cells present in high numbers within lung tissues may also contribute to inflammatory responses relevant to respiratory viral infections associated with allergic disease. Pyle and colleagues[55] demonstrated that monocytes exposed to IgE cross-linking conditions secreted high concentrations of the inflammatory cytokines tumor necrosis factor (TNF)-α and IL-6; this effect was greatest in individuals with elevated serum IgE. Furthermore, monocyte function was critically impaired by this allergic activation, resulting in significant disruption of phagocytosis. Phagocytosis of apoptotic epithelium represents a major component in the resolution of inflammatory responses; crippling of this monocyte function could thus prolong inflammatory responses (see **Fig. 1**). In the setting of aeroallergen sensitization/exposure, coupled with viral-induced apoptosis of respiratory epithelium, cross-linking of allergen-specific IgE on monocytes represents another potential mechanism whereby allergens and viruses may synergistically promote exacerbations of allergic disease.

Enhanced T-Helper 2 Responses

Deficient type I interferon antiviral responses, as demonstrated in epithelial cells,[28] whole blood cultures,[56,57] PBMCs,[30] and purified pDCs[31] isolated from patients with asthma, may indirectly promote the enhancement of Th2 environment through loss of this negative regulatory effect of IFN. Deficient IFN-α/β responses in the context of viral infections could thus promote increased Th2 CD4 inflammatory responses.

Using genomic profiling of PBMC subpopulations isolated from asthmatic patients, Subrata and colleagues[58] demonstrated increased FcϵRI expression and Th2-promoting functions in monocytes and DCs during viral exacerbations of asthma. Of

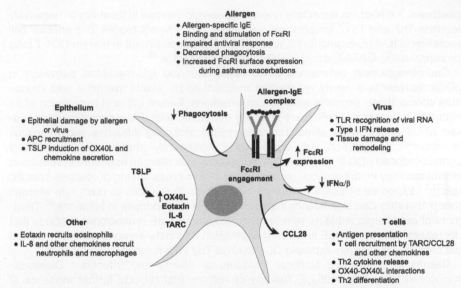

Fig. 1. Antigen-presenting cells (APCs) are key mediators of viral-allergen effects in asthma pathogenesis. Epithelial damage by virus or allergen results in APC recruitment to the lung (myeloid dendritic cells [mDCs], plasmacytoid dendritic cells [pDCs], and monocytes). Virus effects specifically result in type I interferon (IFN) release from APCs, and tissue damage and remodeling of the epithelium. Epithelial thymic stromal lymphopoietin (TSLP) release mediates upregulation of OX40L on DCs and release of multiple chemokines (eotaxin, interleukin [IL]-8, and thymus and activation-regulated chemokine [TARC]). FcεRI engagement by immunoglobulin E (IgE)-allergen complex has multiple downstream effects including inhibition of toll-like receptor (TLR)-mediated antiviral responses (type I IFN secretion from pDCs) and phagocytosis (by monocytes). Chemokines induced by either TSLP- or FcεR-mediated pathways recruit other critical immune cells including eosinophils, macrophages, and T cells. APCs present antigen to T cells either in the tissue or draining lymph node, and drive T-helper 2 (Th2) cell differentiation through OX40L-OX40 interactions.

note, more than 95% of the patients who experienced a severe viral-associated asthma exacerbation were also atopic, adding to the body of evidence linking these 2 factors in asthma.

Viral proteases can also contribute to Th2 inflammatory responses relevant to asthma. Intranasal administration of recombinant RV 2A, a protease of RV, enhanced ovalbumin-induced Th2 inflammation in a murine model.[59] Such enhancement of Th2 responses may further contribute to asthma pathogenesis, promoting the production of IgE, eosinophilic inflammation, and goblet-cell hyperplasia.

Mechanisms Involving the Respiratory Epithelium

Epithelial integrity

Both the integrity of the respiratory epithelium[60] and the mediators released during allergen and viral stimulation may contribute to enhanced disease driven by the synergy of these factors in allergic asthma. Increased airway epithelial damage has been reported in children with allergic sensitization and asthma, and correlated with diminished immune responses to RV infection.[61] This underlying compromise of the epithelial barrier, the site where the host first encounters allergens and viruses, may promote a more rapid loss of epithelial integrity during immune responses to viral infection.

Epithelial mediators: thymic stromal lymphopoietin, interleukin-33, interleukin-25
Mediators secreted by the respiratory epithelium on virus and allergen exposure may also contribute to the pathogenesis of synergistic disease. Thymic stromal lympho-poietin (TLSP), an epithelial-derived cytokine induced by both allergen and viral expo-sure,[62,63] activates dendritic cells to promote Th2 inflammatory responses. Elevated levels of TLSP have been reported in the airway epithelium of atopic asthmatics.[64,65] The amplification of TLR-3–induced TLSP secretion by IL-4 provides evidence that viral infection coupled with the recruitment of Th2 cytokine-producing cells to the airway may further enhance allergic inflammation in the airways of atopic asthmatics.[62]

IL-33, another cytokine that enhances Th2 inflammation, is also increased in lung epithelium from asthmatics.[66] Both allergens[67] and viruses[68] promote increased expression of IL-33. IL-25 also promotes Th2 cytokine release from immune cells and has been detected in lung tissue from asthmatics.[69] The findings that IL-25 is enhanced by viral infection and that Th2 inflammatory responses are reduced by IL-25 blockade and IL-25 receptor knockout (IL-17RB−/−) in a murine model of RSV-induced asthma suggests a potential role for IL-25 in viral allergen-induced asthma exacerbations.[70]

Altered Purinergic Receptor Activation and Signaling

Purines including adenosine triphosphate (ATP) have been implicated in the patho-genesis of allergic inflammation associated with asthma. Both airway allergen chal-lenge and viral exposure result in increased extracellular ATP concentrations in lung tissues, which can lead to activation of purinergic signaling with resulting inflammatory responses.[71] Recently P2X7, a purinergic receptor expressed on epithelial cells and innate immune cells, has been shown to play a role in allergic sensitization and viral-induced asthma exacerbations in both children and adults,[72] suggesting yet another potential mechanism by which viruses and allergens contribute to asthma pathogenesis.

Other mechanisms involving dysregulation of regulatory T-cell and innate lymphoid cell responses,[34] altered IL-15 secretion,[29] and indoleamine 2,3-deoxygenase,[54] a tryptophan-regulating enzyme, are reviewed elsewhere.

Additional Mechanistic Insights from Animal Models

Animal models utilizing mouse pneumovirus I or Sendai virus (SeV) infection provide further insight. SeV infection of mice, which closely mimics the pathology of acute RSV in humans, culminates in chronic airway inflammation, including airway remodel-ing, increased mucous secretion, and airway reactivity.[73] This model, combined with murine allergen models, provides clues in the complex interaction between viruses and allergens. Infection of the respiratory epithelium leads to epithelial-specific cyto-kine and chemokine release.[74,75] This initial inflammatory response recruits IgE recep-tor (FcεRI)-expressing dendritic cells, eosinophils, and CD4 T cells to the lung,[76] resulting in IL-13 release and an "allergic" Th2-mediated response. Paralleling in vivo clinical observations, the antiviral response is critical in controlling viral-induced pathol-ogy, as the absence of TLR-7, a critical component of IFN-α/β signaling, results in dis-ease exacerbation.[75] Following viral infection, reexposure to allergen recapitulates components of human asthma pathology including airway remodeling, mucous cell hyperplasia, and airway reactivity,[77] demonstrating that viral infection can induce an allergic state. These findings, including the role of FcεR expression,[76,77] complement data from human studies, shedding light on potential mechanisms underlying the synergism between the allergic responses and viral infections in asthma (see **Fig. 1**).

FUTURE CONSIDERATIONS AND SUMMARY

The interplay between respiratory viruses and atopy contributes significantly to the development and exacerbation of asthma, thus suggesting that therapeutic strategies aimed at interrupting either the viral or allergic components of disease pathogenesis may provide clinical benefits.

Targeting Viral Infection

Preventing initial viral infection is one approach to halting disease development in high-risk children. For example, treatment of infants with palivizumab, an anti-RSV antibody, decreases infection severity[78] and wheezing episodes during infancy and early childhood.[79,80] Because repetitive, prolonged wheezing increases the risk of developing asthma, these findings suggest that palivizumab treatment in select, high-risk infants might prevent asthma development. Though effective in nonatopic children, palivizumab-mediated reduction in asthma was limited in atopic children.[81] At present there is no approved antiviral treatment of rhinovirus, which plays a more significant role in asthma development. By contrast, effective vaccine and antiviral therapies are available for influenza virus. Influenza vaccination is effective in reducing steroid use, clinic and hospital visits, and exacerbations associated with asthma.[82,83] Furthermore, administration of oseltamivir, an influenza neuraminidase inhibitor, to asthmatic children during acute influenza infection improved lung function over the duration of disease.[84] Despite recommendations from the Centers for Disease Control and Prevention for widespread influenza vaccination in this population, vaccination coverage remains low (~50%) in asthmatic individuals.[85] These studies highlight the importance of promoting both vaccination and continued development of new antiviral agents as strategies to improve asthma-associated morbidity.

Even simple nutritional changes may have effects on prevention of virus-induced disease. A meta-analysis indicates that vitamin D supplementation reduced the incidence of upper respiratory tract infections,[86] and a small trial suggests a positive effect on virus-induced asthma exacerbations in children.[87] Furthermore, targeting the mucosal immune system through the use of probiotics also demonstrated protection from upper respiratory infections.[88] Further analysis revealed a decrease in IgE levels and atopy in children treated with probiotics, but a limited effect on asthma and wheezing.[89]

Targeting Allergic Inflammation

Targeting allergic inflammation represents another therapeutic strategy for preventing virus-induced atopic disease. Although guidelines-based asthma therapy including inhaled corticosteroids and β-agonists do help control exacerbations during seasonal rhinovirus infections,[90] there is a limited effect on viral replication and cytokine release in vitro.[91] Additional therapies, such as targeting IgE with omalizumab, have already been shown to be effective.[53] Development of additional IgE/FcεRI signaling inhibitors that dampen IgE pathways and potentially restore viral-induced IFN-α/β responses may prove useful in preventing allergic airway inflammation associated with viral infections. Additional biologics targeting multiple pathways, including IL-5, IL-4, IL-13, TNF-α, TLR-7 and -9, and Th2 development are being evaluated in clinical trials.[92] Other pathways, such as IL-33, have also been proposed as potential therapeutic targets.[93]

In summary, asthma pathogenesis is complex and multifactorial, and affected by genetic and environmental factors. The interplay between respiratory viral infection and allergic responses dramatically affects disease outcome. While components of the mechanisms underlying these associations are known, many questions remain. Additional research is needed to translate new ideas into effective therapies.

REFERENCES

1. Jackson DJ. Early-life viral infections and the development of asthma: a target for asthma prevention? Curr Opin Allergy Clin Immunol 2014;14(2):131–6.
2. Gern JE. Rhinovirus and the initiation of asthma. Curr Opin Allergy Clin Immunol 2009;9(1):73–8.
3. Jackson DJ, Lemanske RF Jr. The role of respiratory virus infections in childhood asthma inception. Immunol Allergy Clin North Am 2010;30(4):513–22, vi.
4. Henderson J, Granell R, Heron J, et al. Associations of wheezing phenotypes in the first 6 years of life with atopy, lung function and airway responsiveness in mid-childhood. Thorax 2008;63(11):974–80.
5. Lemanske RF Jr. The childhood origins of asthma (COAST) study. Pediatr Allergy Immunol 2002;13(Suppl 15):38–43.
6. Martinez FD, Wright AL, Taussig LM, et al. Asthma and wheezing in the first six years of life. The Group Health Medical Associates. N Engl J Med 1995;332(3): 133–8.
7. Carroll KN, Wu P, Gebretsadik T, et al. The severity-dependent relationship of infant bronchiolitis on the risk and morbidity of early childhood asthma. J Allergy Clin Immunol 2009;123(5):1055–61, 1061.e1.
8. Jackson DJ, Evans MD, Gangnon RE, et al. Evidence for a causal relationship between allergic sensitization and rhinovirus wheezing in early life. Am J Respir Crit Care Med 2012;185(3):281–5.
9. Savenije OE, Granell R, Caudri D, et al. Comparison of childhood wheezing phenotypes in 2 birth cohorts: ALSPAC and PIAMA. J Allergy Clin Immunol 2011;127(6):1505–12.e14.
10. Jackson DJ, Gangnon RE, Evans MD, et al. Wheezing rhinovirus illnesses in early life predict asthma development in high-risk children. Am J Respir Crit Care Med 2008;178(7):667–72.
11. Caliskan M, Bochkov YA, Kreiner-Moller E, et al. Rhinovirus wheezing illness and genetic risk of childhood-onset asthma. N Engl J Med 2013;368(15):1398–407.
12. Daley D, Park JE, He JQ, et al. Associations and interactions of genetic polymorphisms in innate immunity genes with early viral infections and susceptibility to asthma and asthma-related phenotypes. J Allergy Clin Immunol 2012;130(6): 1284–93.
13. Bonnelykke K, Matheson MC, Pers TH, et al. Meta-analysis of genome-wide association studies identifies ten loci influencing allergic sensitization. Nat Genet 2013;45(8):902–6.
14. Savenije OE, Mahachie John JM, Granell R, et al. Association of IL33-IL-1 receptor-like 1 (IL1RL1) pathway polymorphisms with wheezing phenotypes and asthma in childhood. J Allergy Clin Immunol 2014;134:170–7.
15. Torgerson DG, Ampleford EJ, Chiu GY, et al. Meta-analysis of genome-wide association studies of asthma in ethnically diverse North American populations. Nat Genet 2011;43(9):887–92.
16. Gern JE. The ABCs of rhinoviruses, wheezing, and asthma. J Virol 2010;84(15): 7418–26.
17. Johnston NW, Johnston SL, Duncan JM, et al. The September epidemic of asthma exacerbations in children: a search for etiology. J Allergy Clin Immunol 2005;115(1):132–8.

18. Mandelcwajg A, Moulin F, Menager C, et al. Underestimation of influenza viral infection in childhood asthma exacerbations. J Pediatr 2010;157(3):505–6.
19. Atmar RL, Guy E, Guntupalli KK, et al. Respiratory tract viral infections in inner-city asthmatic adults. Arch Intern Med 1998;158(22):2453–9.
20. Beasley R, Coleman ED, Hermon Y, et al. Viral respiratory tract infection and exacerbations of asthma in adult patients. Thorax 1988;43(9):679–83.
21. Johnston SL, Pattemore PK, Sanderson G, et al. Community study of role of viral infections in exacerbations of asthma in 9-11 year old children. BMJ 1995; 310(6989):1225–9.
22. Edwards KM, Zhu Y, Griffin MR, et al. Burden of human metapneumovirus infection in young children. N Engl J Med 2013;368(7):633–43.
23. Dawood FS, Kamimoto L, D'Mello TA, et al. Children with asthma hospitalized with seasonal or pandemic influenza, 2003-2009. Pediatrics 2011;128(1):e27–32.
24. Copenhaver CC, Gern JE, Li Z, et al. Cytokine response patterns, exposure to viruses, and respiratory infections in the first year of life. Am J Respir Crit Care Med 2004;170(2):175–80.
25. Sumino K, Tucker J, Shahab M, et al. Antiviral IFN-gamma responses of monocytes at birth predict respiratory tract illness in the first year of life. J Allergy Clin Immunol 2012;129(5):1267–73.e1.
26. Contoli M, Message SD, Laza-Stanca V, et al. Role of deficient type III interferon-lambda production in asthma exacerbations. Nat Med 2006;12(9):1023–6.
27. Sykes A, Edwards MR, Macintyre J, et al. Rhinovirus 16-induced IFN-alpha and IFN-beta are deficient in bronchoalveolar lavage cells in asthmatic patients. J Allergy Clin Immunol 2012;129(6):1506–14.e6.
28. Wark PA, Johnston SL, Bucchieri F, et al. Asthmatic bronchial epithelial cells have a deficient innate immune response to infection with rhinovirus. J Exp Med 2005; 201(6):937–47.
29. Laza-Stanca V, Message SD, Edwards MR, et al. The role of IL-15 deficiency in the pathogenesis of virus-induced asthma exacerbations. PLoS Pathog 2011; 7(7):e1002114.
30. Durrani SR, Montville DJ, Pratt AS, et al. Innate immune responses to rhinovirus are reduced by the high-affinity IgE receptor in allergic asthmatic children. J Allergy Clin Immunol 2012;130(2):489–95.
31. Gill MA, Bajwa G, George TA, et al. Counterregulation between the FcepsilonRI pathway and antiviral responses in human plasmacytoid dendritic cells. J Immunol 2010;184(11):5999–6006.
32. Grunberg K, Timmers MC, de Klerk EP, et al. Experimental rhinovirus 16 infection causes variable airway obstruction in subjects with atopic asthma. Am J Respir Crit Care Med 1999;160(4):1375–80.
33. Kennedy JL, Shaker M, McMeen V, et al. Comparison of viral load in individuals with and without asthma during infections with rhinovirus. Am J Respir Crit Care Med 2014;189(5):532–9.
34. Gavala ML, Bashir H, Gern JE. Virus/allergen interactions in asthma. Curr Allergy Asthma Rep 2013;13(3):298–307.
35. Gavala ML, Bertics PJ, Gern JE. Rhinoviruses, allergic inflammation, and asthma. Immunol Rev 2011;242(1):69–90.
36. Holt PG, Strickland DH, Sly PD. Virus infection and allergy in the development of asthma: what is the connection? Curr Opin Allergy Clin Immunol 2012;12(2): 151–7.
37. Edwards MR, Bartlett NW, Hussell T, et al. The microbiology of asthma. Nat Rev Microbiol 2012;10(7):459–71.

38. Stein RT, Sherrill D, Morgan WJ, et al. Respiratory syncytial virus in early life and risk of wheeze and allergy by age 13 years. Lancet 1999;354(9178):541–5.
39. Soto-Quiros M, Avila L, Platts-Mills TA, et al. High titers of IgE antibody to dust mite allergen and risk for wheezing among asthmatic children infected with rhinovirus. J Allergy Clin Immunol 2012;129(6):1499–505.e5.
40. Kelly LA, Erwin EA, Platts-Mills TA. The indoor air and asthma: the role of cat allergens. Curr Opin Pulm Med 2012;18(1):29–34.
41. Olenec JP, Kim WK, Lee WM, et al. Weekly monitoring of children with asthma for infections and illness during common cold seasons. J Allergy Clin Immunol 2010; 125(5):1001–6.e1.
42. Murray CS, Poletti G, Kebadze T, et al. Study of modifiable risk factors for asthma exacerbations: virus infection and allergen exposure increase the risk of asthma hospital admissions in children. Thorax 2006;61(5):376–82.
43. Green RM, Custovic A, Sanderson G, et al. Synergism between allergens and viruses and risk of hospital admission with asthma: case-control study. BMJ 2002;324(7340):763.
44. Calhoun WJ, Dick EC, Schwartz LB, et al. A common cold virus, rhinovirus 16, potentiates airway inflammation after segmental antigen bronchoprovocation in allergic subjects. J Clin Invest 1994;94(6):2200–8.
45. Zambrano JC, Carper HT, Rakes GP, et al. Experimental rhinovirus challenges in adults with mild asthma: response to infection in relation to IgE. J Allergy Clin Immunol 2003;111(5):1008–16.
46. Message SD, Laza-Stanca V, Mallia P, et al. Rhinovirus-induced lower respiratory illness is increased in asthma and related to virus load and Th1/2 cytokine and IL-10 production. Proc Natl Acad Sci U S A 2008;105(36):13562–7.
47. Kloepfer KM, Gern JE. Virus/allergen interactions and exacerbations of asthma. Immunol Allergy Clin North Am 2010;30(4):553–63, vii.
48. Gill MA, Long K, Kwon T, et al. Differential recruitment of dendritic cells and monocytes to respiratory mucosal sites in children with influenza virus or respiratory syncytial virus infection. J Infect Dis 2008;198(11):1667–76.
49. Huber JP, Ramos HJ, Gill MA, et al. Cutting edge: type I IFN reverses human Th2 commitment and stability by suppressing GATA3. J Immunol 2010;185(2): 813–7.
50. Moschen AR, Geiger S, Krehan I, et al. Interferon-alpha controls IL-17 expression in vitro and in vivo. Immunobiology 2008;213(9–10):779–87.
51. Schroeder JT, Bieneman AP, Xiao H, et al. TLR9- and FcepsilonRI-mediated responses oppose one another in plasmacytoid dendritic cells by down-regulating receptor expression. J Immunol 2005;175(9):5724–31.
52. Schroeder JT, Bieneman AP, Chichester KL, et al. Decreases in human dendritic cell-dependent T(H)2-like responses after acute in vivo IgE neutralization. J Allergy Clin Immunol 2010;125(4):896–901.e6.
53. Busse WW, Morgan WJ, Gergen PJ, et al. Randomized trial of omalizumab (anti-IgF) for asthma in inner-city children. N Engl J Med 2011;364(11):1005–15.
54. Gill MA. The role of dendritic cells in asthma. J Allergy Clin Immunol 2012;129(4): 889–901.
55. Pyle DM, Yang VS, Gruchalla RS, et al. IgE cross-linking critically impairs human monocyte function by blocking phagocytosis. J Allergy Clin Immunol 2013; 131(2):491–500.e1-e5.
56. Bufe A, Gehlhar K, Grage-Griebenow E, et al. Atopic phenotype in children is associated with decreased virus-induced interferon-alpha release. Int Arch Allergy Immunol 2002;127(1):82–8.

57. Gehlhar K, Bilitewski C, Reinitz-Rademacher K, et al. Impaired virus-induced interferon-alpha2 release in adult asthmatic patients. Clin Exp Allergy 2006; 36(3):331–7.

58. Subrata LS, Bizzintino J, Mamessier E, et al. Interactions between innate antiviral and atopic immunoinflammatory pathways precipitate and sustain asthma exacerbations in children. J Immunol 2009;183(4):2793–800.

59. Singh M, Lee SH, Porter P, et al. Human rhinovirus proteinase 2A induces TH1 and TH2 immunity in patients with chronic obstructive pulmonary disease. J Allergy Clin Immunol 2010;125(6):1369–78.e2.

60. Holgate ST, Roberts G, Arshad HS, et al. The role of the airway epithelium and its interaction with environmental factors in asthma pathogenesis. Proc Am Thorac Soc 2009;6(8):655–9.

61. Baraldo S, Contoli M, Bazzan E, et al. Deficient antiviral immune responses in childhood: distinct roles of atopy and asthma. J Allergy Clin Immunol 2012; 130(6):1307–14.

62. Kato A, Favoreto S Jr, Avila PC, et al. TLR3- and Th2 cytokine-dependent production of thymic stromal lymphopoietin in human airway epithelial cells. J Immunol 2007;179(2):1080–7.

63. Calven J, Yudina Y, Hallgren O, et al. Viral stimuli trigger exaggerated thymic stromal lymphopoietin expression by chronic obstructive pulmonary disease epithelium: role of endosomal TLR3 and cytosolic RIG-I-like helicases. J Innate Immun 2012;4(1):86–99.

64. Shikotra A, Choy DF, Ohri CM, et al. Increased expression of immunoreactive thymic stromal lymphopoietin in patients with severe asthma. J Allergy Clin Immunol 2012;129(1):104–11.e1-e9.

65. Ying S, O'Connor B, Ratoff J, et al. Thymic stromal lymphopoietin expression is increased in asthmatic airways and correlates with expression of Th2-attracting chemokines and disease severity. J Immunol 2005;174(12):8183–90.

66. Prefontaine D, Lajoie-Kadoch S, Foley S, et al. Increased expression of IL-33 in severe asthma: evidence of expression by airway smooth muscle cells. J Immunol 2009;183(8):5094–103.

67. Kouzaki H, Iijima K, Kobayashi T, et al. The danger signal, extracellular ATP, is a sensor for an airborne allergen and triggers IL-33 release and innate Th2-type responses. J Immunol 2011;186(7):4375–87.

68. Le Goffic R, Arshad MI, Rauch M, et al. Infection with influenza virus induces IL-33 in murine lungs. Am J Respir Cell Mol Biol 2011;45(6):1125–32.

69. Wang YH, Angkasekwinai P, Lu N, et al. IL-25 augments type 2 immune responses by enhancing the expansion and functions of TSLP-DC-activated Th2 memory cells. J Exp Med 2007;204(8):1837–47.

70. Petersen BC, Dolgachev V, Rasky A, et al. IL-17E (IL-25) and IL-17RB promote respiratory syncytial virus-induced pulmonary disease. J Leukoc Biol 2014;95: 809–15.

71. Idzko M, Hammad H, van Nimwegen M, et al. Extracellular ATP triggers and maintains asthmatic airway inflammation by activating dendritic cells. Nat Med 2007;13(8):913–9.

72. Denlinger LC, Manthei DM, Seibold MA, et al. P2X7-regulated protection from exacerbations and loss of control is independent of asthma maintenance therapy. Am J Respir Crit Care Med 2013;187(1):28–33.

73. Walter MJ, Morton JD, Kajiwara N, et al. Viral induction of a chronic asthma phenotype and genetic segregation from the acute response. J Clin Invest 2002;110(2):165–75.

74. Nakagome K, Bochkov YA, Ashraf S, et al. Effects of rhinovirus species on viral replication and cytokine production. J Allergy Clin Immunol 2014;134:332–41.
75. Kaiko GE, Loh Z, Spann K, et al. Toll-like receptor 7 gene deficiency and early-life Pneumovirus infection interact to predispose toward the development of asthma-like pathology in mice. J Allergy Clin Immunol 2013;131(5):1331–9.e10.
76. Grayson MH, Cheung D, Rohlfing MM, et al. Induction of high-affinity IgE receptor on lung dendritic cells during viral infection leads to mucous cell metaplasia. J Exp Med 2007;204(11):2759–69.
77. Cheung DS, Ehlenbach SJ, Kitchens T, et al. Development of atopy by severe paramyxoviral infection in a mouse model. Ann Allergy Asthma Immunol 2010; 105(6):437–43.e1.
78. Palivizumab, a humanized respiratory syncytial virus monoclonal antibody, reduces hospitalization from respiratory syncytial virus infection in high-risk infants. The IMpact-RSV Study Group. Pediatrics 1998;102(3 Pt 1):531–7.
79. Blanken MO, Rovers MM, Molenaar JM, et al. Respiratory syncytial virus and recurrent wheeze in healthy preterm infants. N Engl J Med 2013;368(19):1791–9.
80. Yoshihara S, Kusuda S, Mochizuki H, et al. Effect of palivizumab prophylaxis on subsequent recurrent wheezing in preterm infants. Pediatrics 2013;132(5):811–8.
81. Simoes EA, Carbonell-Estrany X, Rieger CH, et al. The effect of respiratory syncytial virus on subsequent recurrent wheezing in atopic and nonatopic children. J Allergy Clin Immunol 2010;126(2):256–62.
82. Kramarz P, Destefano F, Gargiullo PM, et al. Does influenza vaccination prevent asthma exacerbations in children? J Pediatr 2001;138(3):306–10.
83. Ong BA, Forester J, Fallot A. Does influenza vaccination improve pediatric asthma outcomes? J Asthma 2009;46(5):477–80.
84. Johnston SL, Ferrero F, Garcia ML, et al. Oral oseltamivir improves pulmonary function and reduces exacerbation frequency for influenza-infected children with asthma. Pediatr Infect Dis J 2005;24(3):225–32.
85. Centers for Disease Control and Prevention. Vaccination coverage among persons with asthma—United States, 2010-2011 influenza season. MMWR Morb Mortal Wkly Rep 2013;62(48):973–8.
86. Bergman P, Lindh AU, Bjorkhem-Bergman L, et al. Vitamin D and respiratory tract infections: a systematic review and meta-analysis of randomized controlled trials. PLoS One 2013;8(6):e65835.
87. Majak P, Olszowiec-Chlebna M, Smejda K, et al. Vitamin D supplementation in children may prevent asthma exacerbation triggered by acute respiratory infection. J Allergy Clin Immunol 2011;127(5):1294–6.
88. Hao Q, Lu Z, Dong BR, et al. Probiotics for preventing acute upper respiratory tract infections. Cochrane Database Syst Rev 2011;(9):CD006895.
89. Elazab N, Mendy A, Gasana J, et al. Probiotic administration in early life, atopy, and asthma: a meta-analysis of clinical trials. Pediatrics 2013;132(3):e666–76.
90. Reddel HK, Jenkins C, Quirce S, et al. Effect of different asthma treatments on risk of cold-related exacerbations. Eur Respir J 2011;38(3):584–93.
91. Bochkov YA, Busse WW, Brockman-Schneider RA, et al. Budesonide and formoterol effects on rhinovirus replication and epithelial cell cytokine responses. Respir Res 2013;14:98.
92. Bice JB, Leechawengwongs E, Montanaro A. Biologic targeted therapy in allergic asthma. Ann Allergy Asthma Immunol 2014;112(2):108–15.
93. Kim YH, Park CS, Lim DH, et al. Beneficial effect of anti-interleukin-33 on the murine model of allergic inflammation of the lower airway. J Asthma 2012;49(7):738–43.

Pediatric Asthma
Guidelines-Based Care, Omalizumab, and Other Potential Biologic Agents

Michelle Fox Huffaker, MD[a], Wanda Phipatanakul, MD, MS[b],*

KEYWORDS

• Asthma • Asthma management • Pediatric asthma • Biologics • Omalizumab

KEY POINTS

• Current step-up asthma therapy is sufficient for most children with asthma, although physicians must work to ensure medication compliance.
• Phenotypic and genotypic variability in asthma are becoming increasingly important in asthma management, particularly with regard to the use of biologics.
• The future of asthma in children will include earlier diagnosis and even prevention as more is learned about the development of this disease.

INTRODUCTION

Asthma affects more than 6 million children, making it one of the most common chronic diseases of childhood, and the prevalence continues to increase.[1] Asthma accounts for more than 14 million school absences each year and is the leading cause of hospitalizations among children.[2–4] However, advances in medical therapy have reduced the number of asthma-related deaths and improved overall quality of life for many asthmatics.[1,2] Effective management guidelines now exist, with substantial supporting evidence from clinical trials in asthmatic children.[5] However, over the past decade there has been a rapid increase in novel therapies for asthma management and few of these have been studied in children.

Further complicating pediatric asthma management is the diagnosis of asthma. There is significant heterogeneity among children who wheeze, and only a subset of all children who wheeze go on to develop asthma.[6–8] Several studies have evaluated both children who wheeze and those who subsequently develop asthma and have clustered children into distinct phenotypes.[6–9] This phenotypic variability is only a small part of the heterogeneity among asthmatics, as can be seen with the range of

Funding: NIH/NIAID K24 AI106822.
[a] Division of Medicine, Brigham and Women's Hospital, Harvard Medical School, 75 Francis Street, Boston, MA 02115, USA; [b] Division of Immunology, Boston Children's Hospital, Harvard Medical School, 300 Longwood Avenue, Boston, MA 02115, USA
* Corresponding author.
E-mail address: wanda.phipatanakul@childrens.harvard.edu

Immunol Allergy Clin N Am 35 (2015) 129–144
http://dx.doi.org/10.1016/j.iac.2014.09.005
0889-8561/15/$ – see front matter © 2015 Elsevier Inc. All rights reserved.

responses to guidelines-based therapy. Although this heterogeneity causes some difficulty in the diagnosis and management of asthma in children, it also poses the unique opportunity for targeted asthma therapy. In the era of biologics, targeted therapy may become increasingly important and fundamental to management.

This article focuses on (1) the evidence supporting the current guidelines-based therapies, with an emphasis on phenotypic heterogeneity; (2) promising novel therapeutics that have not yet been incorporated into standard care; and (3) potential opportunities for prevention of pediatric asthma.

MEDICATION ADHERENCE

Once the diagnosis of asthma is established, ensuring medication adherence becomes a fundamental component of asthma management.[5,10,11] Poor adherence leads to increased morbidity and unnecessary escalation of treatment regimens.[10,11] In children with asthma, noncompliance with inhalers is a significant problem in all disease severity categories, with some studies citing adherence rates of less than 60%.[12–15]

The reasons for nonadherence are many and differ depending on the child and family.[15–18] Cost, lack of knowledge about asthma, and patient motivation have been cited in multiple studies as the most critical barriers to adherence.[17,18] In several analyses, education of the parent or caregiver on the importance of medication and impact on the underlying disease was a major factor toward improving child medication adherence.[17,18] Providers also play a key role, because appointment time constraints, changes in providers, and barriers to scheduling appointments have all been shown to worsen medication compliance.[17,18] Implementation of the guidelines-based therapy and the development of novel therapies for the refractory asthmatic (discussed later) are only of benefit if clinicians address adherence as a primary component of asthma management.

INHALED CORTICOSTEROIDS

Based on several large trials, inhaled corticosteroids have become the first-line agent in the management of asthma and remain the preferred treatment choice for all levels of persistent asthma in children.[19,20] However, in spite of improving asthma control, inhaled corticosteroids have not been shown to alter the progression of asthma. In a large randomized controlled trial from the childhood asthma management program (CAMP) group, budesonide was not shown to preserve lung function compared with placebo.[21,22] The prevention of early asthma in kids (PEAK) trial showed that inhaled corticosteroids decreased wheezing episodes and need for supplemental inhalers in young children with a positive modified Asthma Predictive Index, but this effect did not last once the inhaled corticosteroids were discontinued.[20] Inhaled corticosteroids similarly have not been shown to alter the progression of intermittent to persistent wheezing in infants.[23] In addition, there is evidence to suggest that well-controlled asthmatic children on inhaled corticosteroids with normal spirometry continue to have abnormalities in lung clearance indices, suggesting that abnormalities persist despite not being detectable using standard office measurements.[24]

Newer data suggest that inhaled corticosteroids may hold greater benefit in certain subpopulations. Numerous studies have shown heterogeneity in response to inhaled corticosteroids.[20,25–28] For example, some studies have shown that treatment with fluticasone propionate has greatest benefit in children with frequent symptoms, family history of asthma, and a positive Asthma Predictive Index.[20,25] Another study found better outcomes with inhaled corticosteroids in white children, boys, and those with aeroallergen sensitization.[27] More recently, benefit from fluticasone propionate has been associated with specific genetic polymorphisms.[26,28]

Furthermore, the newer generation of inhaled corticosteroids may improve control for the asthmatic population. The newer inhaled corticosteroids ciclesonide and mometasone generate smaller particles and thus better reach the peripheral airways at lower doses. Although there is evidence to suggest that children on traditional long-term inhaled corticosteroids may have increased risk for delayed growth, studies support that most children achieve their predicted adult heights when treated with recommended doses.[22,29] Nevertheless, studies suggest that the newer generation of inhaled corticosteroids have a smaller side effect profile because of lower daily doses.[16,30–35] However, a 2013 Cochrane Review found no difference in control of asthma symptoms, exacerbations, or side effects between ciclesonide, budesonide, and fluticasone.[36] An additional potential benefit of these newer agents is that both ciclesonide and mometasone are effective as once-daily dosing, and thus may improve medication adherence.[16,34,37]

ALTERNATIVES TO INHALED CORTICOSTEROIDS

Other agents, including cromolyn and leukotriene receptor antagonists, have also shown some benefit in children but overall have not performed as well as inhaled corticosteroids and thus are not considered first-line therapy.[5,38–44] As with inhaled corticosteroids, there may be some phenotypic variability in response to leukotriene receptor antagonists. Evidence suggests that the differential response to inhaled corticosteroids and leukotriene receptor antagonists is greatest in children with lower lung function, allergic airway inflammation, and increased FeNO levels, and children with higher ratios of urinary leukotriene E4 to FeNO may respond better to leukotriene receptor antagonists.[38–45] The data are inconsistent and thus these biomarkers have not yet been included in the guidelines for clinical practice.[5]

Theophylline, an agent with a long history in the management of asthma, has been shown to be inferior to inhaled corticosteroids and inferior to montelukast as add-on therapy.[46,47] One small trial showed that the addition of theophylline to inhaled corticosteroids resulted in improvement in peak expiratory flow, but did not improve forced expiratory volume in 1 second (FEV_1) or bronchial reactivity.[48] Given the lack of substantial supporting evidence, potential toxicity, and need for frequent monitoring, theophylline is not part of first-line therapy for children with asthma and is not recommended for children less than 5 years of age.[5]

STEP-UP THERAPY

If inhaled corticosteroids do not adequately manage a child's asthma, the guidelines suggest that the next step in therapy should be the addition of a long-acting beta agonist.[5] The addition of a long-acting beta agonist to inhaled corticosteroids has been shown to improve lung function for most children, but many studies have shown that there is significant variability in response and resulting asthma control.[44,49–54] The Best Add-On Giving Effective Response (BADGER) study showed that, although the addition of long-acting beta agonists to low-dose inhaled corticosteroids was most likely to reduce exacerbations and improve FEV_1 and the number of asthma control days compared with medium-dose inhaled corticosteroids or the addition of a leukotriene receptor antagonist, the study also showed that there was significant variability among the children with regard to these results.[54] As many as 26.7% of children in the study responded better to a medium dose of inhaled corticosteroids and 29.2% to leukotriene receptor antagonists.[54] In a recent post-hoc analysis of the BADGER study, Rabinovitch and colleagues[44] identified phenotypic variables that differentiate these populations of children. Higher impulse oscillometry reactance area, suggesting peripheral airway obstruction, corresponded with better response to the addition of long-acting beta agonists to low-dose inhaled corticosteroids than increasing the dose of inhaled corticosteroids or adding a leukotriene receptor antagonist.[44] In addition, higher urinary leukotriene E_4 levels predicted better response to the addition of leukotriene receptor antagonists.[44] Additionally, genetic variants have been identified in certain populations that lead to differential responses to bronchodilators.[55-57] Thus, as with inhaled corticosteroids and leukotriene receptor antagonists (discussed earlier), there is phenotypic variability in response to beta agonists. Further work is needed before genetics or biomarkers are used to guide asthma management in clinical practice.

NOVEL USES FOR OLD THERAPIES

Macrolides have been broadly studied in adult chronic pulmonary diseases as well as in children with cystic fibrosis, and have shown significant benefits in some patients.[16,58-61] The observed improvement is thought to be related to the immunomodulatory role of macrolides and resulting decrease in airway neutrophils.[16,58-61] Initial optimism surrounding the benefit of macrolides in management of refractory asthma was moderated by the discovery that many macrolides decrease the clearance of steroids.[16,62,63] More recently, several small studies have suggested that the use of macrolides in children with asthma may reduce bronchial hyperresponsiveness and airway neutrophils, and shorten the duration of symptoms.[64,65] There is also some evidence to suggest that asthmatics with colonization by *Chlamydia pneumoniae* or *Mycoplasma pneumoniae* may have more benefit from macrolides.[16,66,67] Some clinicians have argued that, given the low risk nature of macrolides, a trial of therapy in refractory asthmatics is reasonable, although this recommendation has yet to become part of the US guidelines for pediatric asthma management.[5,10] The National Heart, Lung and Blood Institute (NHLBI) AsthmaNet is currently investigating whether azithromycin initiated at the start of upper respiratory infection in preschool children who wheeze will alter the development of lower respiratory illness and exacerbation (NCT01272635).

Vitamin D is also known to have immunomodulatory effects and may play a role in the management of asthma.[16,68,69] Vitamin D has been shown in vitro to stimulate T-regulatory cells and the production of interleukin (IL)-10 in response to steroids, which then inhibits allergen-specific Th2 cells.[16,68] Furthermore, a study from the Childhood Asthma Management Program found that children with vitamin D deficiency were likely to have poorer lung function and less response to inhaled corticosteroids.[69] A recent study published in the *Journal of the American Medical Association* found that vitamin D did not reduce the rate of exacerbation in adults with asthma.[70] Further analysis is needed to determine the utility of vitamin D supplementation in asthmatic children as well as other specific subgroups.[70]

THE ERA OF BIOLOGICS

A subset of asthmatics remains severely symptomatic despite the therapies discussed earlier, and before the introduction of biologics, these patients were relegated to long-term oral corticosteroids. With the advent of biologics, there is now hope that these severe steroid-dependent asthmatics may have alternative options for treatment.

Furthermore, biologics provide the perfect opportunity to selectively choose therapy based on asthma phenotype. The first of these agents to be accepted in the national guidelines is omalizumab. Omalizumab, an anti–immunoglobulin (Ig) E monoclonal antibody, is now recommended by the most recent guidelines from the National Asthma Education and Prevention Program for children 12 years of age and older with moderate to severe asthma. These recommendations are supported by more than a decade of work showing that omalizumab reduces the frequency of asthma exacerbations, emergency department visits, and hospitalizations, and decreases the need for rescue medications and steroids in children with asthma.[71-77] There are limited data at this point on the safety and efficacy of long-term use; some of the longest studies have shown that the medication was tolerated for at least 3 years with improvement in both symptoms and lung function.[78] In addition, data are limited for children less than 12 years of age.

Omalizumab has been further studied in specific patient populations and has shown significant benefit for asthmatics of certain phenotypes. A major randomized controlled trial of omalizumab in inner-city children with asthma of any severity showed significant reduction in asthma exacerbations and symptoms.[79] Omalizumab had the greatest benefit in children with sensitization and exposure to cockroach and dust mites.[79] Post-hoc analysis further supported the concept that anti-IgE therapy may be of particular benefit in children with seasonal exacerbations.[79] Studies of omalizumab in other clinical phenotypes that are thought to be Th2 driven, including patients with chronic rhinosinusitis and those with nasal polyps, have shown promise as well.[80,81] Given the cost of omalizumab, many clinicians have argued for the importance of identifying populations that will have significant benefit and of using the drug selectively in those groups, although newer indications in other allergic diseases, including the recent new indication for chronic urticaria, may expand its utility and control costs.[79,82,83] In the past, the populations identified have been those with increased IgE levels and more severe asthma, although recent work has begun to investigate the impact of anti-IgE on specific biomarkers in allergic asthmatics, including FeNO, eosinophilia, and periostin.[79,84-87] In the future, anti-IgE therapy may even play a role in asthma prevention, as is discussed in more detail below.[88]

Although omalizumab is the only biologic that has been approved for asthma in children, there are several others that have shown promise in clinical trials in adults and thus may eventually be incorporated into pediatric asthma management as well. In addition, there are ongoing clinical trials for many of biologics in adolescents aged 12 years and older. Many of these newer biologics target T cells or T-cell cytokines. The role of T cells in asthma is well established and is discussed in detail elsewhere.[89] This article discusses several of the newer biologics, but this list is only intended to be illustrative of the numerous and varied biologics in existence for asthma and is not meant to be a comprehensive list of all biologics trialed in asthma to date.

One such biologic targeting T cells is keliximab, a monoclonal antibody to the CD4 receptor. In phase II trails, keliximab seemed to improve peak expiratory flow, but resulted in diminished CD4 counts.[90,91] Several of the other biologics under investigation target the cytokines involved in Th2-mediated allergic and asthmatic inflammation, including IL-2, IL-5, IL-4, and IL-13. IL-2 leads to the activation of Th2 cells, and symptomatic asthmatics have long been known to have increased levels of the IL-2 receptor.[92] Daclizumab, a monoclonal antibody to the IL-2 receptor, has been shown in phase II trials to improve lung function in adults with moderate to severe asthma on inhaled corticosteroids.[93] No trials have been done on daclizumab in children or adolescents with asthma.

There are several new monoclonal antibodies targeting IL-5, a cytokine linked directly with sputum eosinophilia and airway hyper-responsiveness in asthma.[94] Mepolizumab, a monoclonal antibody targeting IL-5, has had very promising results thus far.[95,96] IL-5 is a cytokine that has been linked directly with sputum eosinophilia and airway hyper-responsiveness in asthma.[94] Early work showed that mepolizumab reduced exacerbations and improved quality of life scores in adults with eosinophilic asthma in phase III clinical trials.[97-99] Two studies recently published in the *New England Journal of*

Medicine showed that mepolizumab reduced asthma exacerbations, improved asthma morbidity, and had a significant steroid-sparing effect in subjects with eosinophilic asthma.[95,96] While both of these studies included adolescent asthmatic patients, the total number of children in these studies was small. There are ongoing clinical trials recruiting children ages 12 and older, including NCT01842607, designed to examine the long-term safety of this drug. Reslizumab, another monoclonal antibody to IL-5, has shown promise in phase II trials in improving asthma quality of life scores and lung function.[100,101] Interestingly, the greatest benefit was seen in those patients with asthma and nasal polyps.[101] The efficacy and safety of reslizumab in children ages 12 and older with eosinophilic asthma is currently being examined in the following clinical trials: NCT01270464, NCT01287039, NCT01285323, and NCT01290887.

IL-4 and IL-13 are directly involved in IgE-mediated mast cell degranulation and mucus hypersecretion and plays a role in airways remodeling in asthma.[102] Dupilumab, a human monoclonal antibody to IL-4, has been shown to reduce the frequency of asthma exacerbations and improve lung function in adults with persistent moderate to severe asthma and increased sputum eosinophil levels.[103] No trials have been done on dupilumab in children or adolescents with asthma. Pitrakinra, a recombinant form of IL-4 that blocks IL-4 receptor signaling, decreased asthma exacerbations and symptoms in patients with specific IL-4 receptor polymorphisms.[104] No trials have been done on pitrakinra in children or adolescents. Lebrikizumab, a monoclonal antibody to IL-13, has been shown in a phase II trial to improve lung function in adult asthmatics, particularly those with increased serum periostin levels.[105] Periostin, a matricellular protein, is secreted by bronchial epithelial cells in response to IL-13 and results in airway remodeling.[106] Lebrikizumab is currently being studied in children in several different clinical trials, including adolescents aged 12 to 17 years on both an inhaled corticosteroid and a second controller agent, steroid-dependent children aged 12 years and older, and steroid-dependent children aged 12 years and older with a trial design focused on changes in biomarkers. Another anti–IL-13 antibody, tralokinumab, was found in phase IIa trials to also improve lung function, and most dramatically in those with high levels of airway eosinophils.[107] Tralokinumab is currently undergoing pharmacokinetic studies in children aged 12 to 17 years.

POTENTIAL THERAPEUTIC TARGETS

In addition to the cytokines mentioned earlier, numerous other cytokines have been suggested as targets for biologics in the treatment of asthma (**Table 1**).[108,109] Studies in mice suggest that IL-9 may play a role in airway hyperresponsiveness, airway eosinophilia, and mucus secretion.[110] Medi-528, a monoclonal antibody to IL-9, is under investigation, and has reached phase 2 trials with some promise.[111] Work is also ongoing to develop an anti–IL-25 antibody for use in allergic asthmatics, because IL-25 plays a role in the activation of Th2 lymphocytes and the development of allergic asthmatic traits.[112] IL-33 was also recently identified as an important potential target, because it was found to promote airway remodeling in pediatric patients with steroid-resistant asthma.[113] Preclinical studies have shown that anti–IL-33 can prevent the development of allergic asthma in mice.[114] Tumor necrosis factor (TNF) alpha, which has shown great success in many chronic inflammatory diseases, is known to be upregulated in the airways of severe asthmatics.[115,116] However, anti-TNF agents, such as infliximab and golimumab, have not had significant success in asthma secondary to significant risk with limited benefit.[117,118]

Tyrosine kinase inhibitors, which have become part of the standard of care in the management of many malignancies, have recently come under investigation for use

Table 1
Potential therapeutic targets and ongoing studies to establish their roles in asthma

Therapeutic Target	Role in Asthma	Current Investigation
IL-9	AHR, airway eosinophilia, mucus secretion[110]	Medi-528, phase II trials[111]
IL-25	Activation of Th2 cells, allergic asthma[112]	Preclinical studies,[112] development of anti–IL-25 antibody
IL-33	Airway remodeling[113]	Preclinical studies[114]
Tyrosine kinase inhibitors	Inflammatory gene expression[16,119]	Masitinib,[119] phase III clinical trial currently recruiting (NCT01449162)
CCR3	Airway eosinophilia, airway remodeling[123,124]	GW766994, phase II clinical trial (NCT01160224)
CCR4	Airway inflammation[108,125]	AMG 761, phase I clinical trial (NCT01514981)

Abbreviation: AHR, airway hyperresponsiveness.

in asthma given their role in inflammatory gene expression.[16,119] A preliminary study of masitinib, a c-kit/platelet-derived growth factor (PDGF) receptor tyrosine kinase inhibitor, showed promise in reducing asthma symptoms in severe steroid-dependent asthmatics.[119] Further work is needed to determine whether the benefits outweigh the potential side effects of such therapy, and a phase III clinical trial of masitinib in severe steroid-dependent asthmatics is currently underway.

Chemokines involved in the homing of inflammatory cells have also attracted attention as being potential targets in the treatment of asthma.[108] C-C chemokine receptor type 3 (CCR3) and eotaxin are involved in eosinophil infiltration in the airways, and their presence and level in induced sputum correlates with asthma severity.[120,121] Furthermore, additional work suggests that CCR3 may play a role in smooth muscle remodeling in asthmatic airways.[122] There has been some investigation into CCR3 and eotaxin antagonists, and results of a clinical trial of a CCR3 receptor antagonist in adults with mild to moderate asthma are currently pending publication.[123,124] CCR4 is overexpressed in Th2 lymphocytes in asthma, and RS-1748, a CCR4 antagonist, has been shown to reduce airway inflammation in animal models.[108,125] Another CCR4 antagonist, AMG 761, is currently undergoing phase I clinical trials in asthmatics. Other chemokines may eventually be targeted for asthma therapy as well.

There are many other potential targets under investigation, including phospholipase A2, 5′-lipoxygensase, phosphodiesterase-4, thymic stromal lymphopoietin, OX40 ligand, and tissue kallikrein-1. Discussion of these targets is beyond the scope of this article, but are discussed in more detail elsewhere.[16,108]

PREVENTION

Prevention is the goal of any chronic disease management, including for asthma, and there is currently no known agent that has been proven modify disease progression in early disease or even prevent the onset of disease. With tools such as the Asthma Predictive Index to predict which children will develop asthma, improved asthma phenotyping, and even asthma genotyping, prevention may be a possibility for the future.[126] One phenotype that has been targeted for prevention already is the allergic atopic phenotype. There is a strong association between exposure to allergen sensitization and asthma, and early exposure to allergens in sensitized atopic children has been shown to reduce lung function.[127,128] Prophylactic interventions have thus been aimed at reducing allergen exposure and inducing tolerance. The Inner City Asthma Study showed that reducing cockroach and dustmite allergen in the home significantly reduced asthma symptoms in inner-city asthmatic children.[129] Jacobsen et al showed that open label treatment with subcutaneous specific immunotherapy potentially altered the course of asthma in atopic children.[130,131] Sublingual immunotherapy may also have similar effects, but the results have been mixed.[132–136] Omalizumab (anti-IgE), is a well-established therapy for asthma and being extensively evaluated in children. With its role in complete blockade of all IgE regardless of idiotype, given the critical role of atopy and the atopic march in asthma development and persistence, it is still in need of evaluation in its role in potential prevention and disease modification of asthma in young children.[88]

There is also a strong association between RSV bronchiolitis, other viral respiratory infections, and the development of asthma.[127,137–141] Palivizumab, an anti-RSV monoclonal antibody, has been shown to reduce wheezing in premature infants, suggesting that perhaps it may prevent the development of asthma in this population.[142,143] The impact of palivizumab on wheezing in term infants remains to be determined. Other anti-virals could also be considered, but none of the available agents so far have proven consistent effectiveness in lower respiratory disease. Furthermore, the Inner City Asthma Consortium demonstrated that the use of omalizumab during the common cold season reduced rates of exacerbation.[79] Clinical trial NCT01430403 investigating the role of omalizumab in prevention of asthma exacerbations in asthmatic children during the fall season has been completed and is awaiting publication. As discussed in detail elsewhere, perhaps in the future, anti-IgE may be used during the cold season to prevent the development of asthma in at risk populations.[88]

In addition, given the growing evidence for the role of gut flora in the development of allergic and atopic disease, probiotics have become of interest in preventing not only asthma, but other allergic diseases as well. Unfortunately, the data have not supported the use of probiotics in the prevention of asthma thus far. Multiple studies have had limited if any positive results and a recent meta-analysis of trials of probiotic supplementation in pregnancy and infancy found no evidence that probiotics prevented the development of asthma.[144,145] Some studies suggest that there may be a role for probiotics in preventing asthma in children that are otherwise atopic, although further work is needed in this area.[146] Clinical trials of probiotics to prevent asthma in infants are currently ongoing: NCT00113659, NCT01285830. Further, a killed bacterial lysate, OM-85 BV, has been demonstrated to decrease the frequency and duration of wheezing episodes in young children, and could also be considered in prevention.[147]

SUMMARY

The management of asthma is becoming more patient specific as more is learned about the biology of the development and progression of asthma. The future of asthma management is likely to involve phenotypic characterization and potentially even genotypic characterization in certain cases to determine appropriate therapy. Until that time, the current therapies are sufficient for most pediatric asthmatic patients and the focus should remain on ensuring adherence to the guidelines through education of both patients and providers.

REFERENCES

1. National Health Interview Survey. Current asthma prevalence. Atlanta, Georgia: National Center for Health Statistics; Centers for Disease Control and Prevention; 2005.

2. Department of Health and Human Services. Healthy People 2010 Midcourse Review. In: Health and Human Services, editor. Washington, DC: US Government Printing Office; 2007. p. 3–27.
3. Akinbami LJ, Schoendorf KC. Trends in childhood asthma: prevalence, health care utilization, and mortality. Pediatrics 2002;110(2 Pt 1):315–22.
4. National Center for Education Statistics. Condition of education. Washington: US Department of Education; 2001.
5. Expert Panel Report 3. Guidelines for the diagnosis and management of asthma. National Heart, Lung, and Blood Institute. US Department of Health and Human Services. Washington. 2007.
6. Martinez FD, Wright AL, Taussig LM, et al. Asthma and wheezing in the first six years of life. The Group Health Medical Associates. N Engl J Med 1995;332(3):133–8.
7. Henderson J, Granell R, Heron J, et al. Associations of wheezing phenotypes in the first 6 years of life with atopy, lung function and airway responsiveness in mid-childhood. Thorax 2008;63(11):974–80.
8. Spycher BD, Silverman M, Brooke AM, et al. Distinguishing phenotypes of childhood wheeze and cough using latent class analysis. Eur Respir J 2008;31(5):974–81.
9. Just J, Gouvis-Echraghi R, Rouve S, et al. Two novel, severe asthma phenotypes identified during childhood using a clustering approach. Eur Respir J 2012;40(1):55–60.
10. Halterman JS, Aligne CA, Auinger P, et al. Inadequate therapy for asthma among children in the United States. Pediatrics 2000;105(1 Pt 3):272–6.
11. DiMatteo MR, Giordani PJ, Lepper HS, et al. Patient adherence and medical treatment outcomes: a meta-analysis. Med Care 2002;40(9):794–811.
12. Sawicki GS, Strunk RC, Schuemann B, et al. Patterns of inhaled corticosteroid use and asthma control in the Childhood Asthma Management Program Continuation Study. Ann Allergy Asthma Immunol 2010;104(1):30–5.
13. Milgrom H, Bender B, Ackerson L, et al. Noncompliance and treatment failure in children with asthma. J Allergy Clin Immunol 1996;98(6 Pt 1):1051–7.
14. Gamble J, Stevenson M, McClean E, et al. The prevalence of nonadherence in difficult asthma. Am J Respir Crit Care Med 2009;180(9):817–22.
15. Bauman LJ, Wright E, Leickly FE, et al. Relationship of adherence to pediatric asthma morbidity among inner-city children. Pediatrics 2002;110(1 Pt 1):e6.
16. Robinson PD, Van Asperen P. Newer treatments in the management of pediatric asthma. Paediatr Drugs 2013;15(4):291–302.
17. Bender BG. Overcoming barriers to nonadherence in asthma treatment. J Allergy Clin Immunol 2002;109(Suppl 6):S554–9.
18. Grover C, Armour C, Asperen PP, et al. Medication use in children with asthma: not a child size problem. J Asthma 2011;48(10):1085–103.
19. Bisgaard H, Allen D, Milanowski J, et al. Twelve-month safety and efficacy of inhaled fluticasone propionate in children aged 1 to 3 years with recurrent wheezing. Pediatrics 2004;113(2):e87–94.
20. Guilbert TW, Morgan WJ, Zeiger RS, et al. Long-term inhaled corticosteroids in preschool children at high risk for asthma. N Engl J Med 2006;354(19):1985–97.
21. Long-term effects of budesonide or nedocromil in children with asthma. The Childhood Asthma Management Program Research Group. N Engl J Med 2000;343(15):1054–63.
22. Covar RA, Spahn JD, Murphy JR, et al. Progression of asthma measured by lung function in the childhood asthma management program. Am J Respir Crit Care Med 2004;170(3):234–41.

23. Bisgaard H, Hermansen MN, Loland L, et al. Intermittent inhaled corticosteroids in infants with episodic wheezing. N Engl J Med 2006;354(19):1998–2005.

24. Macleod KA, Horsley AR, Bell NJ, et al. Ventilation heterogeneity in children with well controlled asthma with normal spirometry indicates residual airways disease. Thorax 2009;64(1):33–7.

25. Roorda RJ, Mezei G, Bisgaard H, et al. Response of preschool children with asthma symptoms to fluticasone propionate. J Allergy Clin Immunol 2001; 108(4):540–6.

26. Stockmann C, Fassl B, Gaedigk R, et al. Fluticasone propionate pharmacogenetics: CYP3A4*22 polymorphism and pediatric asthma control. J Pediatr 2013;162(6):1222–7, 1227.e1–2.

27. Bacharier LB, Guilbert TW, Zeiger RS, et al. Patient characteristics associated with improved outcomes with use of an inhaled corticosteroid in preschool children at risk for asthma. J Allergy Clin Immunol 2009;123(5):1077–82, 1082.e1–5.

28. Jin Y, Hu D, Peterson EL, et al. Dual-specificity phosphatase 1 as a pharmacogenetic modifier of inhaled steroid response among asthmatic patients. J Allergy Clin Immunol 2010;126(3):618–25 e1–2.

29. Agertoft L, Pedersen S. Effect of long-term treatment with inhaled budesonide on adult height in children with asthma. N Engl J Med 2000;343(15): 1064–9.

30. Robinson PD, Van Asperen P. Asthma in childhood. Pediatr Clin North Am 2009; 56(1):191–226, xii.

31. Milgrom H. Mometasone furoate in children with mild to moderate persistent asthma: a review of the evidence. Paediatr Drugs 2010;12(4):213–21.

32. Skoner DP, Meltzer EO, Milgrom H, et al. Effects of inhaled mometasone furoate on growth velocity and adrenal function: a placebo-controlled trial in children 4-9 years old with mild persistent asthma. J Asthma 2011;48(8):848–59.

33. Gelfand EW, Georgitis JW, Noonan M, et al. Once-daily ciclesonide in children: efficacy and safety in asthma. J Pediatr 2006;148(3):377–83.

34. Pedersen S, Garcia Garcia ML, Manjra A, et al. A comparative study of inhaled ciclesonide 160 microg/day and fluticasone propionate 176 microg/day in children with asthma. Pediatr Pulmonol 2006;41(10):954–61.

35. Skoner DP, Maspero J, Banerji D. Assessment of the long-term safety of inhaled ciclesonide on growth in children with asthma. Pediatrics 2008;121(1): e1–14.

36. Kramer S, Rottier BL, Scholten RJ, et al. Ciclesonide versus other inhaled corticosteroids for chronic asthma in children. Cochrane Database Syst Rev 2013;(2):CD010352.

37. Friedman HS, Navaratnam P, McLaughlin J. Adherence and asthma control with mometasone furoate versus fluticasone propionate in adolescents and young adults with mild asthma. J Asthma 2010;47(9):994–1000.

38. Knuffman JE, Sorkness CA, Lemanske RF Jr, et al. Phenotypic predictors of long-term response to inhaled corticosteroid and leukotriene modifier therapies in pediatric asthma. J Allergy Clin Immunol 2009;123(2):411–6.

39. Chauhan BF, Ducharme FM. Anti-leukotriene agents compared to inhaled corticosteroids in the management of recurrent and/or chronic asthma in adults and children. Cochrane Database Syst Rev 2012;(5):CD002314.

40. Sorkness CA, Lemanske RF Jr, Mauger DT, et al. Long-term comparison of 3 controller regimens for mild-moderate persistent childhood asthma: the Pediatric Asthma Controller Trial. J Allergy Clin Immunol 2007;119(1):64–72.

41. Szefler SJ, Phillips BR, Martinez FD, et al. Characterization of within-subject responses to fluticasone and montelukast in childhood asthma. J Allergy Clin Immunol 2005;115(2):233–42.
42. Zeiger RS, Szefler SJ, Phillips BR, et al. Response profiles to fluticasone and montelukast in mild-to-moderate persistent childhood asthma. J Allergy Clin Immunol 2006;117(1):45–52.
43. Meyer KA, Arduino JM, Santanello NC, et al. Response to montelukast among subgroups of children aged 2 to 14 years with asthma. J Allergy Clin Immunol 2003;111(4):757–62.
44. Rabinovitch N, Mauger DT, Reisdorph N, et al. Predictors of asthma control and lung function responsiveness to step 3 therapy in children with uncontrolled asthma. J Allergy Clin Immunol 2014;133(2):350–6.
45. Rabinovitch N, Graber NJ, Chinchilli VM, et al. Urinary leukotriene E4/exhaled nitric oxide ratio and montelukast response in childhood asthma. J Allergy Clin Immunol 2010;126(3):545–51.e1-4.
46. Seddon P, Bara A, Ducharme FM, et al. Oral xanthines as maintenance treatment for asthma in children. Cochrane Database Syst Rev 2006;(1): CD002885.
47. Kondo N, Katsunuma T, Odajima Y, et al. A randomized open-label comparative study of montelukast versus theophylline added to inhaled corticosteroid in asthmatic children. Allergol Int 2006;55(3):287–93.
48. Suessmuth S, Freihorst J, Gappa M. Low-dose theophylline in childhood asthma: a placebo-controlled, double-blind study. Pediatr Allergy Immunol 2003;14(5):394–400.
49. Russell G, Williams DA, Weller P, et al. Salmeterol xinafoate in children on high dose inhaled steroids. Ann Allergy Asthma Immunol 1995;75(5):423–8.
50. Zimmerman B, D'Urzo A, Berube D. Efficacy and safety of formoterol Turbuhaler when added to inhaled corticosteroid treatment in children with asthma. Pediatr Pulmonol 2004;37(2):122–7.
51. Bisgaard H. Effect of long-acting beta2 agonists on exacerbation rates of asthma in children. Pediatr Pulmonol 2003;36(5):391–8.
52. Van den Berg NJ, Ossip MS, Hederos CA, et al. Salmeterol/fluticasone propionate (50/100 microg) in combination in a Diskus inhaler (Seretide) is effective and safe in children with asthma. Pediatr Pulmonol 2000;30(2): 97–105.
53. Lenney W, McKay AJ, Tudur Smith C, et al. Management of Asthma in School age Children On Therapy (MASCOT): a randomised, double-blind, placebo-controlled, parallel study of efficacy and safety. Health Technol Assess 2013; 17(4):1–218.
54. Lemanske RF Jr, Mauger DT, Sorkness CA, et al. Step-up therapy for children with uncontrolled asthma receiving inhaled corticosteroids. N Engl J Med 2010;362(11):975–85.
55. Drake KA, Torgerson DG, Gignoux CR, et al. A genome-wide association study of bronchodilator response in Latinos implicates rare variants. J Allergy Clin Immunol 2014;133(2):370–8.
56. Tcheurekdjian H, Via M, De Giacomo A, et al. ALOX5AP and LTA4H polymorphisms modify augmentation of bronchodilator responsiveness by leukotriene modifiers in Latinos. J Allergy Clin Immunol 2010;126(4):853–8.
57. Choudhry S, Que LG, Yang Z, et al. GSNO reductase and beta2-adrenergic receptor gene-gene interaction: bronchodilator responsiveness to albuterol. Pharmacogenet Genomics 2010;20(6):351–8.

58. Wong C, Jayaram L, Karalus N, et al. Azithromycin for prevention of exacerbations in non-cystic fibrosis bronchiectasis (EMBRACE): a randomised, double-blind, placebo-controlled trial. Lancet 2012;380(9842):660–7.
59. Saiman L, Marshall BC, Mayer-Hamblett N, et al. Azithromycin in patients with cystic fibrosis chronically infected with *Pseudomonas aeruginosa*: a randomized controlled trial. JAMA 2003;290(13):1749–56.
60. Equi A, Balfour-Lynn IM, Bush A, et al. Long term azithromycin in children with cystic fibrosis: a randomised, placebo-controlled crossover trial. Lancet 2002; 360(9338):978–84.
61. Clement A, Tamalet A, Leroux E, et al. Long term effects of azithromycin in patients with cystic fibrosis: a double blind, placebo controlled trial. Thorax 2006; 61(10):895–902.
62. Flotte TR, Loughlin GM. Benefits and complications of troleandomycin (TAO) in young children with steroid-dependent asthma. Pediatr Pulmonol 1991;10(3): 178–82.
63. Ball BD, Hill MR, Brenner M, et al. Effect of low-dose troleandomycin on glucocorticoid pharmacokinetics and airway hyperresponsiveness in severely asthmatic children. Ann Allergy 1990;65(1):37–45.
64. Koutsoubari I, Papaevangelou V, Konstantinou GN, et al. Effect of clarithromycin on acute asthma exacerbations in children: an open randomized study. Pediatr Allergy Immunol 2012;23(4):385–90.
65. Piacentini GL, Peroni DG, Bodini A, et al. Azithromycin reduces bronchial hyperresponsiveness and neutrophilic airway inflammation in asthmatic children: a preliminary report. Allergy Asthma Proc 2007;28(2):194–8.
66. Kraft M, Cassell GH, Pak J, et al. *Mycoplasma pneumoniae* and *Chlamydia pneumoniae* in asthma: effect of clarithromycin. Chest 2002;121(6):1782–8.
67. Chu HW, Kraft M, Rex MD, et al. Evaluation of blood vessels and edema in the airways of asthma patients: regulation with clarithromycin treatment. Chest 2001;120(2):416–22.
68. Xystrakis E, Kusumakar S, Boswell S, et al. Reversing the defective induction of IL-10-secreting regulatory T cells in glucocorticoid-resistant asthma patients. J Clin Invest 2006;116(1):146–55.
69. Wu AC, Tantisira K, Li L, et al. Effect of vitamin D and inhaled corticosteroid treatment on lung function in children. Am J Respir Crit Care Med 2012;186(6): 508–13.
70. Castro M, King TS, Kunselman SJ, et al. Effect of vitamin D3 on asthma treatment failures in adults with symptomatic asthma and lower vitamin D levels: the VIDA randomized clinical trial. JAMA 2014;311(20):2083–91.
71. Busse W, Corren J, Lanier BQ, et al. Omalizumab, anti-IgE recombinant humanized monoclonal antibody, for the treatment of severe allergic asthma. J Allergy Clin Immunol 2001;108(2):184–90.
72. Grimaldi-Bensouda L, Zureik M, Aubier M, et al. Does omalizumab make a difference to the real-life treatment of asthma exacerbations?: results from a large cohort of patients with severe uncontrolled asthma. Chest 2013;143(2): 398–405.
73. Lafeuille MH, Dean J, Zhang J, et al. Impact of omalizumab on emergency-department visits, hospitalizations, and corticosteroid use among patients with uncontrolled asthma. Ann Allergy Asthma Immunol 2012;109(1):59–64.
74. Brodlie M, McKean MC, Moss S, et al. The oral corticosteroid-sparing effect of omalizumab in children with severe asthma. Arch Dis Child 2012;97(7): 604–9.

75. Humbert M, Beasley R, Ayres J, et al. Benefits of omalizumab as add-on therapy in patients with severe persistent asthma who are inadequately controlled despite best available therapy (GINA 2002 step 4 treatment): INNOVATE. Allergy 2005;60(3):309–16.
76. Lanier B, Bridges T, Kulus M, et al. Omalizumab for the treatment of exacerbations in children with inadequately controlled allergic (IgE-mediated) asthma. J Allergy Clin Immunol 2009;124(6):1210–6.
77. Soler M, Matz J, Townley R, et al. The anti-IgE antibody omalizumab reduces exacerbations and steroid requirement in allergic asthmatics. Eur Respir J 2001; 18(2):254–61.
78. Ozgur ES, Ozge C, Ilvan A, et al. Assessment of long-term omalizumab treatment in patients with severe allergic asthma long-term omalizumab treatment in severe asthma. J Asthma 2013;50(6):687–94.
79. Busse WW, Morgan WJ, Gergen PJ, et al. Randomized trial of omalizumab (anti-IgE) for asthma in inner-city children. N Engl J Med 2011;364(11):1005–15.
80. Gevaert P, Calus L, Van Zele T, et al. Omalizumab is effective in allergic and nonallergic patients with nasal polyps and asthma. J Allergy Clin Immunol 2013;131(1):110–6.e1.
81. Tajiri T, Matsumoto H, Hiraumi H, et al. Efficacy of omalizumab in eosinophilic chronic rhinosinusitis patients with asthma. Ann Allergy Asthma Immunol 2013;110(5):387–8.
82. Oba Y, Salzman GA. Cost-effectiveness analysis of omalizumab in adults and adolescents with moderate-to-severe allergic asthma. J Allergy Clin Immunol 2004;114(2):265–9.
83. Campbell JD, Spackman DE, Sullivan SD. The costs and consequences of omalizumab in uncontrolled asthma from a USA payer perspective. Allergy 2010; 65(9):1141–8.
84. Hanania NA, Wenzel S, Rosen K, et al. Exploring the effects of omalizumab in allergic asthma: an analysis of biomarkers in the EXTRA study. Am J Respir Crit Care Med 2013;187(8):804–11.
85. Maselli DJ, Singh H, Diaz J, et al. Efficacy of omalizumab in asthmatic patients with IgE levels above 700 IU/mL: a retrospective study. Ann Allergy Asthma Immunol 2013;110(6):457–61.
86. Bousquet J, Wenzel S, Holgate S, et al. Predicting response to omalizumab, an anti-IgE antibody, in patients with allergic asthma. Chest 2004;125(4): 1378–86.
87. Wahn U, Martin C, Freeman P, et al. Relationship between pretreatment specific IgE and the response to omalizumab therapy. Allergy 2009;64(12): 1780–7.
88. Holt PG, Sly PD. Viral infections and atopy in asthma pathogenesis: new rationales for asthma prevention and treatment. Nat Med 2012;18(5):726–35.
89. Lloyd CM, Hessel EM. Functions of T cells in asthma: more than just T(H)2 cells. Nat Rev Immunol 2010;10(12):838–48.
90. Kon OM, Sihra BS, Compton CH, et al. Randomised, dose-ranging, placebo-controlled study of chimeric antibody to CD4 (keliximab) in chronic severe asthma. Lancet 1998;352(9134):1109–13.
91. Kon OM, Sihra BS, Loh LC, et al. The effects of an anti-CD4 monoclonal antibody, keliximab, on peripheral blood CD4+ T-cells in asthma. Eur Respir J 2001;18(1):45–52.
92. Corrigan CJ, Hartnell A, Kay AB. T lymphocyte activation in acute severe asthma. Lancet 1988;1(8595):1129–32.

93. Busse WW, Israel E, Nelson HS, et al. Daclizumab improves asthma control in patients with moderate to severe persistent asthma: a randomized, controlled trial. Am J Respir Crit Care Med 2008;178(10):1002–8.

94. Molfino NA, Gossage D, Kolbeck R, et al. Molecular and clinical rationale for therapeutic targeting of interleukin-5 and its receptor. Clin Exp Allergy 2012; 42(5):712–37.

95. Bel EH, Wenzel SE, Thompson PJ, et al. Oral glucocorticoid-sparing effect of mepolizumab in eosinophilic asthma. N Engl J Med 2014;371(13): 1189–97.

96. Ortega HG, Liu MC, Pavord ID, et al. Mepolizumab treatment in patients with severe eosinophilic asthma. N Engl J Med 2014;371(13):1198–207.

97. Haldar P, Brightling CE, Hargadon B, et al. Mepolizumab and exacerbations of refractory eosinophilic asthma. N Engl J Med 2009;360(10):973–84.

98. Nair P, Pizzichini MM, Kjarsgaard M, et al. Mepolizumab for prednisone-dependent asthma with sputum eosinophilia. N Engl J Med 2009;360(10): 985–93.

99. Pavord ID, Korn S, Howarth P, et al. Mepolizumab for severe eosinophilic asthma (DREAM): a multicentre, double-blind, placebo-controlled trial. Lancet 2012;380(9842):651–9.

100. Kips JC, O'Connor BJ, Langley SJ, et al. Effect of SCH55700, a humanized anti-human interleukin-5 antibody, in severe persistent asthma: a pilot study. Am J Respir Crit Care Med 2003;167(12):1655–9.

101. Castro M, Mathur S, Hargreave F, et al. Reslizumab for poorly controlled, eosinophilic asthma: a randomized, placebo-controlled study. Am J Respir Crit Care Med 2011;184(10):1125–32.

102. Steinke JW, Borish L. Th2 cytokines and asthma. Interleukin-4: its role in the pathogenesis of asthma, and targeting it for asthma treatment with interleukin-4 receptor antagonists. Respir Res 2001;2(2):66–70.

103. Wenzel S, Ford L, Pearlman D, et al. Dupilumab in persistent asthma with elevated eosinophil levels. N Engl J Med 2013;368(26):2455–66.

104. Slager RE, Otulana BA, Hawkins GA, et al. IL-4 receptor polymorphisms predict reduction in asthma exacerbations during response to an anti-IL-4 receptor alpha antagonist. J Allergy Clin Immunol 2012;130(2):516–22.e4.

105. Corren J, Lemanske RF, Hanania NA, et al. Lebrikizumab treatment in adults with asthma. N Engl J Med 2011;365(12):1088–98.

106. Sidhu SS, Yuan S, Innes AL, et al. Roles of epithelial cell-derived periostin in TGF-beta activation, collagen production, and collagen gel elasticity in asthma. Proc Natl Acad Sci U S A 2010;107(32):14170–5.

107. Piper E, Brightling C, Niven R, et al. A phase II placebo-controlled study of tralokinumab in moderate-to-severe asthma. Eur Respir J 2012;41(2):330–8.

108. Antoniu SA. Monoclonal antibodies for asthma and chronic obstructive pulmonary disease. Expert Opin Biol Ther 2013;13(2):257–68.

109. Hansbro PM, Scott GV, Essilfie AT, et al. Th2 cytokine antagonists: potential treatments for severe asthma. Expert Opin Investig Drugs 2012;22(1):49–69.

110. Temann UA, Geba GP, Rankin JA, et al. Expression of interleukin 9 in the lungs of transgenic mice causes airway inflammation, mast cell hyperplasia, and bronchial hyperresponsiveness. J Exp Med 1998;188(7):1307–20.

111. Parker JM, Oh CK, LaForce C, et al. Safety profile and clinical activity of multiple subcutaneous doses of MEDI-528, a humanized anti-interleukin-9 monoclonal antibody, in two randomized phase 2a studies in subjects with asthma. BMC Pulm Med 2011;11:14.

112. Suzukawa M, Morita H, Nambu A, et al. Epithelial cell-derived IL-25, but not Th17 cell-derived IL-17 or IL-17F, is crucial for murine asthma. J Immunol 2012;189(7):3641–52.
1,13. Saglani S, Lui S, Ullmann N, et al. IL-33 promotes airway remodeling in pediatric patients with severe steroid-resistant asthma. J Allergy Clin Immunol 2013; 132(3):676–85.e13.
114. Liu X, Li M, Wu Y, et al. Anti-IL-33 antibody treatment inhibits airway inflammation in a murine model of allergic asthma. Biochem Biophys Res Commun 2009; 386(1):181–5.
115. Howarth PH, Babu KS, Arshad HS, et al. Tumour necrosis factor (TNFalpha) as a novel therapeutic target in symptomatic corticosteroid dependent asthma. Thorax 2005;60(12):1012–8.
116. Berry MA, Hargadon B, Shelley M, et al. Evidence of a role of tumor necrosis factor alpha in refractory asthma. N Engl J Med 2006;354(7):697–708.
117. Erin EM, Leaker BR, Nicholson GC, et al. The effects of a monoclonal antibody directed against tumor necrosis factor-alpha in asthma. Am J Respir Crit Care Med 2006;174(7):753–62.
118. Wenzel SE, Barnes PJ, Bleecker ER, et al. A randomized, double-blind, placebo-controlled study of tumor necrosis factor-alpha blockade in severe persistent asthma. Am J Respir Crit Care Med 2009;179(7):549–58.
119. Humbert M, de Blay F, Garcia G, et al. Masitinib, a c-kit/PDGF receptor tyrosine kinase inhibitor, improves disease control in severe corticosteroid-dependent asthmatics. Allergy 2009;64(8):1194–201.
120. Taha RA, Laberge S, Hamid Q, et al. Increased expression of the chemoattractant cytokines eotaxin, monocyte chemotactic protein-4, and interleukin-16 in induced sputum in asthmatic patients. Chest 2001;120(2):595–601.
121. Fulkerson PC, Fischetti CA, McBride ML, et al. A central regulatory role for eosinophils and the eotaxin/CCR3 axis in chronic experimental allergic airway inflammation. Proc Natl Acad Sci U S A 2006;103(44):16418–23.
122. Joubert P, Lajoie-Kadoch S, Labonte I, et al. CCR3 expression and function in asthmatic airway smooth muscle cells. J Immunol 2005;175(4):2702–8.
123. Dent G, Hadjicharalambous C, Yoshikawa T, et al. Contribution of eotaxin-1 to eosinophil chemotactic activity of moderate and severe asthmatic sputum. Am J Respir Crit Care Med 2004;169(10):1110–7.
124. Erin EM, Williams TJ, Barnes PJ, et al. Eotaxin receptor (CCR3) antagonism in asthma and allergic disease. Curr Drug Targets Inflamm Allergy 2002;1(2): 201–14.
125. Nakagami Y, Kawase Y, Yonekubo K, et al. RS-1748, a novel CC chemokine receptor 4 antagonist, inhibits ovalbumin-induced airway inflammation in guinea pigs. Biol Pharm Bull 2010;33(6):1067–9.
126. Huffaker MF, Phipatanakul W. Utility of the Asthma Predictive Index in predicting childhood asthma and identifying disease-modifying interventions. Ann Allergy Asthma Immunol 2014;112(3):188–90.
127. Murray CS, Poletti G, Kebadze T, et al. Study of modifiable risk factors for asthma exacerbations: virus infection and allergen exposure increase the risk of asthma hospital admissions in children. Thorax 2006;61(5):376–82.
128. Illi S, von Mutius E, Lau S, et al. Perennial allergen sensitisation early in life and chronic asthma in children: a birth cohort study. Lancet 2006;368(9537):763–70.
129. Morgan WJ, Crain EF, Gruchalla RS, et al. Results of a home-based environmental intervention among urban children with asthma. N Engl J Med 2004; 351(11):1068–80.

130. Jacobsen L, Niggemann B, Dreborg S, et al. Specific immunotherapy has long-term preventive effect of seasonal and perennial asthma: 10-year follow-up on the PAT study. Allergy 2007;62(8):943–8.

131. Jacobsen L. Preventive aspects of immunotherapy: prevention for children at risk of developing asthma. Ann Allergy Asthma Immunol 2001;87(1 Suppl 1):43–6.

132. Marogna M, Tomassetti D, Bernasconi A, et al. Preventive effects of sublingual immunotherapy in childhood: an open randomized controlled study. Ann Allergy Asthma Immunol 2008;101(2):206–11.

133. De Castro G, Zicari AM, Indinnimeo L, et al. Efficacy of sublingual specific immunotherapy on allergic asthma and rhinitis in children's real life. Eur Rev Med Pharmacol Sci 2013;17(16):2225–31.

134. Kim JM, Lin SY, Suarez-Cuervo C, et al. Allergen-specific immunotherapy for pediatric asthma and rhinoconjunctivitis: a systematic review. Pediatrics 2013; 131(6):1155–67.

135. Lin SY, Erekosima N, Kim JM, et al. Sublingual immunotherapy for the treatment of allergic rhinoconjunctivitis and asthma: a systematic review. JAMA 2013; 309(12):1278–88.

136. Holt PG, Sly PD, Sampson HA, et al. Prophylactic use of sublingual allergen immunotherapy in high-risk children: a pilot study. J Allergy Clin Immunol 2013;132(4):991–3 e1.

137. Stensballe LG, Simonsen JB, Thomsen SF, et al. The causal direction in the association between respiratory syncytial virus hospitalization and asthma. J Allergy Clin Immunol 2009;123(1):131–7.e1.

138. Henderson J, Hilliard TN, Sherriff A, et al. Hospitalization for RSV bronchiolitis before 12 months of age and subsequent asthma, atopy and wheeze: a longitudinal birth cohort study. Pediatr Allergy Immunol 2005;16(5):386–92.

139. Bacharier LB, Cohen R, Schweiger T, et al. Determinants of asthma after severe respiratory syncytial virus bronchiolitis. J Allergy Clin Immunol 2012;130(1): 91–100.e3.

140. Stein RT, Sherrill D, Morgan WJ, et al. Respiratory syncytial virus in early life and risk of wheeze and allergy by age 13 years. Lancet 1999;354(9178):541–5.

141. Sigurs N, Aljassim F, Kjellman B, et al. Asthma and allergy patterns over 18 years after severe RSV bronchiolitis in the first year of life. Thorax 2010; 65(12):1045–52.

142. Simoes EA, Groothuis JR, Carbonell-Estrany X, et al. Palivizumab prophylaxis, respiratory syncytial virus, and subsequent recurrent wheezing. J Pediatr 2007;151(1):34–42.e1.

143. Blanken MO, Rovers MM, Molenaar JM, et al. Respiratory syncytial virus and recurrent wheeze in healthy preterm infants. N Engl J Med 2013;368(19):1791–9.

144. Azad MB, Coneys JG, Kozyrskyj AL, et al. Probiotic supplementation during pregnancy or infancy for the prevention of asthma and wheeze: systematic review and meta-analysis. BMJ 2013;347:f6471.

145. Rose MA, Stieglitz F, Koksal A, et al. Efficacy of probiotic Lactobacillus GG on allergic sensitization and asthma in infants at risk. Clin Exp Allergy 2010; 40(9):1398–405.

146. van der Aa LB, van Aalderen WM, Heymans HS, et al. Synbiotics prevent asthma-like symptoms in infants with atopic dermatitis. Allergy 2011;66(2):170–7.

147. Razi CH, Harmanci K, Abaci A, et al. The immunostimulant OM-85 BV prevents wheezing attacks in preschool children. J Allergy Clin Immunol 2010;126(4): 763–9.

Eosinophilic Esophagitis

Seema S. Aceves, MD, PhD

KEYWORDS

- Eosinophilic esophagitis • Pathogenesis • Clinical features • Treatment options
- Fibrosis • Remodeling

KEY POINTS

- Eosinophilic esophagitis (EoE) is a clinicopathologic disease of increasing prevalence in adults and children.
- EoE is a chronic disease and as such its prevalence will continue to rise.
- Antigen triggers drive eosinophilic and T helper cell type 2 inflammation, resulting in subepithelial fibrosis; this esophageal remodeling is the likely underlying pathogenesis for complications.
- Management strategies include dietary antigen elimination and topical corticosteroids.
- Long-term therapy and repeated endoscopy are needed in most subjects so consideration must be given to maintenance regimens and side effects.

INTRODUCTION

Eosinophilic esophagitis (EoE) is a chronic, antigen-mediated immune disease leading to esophageal stricture and dysmotility.[1,2] EoE is a clinicopathologic diagnosis that requires endoscopy with biopsy that demonstrates more than 15 eosinophils per high power field.[1] Other causes of esophageal eosinophilia including acid-induced eosinophilia, drug reaction, hypereosinophilic syndrome, infection, and celiac disease, and must be ruled out before making a diagnosis of primary EoE.[1,3–7]

Complications of EoE include stricture formation and adult studies clearly demonstrate that the absence of inflammatory control leads to progressive fibrostenosis with reduced esophageal compliance, increased esophageal rigidity, and risk of food impactions.[8–11] Symptoms in adults, adolescents, and children with longstanding or difficult-to-control EoE include dysphagia; younger children have vomiting, poor appetite, poor weight gain, and abdominal pain.[1,12] The mechanisms of fibrostenosis lie in esophageal remodeling with epithelial–mesenchymal transformation,[13] increased collagen and fibronectin deposition,[14,15] subepithelial fibrosis, inflammation and angiogenesis,[14,16] and altered smooth muscle function.[15,17]

Funding Sources: NIH/NIAID AI 092135, DOD FA100044.
Department of Pediatrics and Medicine, Division of Allergy and Immunology, Center for Infection, Inflammation, and Immunology, 9500 Gilman Drive, MC-0760, La Jolla, CA 92093, USA
E-mail address: saceves@ucsd.edu

Immunol Allergy Clin N Am 35 (2015) 145–159
http://dx.doi.org/10.1016/j.iac.2014.09.007
0889-8561/15/$ – see front matter © 2015 Elsevier Inc. All rights reserved.

This review describes the clinical features, treatment options, epidemiology, and pathogenesis of EoE in children and adults.

CLINICAL FEATURES

The EoE population is clinically allergic in multiple end organs.[1] Up to 70% of subjects have asthma, 4% to 75% have allergic rhinitis, up to 5% to 43% have reported food allergies with anaphylaxis, and more than 80% have sensitization to foods using serum, skin prick, or atopy patch tests to foods.[1] This high predisposition to other allergic diatheses must be considered during disease management. Symptoms of EoE shift with age—the youngest children have subjective symptoms of vomiting, poor appetite, and poor growth; older children complain of abdominal pain; and adolescents and adults complain mainly of dysphagia.[1,18] Dysphagia is the single most common reason for endoscopy in EoE adults and EoE accounts for 46% to 63% of subjects who are evaluated for food impactions.[19] Although EoE can be diagnosed at any age, it is most common in a younger population (<50 years old).[19]

EoE is a male-predominant disease.[1] This has been recapitulated in multiple studies in both children and adults. In addition, EoE is more commonly found in the Caucasian population.[19] Whether this is a referral or socioeconomic bias remains to be fully explored, but current studies are consistent in showing that the majority of EoE subjects are white males.[19] However, EoE can affect all ethnicities and limited studies in African Americans demonstrate that younger age, eczema, and failure to thrive may be more common in black as opposed to white EoE subjects.[19–22]

Current studies in adults clearly show that EoE is a stricturing disease with food impaction risk that increases proportionally with esophageal rigidity and stricture risk that doubles with each decade of untreated inflammation.[8–10] Whereas 17% of subjects with 2 years of EoE duration have strictures, 71% of subjects with 20 years of EoE duration have strictures.[8] This point is particularly salient when considering EoE management in children and begs the question of whether keeping sustained control of inflammation will obviate esophageal narrowing, strictures, or both. In addition, it will be important to understand the degree of inflammatory control that is required to diminish stricture risk.

EPIDEMIOLOGY, GENETICS, AND ANTIGENIC TRIGGERS

Like other allergic disorders, EoE seems to have an etiology that involves gene–environment interactions. Because EoE is a chronic disease that relapses when treatment is removed, it is not surprising that population-based studies show that the prevalence of EoE is increasing with current estimates of up to 1 per 1000.[18,19,23–26] The prevalence seems to increase until 35 to 45 years of age, at which time the prevalence begins to decrease. It is possible that this age shift may not have longevity if the incidence of this chronic disorder continues to rise. The incidence does seem to be on the rise and does not seem to be owing merely to increased recognition. Estimated incidences are 1.3 to 12.8 per 100,000 in children and adults in the United States and Europe.[19] The observed rise in incidence would certainly align with that seen in other allergic disorders such as immunoglobulin (Ig)E-mediated food allergy.

Current epidemiologic studies in EoE suggest that there are environmental risk factors, although none except aeroallergens have been studied in mechanistic detail.[19] Aeroallergens including pollens have been shown to cause EoE both in human subjects and in animal models. Some studies demonstrate that EoE diagnosis and complications can have seasonality.[27–31] Interestingly, the prevalence of esophageal eosinophilia varies by climate zone with more EoE in arid, cold climates.[32] In addition, epidemiologic association studies show that antibiotic use, prematurity, nonexclusive breast feeding, and Caesarian section tend to be associated with increased EoE rates.[19,33] In contrast, *Helicobacter pylori* infection was associated with lower rates of esophageal eosinophilia, which may suggest that infections could be protective for EoE.[34]

Given the recent increase in EoE, it is unlikely that classical genetics are the explanation and the role of epigenetic changes in EoE remains to be studied. Certainly, EoE risk factors include those that are associated with atopy in general, including polymorphisms in thymic stromal lymphopoeitin and its receptor, which is located on the Y chromosome.[35,36] A functional single nucleotide polymorphism in the transforming growth factor (TGF)β1 gene seems to associate with EoE that is more difficult to treat.[37]

EoE triggers have been definitively proven using both animal models and human studies. Aeroallergens including dust mites, molds, and pollens induce EoE.[31,38,39] Ovalbumin (egg protein) is sufficient to drive murine EoE, as is peanut antigen.[40–42] Human elimination and re-introduction diets have shown that milk and wheat are the most common antigenic triggers, as are egg, soy, meats, grains, and to lesser degrees, peanuts/tree nuts, fish, and shellfish.

PATHOPHYSIOLOGY
Inflammatory Cells and Interleukins

Like many eosinophil-associated diseases, EoE has a predominantly T helper cell type 2 inflammatory profile. Interleukin (IL)-13 is a master regulator of EoE and can affect the function of multiple esophageal cell types, including epithelial cells and fibroblasts.[43–45] Epithelial cells increase production of eotaxin-3 and fibroblasts induce periostin in response to IL-13 treatment.[45] Clinical therapeutic trials using anti–IL-13 have been recently completed, but the results have not yet been published.

IL-5 is an eosinophiliopoeitic IL that is increased in adult and pediatric EoE subjects.[46–48] Although likely to be important in EoE pathogenesis, isolated blockade of IL-5 using humanized anti–IL-5 antibodies was not sufficient to cause EoE remission in most patients.[49,50] Although esophageal eosinophil counts were decreased after anti–IL-5, symptoms did not change.[49,50] A few pediatric subjects continue on anti–IL-5 on a compassionate use basis.

Innate Immune Cells

Eosinophils seem to be integral to EoE disease pathogenesis.[44,48,51] Eosinophil products such as TGF-β1 can increase gene expression of collagen and fibronectin in the esophagus.[15] Animal models that have increased IL-13 expression have a propensity toward food impaction and stricture.[51] This predilection is mitigated by eosinophil deficiency, demonstrating that eosinophils are an important driving force for fibrosis and strictures.[51] Similarly, basophil-deficient mice are protected from experimental EoE and food impactions.[52]

Although defined by the presence of eosinophils, there is a significant degree of noneosinophilic inflammation in the EoE esophagus. Mast cells are found in abundance both in the epithelium, subepithelium, and muscularis mucosa in EoE.[17,53–57] In addition, autopsy reports find increased levels of mast cells through the full thickness of the esophagus.[58] Unlike eosinophil-deficient mice, mast cell–deficient mice are not protected from strictures.[51] They do, however, have decreased smooth muscle proliferation, as well as decreased dysmotility, indicating that mast cells affect esophageal motor function.[51]

The mechanisms by which inflammatory cells affect esophageal motility are beginning to be elucidated. Eosinophil granule products such as major basic protein (MBP) can alter esophageal smooth muscle function in a model that relies on neuron-mediated contraction.[15] Mast cell and eosinophils both make TGF-β1, which can directly alter the contraction of collagen gels impregnated with esophageal smooth muscle cells.[17,59] Recently, this has been demonstrated to rely on the expression of phospholamban (PLN), a sarcoplasmic reticulum protein that regulates calcium flux.[59] Although biopsies from control subjects do not express PLN, EoE esophageal smooth muscle expresses PLN. Inhibiting PLN gene expression and signals through TGF-β receptor I both significantly decrease esophageal smooth muscle contraction in response to TGF-β1.[59]

In the context of innate immunity, recent studies have shown increased messenger RNA for CXCL16, CD1d, and va23, consistent with increased numbers of invariant natural killer T (iNKT) cells. Studies in murine models show that iNKT are necessary for EoE.[60] Human studies also demonstrate that iNKT cells are present at elevated levels in the esophagus but at decreased levels in the peripheral blood of pediatric EoE subjects. These iNKT cells proliferate in the presence of milk sphingolipid, thereby providing a potential mechanism by which milk could initiate or propagate esophageal inflammation.[61] IL-15 is elevated in EoE and may be important for iNKT regulation.[62,63]

Adaptive Immune Cells

Allergic inflammation relies on both innate and adaptive immunity. In general, T-cell phenotypes in EoE esophagi have not been well characterized. However, reports from multiple groups demonstrate that there are increased numbers of CD3$^+$, CD8$^+$, and CD45RO$^+$ cells the EoE esophagus.[64,65] Animal models show that CD4$^+$ cells are required for EoE instigation.[66] Food-antigen–specific CD4$_+$ cells that produce IL-5 are present at elevated levels in the periphery of patients with eosinophilic gastroenteritis compared with subjects who have anaphylaxis whose cells produce mainly IL-4.[67] In vitro, IL-5–producing cells require long-term culture, chronic antigen exposure, and have chromatin changes at the IL-5 gene.[68] These data suggest that chronic disease that involve food antigens, such as EoE, may drive T cells toward an IL-5–producing phenotype and could explain the delayed hypersensitivity mechanism in EoE.

In terms of T cells and shifts in the distinct mechanisms that underlie anaphylaxis versus EoE, it is interesting that subjects with IgE-mediated anaphylaxis can have EoE onset while undergoing oral desensitization trials.[69,70] This observation suggests that the reaction to foods can shift from being IgE mediated to being cell mediated in the same person. Indeed, this has now been clearly documented in children with milk allergy who outgrew their milk anaphylaxis but later developed EoE owing to milk.[71] As such, new-onset abdominal pain, dysphagia, or reflux symptoms in a subject with a history of food allergies should trigger a consideration of EoE.

Recently increased TGF-β signaling has been linked with allergies, including food allergies and EoE in people with the connective tissue disorder, Loeys–Dietz syndrome.[72] Loeys–Dietz syndrome is caused by mutations in genes encoding the TGF-β receptor, which allows for increased signals via TGF-β1. In Loeys–Dietz syndrome, FoxP3-positive regulatory T cells seem to enhance, rather than suppress, allergic inflammation by producing T helper cell type 2 cytokines, including IL-13.[72] Interestingly, a recent link between connective tissue disorders and EoE has been made, specifically with Marfan syndrome, which also involves a gain of function in TGF-β1 signals via mutations in the fibrillin gene.[73] Given the increased levels of TGF-β1 in EoE, it is intriguing to speculate that one source of TGF-β1 could be activated regulatory T cells in the EoE esophagus.

THE ROLE OF IMMUNOGLOBULIN E IN EOSINOPHILIC ESOPHAGITIS

Murine models have shown that EoE does not rely on B cells.[66,74] However, whether the presence of IgE can propagate or exacerbate disease is not clear. There are increased numbers of IgE receptor–positive cells in the esophagus of EoE subjects, consistent with the observation that there are both mast cells and basophils present at higher numbers in EoE.[52,75] In addition, there is an abundance of B cells in the lamina propria in EoE and increased expression of class switch genes.[76] Consistent with the concept that IgE is dispensable for EoE pathogenesis, treatment with omalizumab does not alter esophageal eosinophilia in adults.[74]

The role of cross-reactive IgE in EoE is beginning to be studied. A study of European adult EoE subjects demonstrated that 20% were sensitized to *Candida* (all had been treated successfully with esophageal topical corticosteroids (TCS) and none had evidence of superinfection).[77] In addition, a significant number of subjects had sensitization to cross-reacting plant allergens, with profilins being the most common, followed by pathogenesis related 10 proteins and lipid transfer proteins. Interestingly, profilin sensitization was associated with dysphagia owing to rice and bread.[77]

PATHOGENESIS OF REMODELING

The pathogenesis of EoE complications, including fibrosis and strictures, relies on esophageal tissue remodeling. It was initially observed that adult EoE subjects had increased fibrosis and the potential mechanisms that drive remodeling have been elucidated more recently.[2] TGF-β1 can have multiple effects on esophageal cell function. Studies using human epithelial cells show that TGF-β1 induces epithelial mesenchymal transformation with increased vimentin expression.[13] The degree of epithelial mesenchymal transformation correlates positively with both TGF-β1 expression and with eosinophil numbers. Because mast cells and eosinophils make TGF-β1,[14,17] this suggests a mechanism whereby infiltrating inflammatory cells could induce changes in epithelial cell phenotype.

TGF-β1 can also have profibrotic effects on esophageal fibroblasts. Treatment of fibroblasts with EoE esophageal lysates induces expression of fibronectin and collagen, an effect that can be blocked using a TGF-β1–neutralizing antibody.[15] TGF-β1 can also directly induce the expression of profibrotic genes, such as fibronectin, collagen I, periostin, and smooth muscle actin in EoE fibroblasts.[15,78] Murine models have shown that signals through Smad2/3, the canonical TGF-β1 pathway, are important in esophageal fibrosis and animals that lack Smad3 are largely protected from EoE-associated fibrosis.[40] In addition to effects on gene expression, TGF-β1 can change cellular function. TGF-β1 treatment of collagen gels impregnated with EoE fibroblasts or primary esophageal smooth muscle causes transcription-dependent contraction.[17,59] This effect relies on TGF-β receptor I signals and PLN, and it possible that such morphologic changes in EoE fibroblasts are akin to those seen in the tissue contractures associated with wound healing.[59]

TGF-β1 expression and fibrosis are increased in children with EoE and can decrease after successful therapy with TCS and/or dietary elimination.[37,79,80] However, adult studies have had more variable results, with some studies demonstrating elevated TGF-β1 that resolves and others showing variability in TGF-β1 expression and its resolution.[81,82] It is important to note that studies that show more variable expression have relied on assessing messenger RNA rather than protein.[81] Because TGF-β1 is a complex molecule that associates with 2 latency peptides, interacts with the extracellular matrix, and dimerizes before initiating signaling, the levels of messenger RNA may not reflect TGF-β1 protein levels or activity. In contrast with pediatric studies, some adult studies have demonstrated increased levels of chemokine ligand 18, a profibrotic factor whose receptor, chemokine receptor-8, has been recently identified and also shown to be expressed at elevated levels in EoE.[83]

TREATMENT OPTIONS
Acute Management

As a new disease with no therapies approved by the US Food and Drug Administration[84] and for which we continue to have more questions than answers, the initial diagnosis of EoE can be overwhelming. As such, any new EoE diagnosis must be accompanied by a significant amount of education on the natural history of the disease, the likely need for chronic therapy, and the potential therapeutic options and their side effects.

First-line management for esophageal eosinophilia should include confirmation of the clinicopathologic diagnosis of EoE. This includes a careful medication history for agents such as anticonvulsants, ruling out infection and other systemic diseases that can cause esophageal eosinophilia, review of the upper (and lower if available) intestinal biopsies to ascertain for other gastrointestinal diseases that can be associated with esophageal eosinophilia such as inflammatory bowel and celiac disease, and treatment of gastroesophageal reflux disease to discern primary EoE from acid-induced or proton pump inhibitor (PPI)–responsive eosinophilia.[1] The interplay between acid and EoE is particularly complex and it seems that acid alone can initiate a robust, panesophageal eosinophilia with clinical and endoscopic features of EoE in some people.[85] Indeed, treatment with twice daily PPI therapy resolves all of the clinicopathologic features in these subjects, leading to the current nomenclature of PPI-responsive esophageal eosinophilia.[1] Whether this particular entity represents pure acid-induced eosinophilia is not clear. Indeed, it seems that a subset of these subjects may represent a subphenotype of EoE with PPI response being transient in some subjects.[65,86]

Once a diagnosis has been established, optimal control of all other atopic diatheses is recommended.[1] This includes skin prick testing for aeroallergen triggers with a thought to whether EoE could be a seasonal manifestation of pollen allergy; pulmonary function testing to control underlying asthma; and management of eczema.[1] Information regarding aeroallergen sensitization can also be important when designing management strategies. For example, a recent case report demonstrated successful EoE therapy using specific immunotherapy for house dust mites.[87] In addition, if pollen sensitization is playing a role in EoE flares, then certain seasons may warrant more aggressive management and/or consideration of pollen load when analyzing biopsy results demonstrating esophageal eosinophilia.[27,28,30,31] Skin prick testing for foods should be considered, especially if elimination diet will be utilized. The best approach to EoE management is multidisciplinary that involves a gastroenterologist, allergist/immunologist, dietician, and nurse/clinical coordinator.

Successful therapeutic options for EoE management include esophageal TCS or diet. TCS therapy can consist of fluticasone or ciclesonide puffed and swallowed without a spacer. Doses of 440 μg of fluticasone twice daily induced remission in 50% of pediatric subjects and 880 μg of fluticasone twice daily induced remission in 65% of subjects (pediatric + adult subjects).[53,88] Oral viscous budesonide 1 to 2 mg combined with a PPI demonstrated 87% efficacy in pediatric subjects; oral budesonide suspension 1.4 to 2 mg in the absence of PPI resulted in 53% efficacy at medium dose in pediatric subjects.[89,90] Adult subjects treated with oral viscous budesonide had greater response rates than those given nebulized budesonide in a

US trial.[91] In contrast, large particle nebulization (not available in the United States) was successful in 72% of adult subjects.[82] As such, esophageal TCS can be considered an effective therapy for EoE in adults and children. The most common side effect of short-term therapy is esophageal candidiasis.[1]

Dietary elimination is also highly effective in EoE. Other than prednisone, the single most effective therapy in EoE is amino acid–based formula, which has remission rates of greater than 90%.[92–95] However, owing to its unpalatable nature and the difficulty in consuming a liquid diet in the long term, it is a difficult maintenance regimen for the majority of subjects.[95] Fortunately, directed elimination diet is also successful in EoE with remission rates of 50% to 70%.[93,94,96–100]

Directed elimination diet can be done using a targeted diet that is based on skin prick testing and atopy patch testing to foods. Although this has been successful in creating a targeted elimination diet in children at 2 different centers, the adult data have not shown the same success rate.[93,94,101,102] Reported negative predictive values (overall 92%) exceed positive predictive values and overall success rates for skin prick testing/atopy patch testing–based diets are on average 44%.[93] Success rates can be substantially improved when skin prick testing/atopy patch testing–based diets are combined with empiric milk elimination, which has poor predictive value on its own.[93]

Another successful route of elimination diet is an empiric approach that eliminates commonly ingested foods. Specifically, milk, egg, soy, wheat, peanuts/tree nuts, and fish/shellfish are avoided in the US population, leading to remission rates of 70% in adults and children in prospective and retrospective clinical trials, respectively.[96,99] Ongoing trials will help to determine the success rates of four and fewer food elimination diets. Current limited studies suggest that pediatric subjects may tolerate milk baked into foods even when milk is an instigator for their EoE.[103] In addition, a single adult study demonstrated that up to 400 mL of a partially hydrolyzed milk-based formula is tolerated by 88% of subjects with milk-induced EoE.[104]

Last, acute management of EoE can involve mechanical removal of a food bolus. Indeed, EoE is among the leading causes of emergency room visits for food impaction.[19,105] Acute complications of food impactions and strictures include spontaneous or iatrogenic esophageal rupture.[106–108] In addition, esophageal dilation in EoE is frequently accompanied by linear rents, bleeding, and postoperative chest pain.[1]

Maintenance Therapy

In general, there is a paucity of data on maintenance regimens for EoE. It is clear that EoE is a chronic disease and that addition of a triggering antigen or removal of esophageal TCS results in disease recurrence.[1,109] A prospective, 50-week maintenance trial in adult subjects successfully treated with large particle nebulized budesonide demonstrated that lowering the dose from 2 to 0.5 mg was not successful in maintaining disease remission.[110] Although EoE recurred more slowly in those subjects treated with budesonide compared with placebo, both groups had recrudescence of significant esophageal eosinophilia. In addition, both groups had recurrence of fibrosis, albeit significantly less in the budesonide-treated group. As such, chronic therapy is required and a 4-fold decrease in the dose will not maintain initial control on esophageal eosinophilia or fibrosis.

Recently, a high dose followed by dose reduction trial was reported in pediatric and adult EoE subjects.[88] Lowering the dose of fluticasone from an initial dose of 1760 to 880 μg in subjects who attained remission resulted in continued EoE control for an additional 3 months (93% of subjects, 73% with continued complete remission,

20% with partial remission).[88] As such, it is possible that reducing the dose by one half but not by one quarter could be a successful maintenance regimen in EoE. Interestingly, recent studies in adults show that treatment with TCS associates with decreased risk of food impactions.[111]

In terms of dietary elimination, foods are usually reintroduced 1 by 1 with repeat endoscopy with biopsy to prove retained inflammatory control.[1] As such, multiple endoscopies can be required to find a "safe" diet. The more foods that are eliminated initially, the greater the number of endoscopies required. Generally foods are avoided for 6 to 8 weeks and then reintroduced for about 8 weeks before repeat biopsy. In children, it has been reported that only 8% developed tolerance to some or all of their avoided foods over 1 to 14 years.[112]

The need for chronic treatment warrants that consideration be given to the best therapeutic strategy and the side effects that accompany each.[8,9,19,109] Height and weight should be checked to monitor growth velocity, both for nutritional and TCS side effect reasons.[113,114] It is reasonable to consider assessing the effects of both esophageal TCS and PPI on bone mineralization using bone density studies and to assess the absorption of esophageal TCS by checking cortisol levels.[115–117] With regard to elimination diets, nutritional guidance should be instituted to gauge whether there is adequate caloric intake and proper vitamin and mineral consumption. Because foods are being eliminated in a population that is allergic and has increased rates of anaphylaxis and food sensitization, the treating clinician should consider the possibility of loss of tolerance to food to which a subject is sensitized.[1,118] The onset of immediate hypersensitivity reactions upon food avoidance has been well documented in patients with eczema.[119–121] Last, the data on the effects of repeated anesthesia on growth and development in otherwise healthy children are limited, but the discovery and utilization of less invasive techniques for EoE management would have significant clinical impact.[122,123]

CONTROVERSIES AND SUMMARY

The controversies in EoE are numerous and a complete discussion is beyond the scope of this article.[124] The numbers of eosinophils required to make the diagnosis of EoE is based on expert opinion rather than experimental evidence and, as such, the degree of inflammatory control that is required to avoid disease complications is not clear. In addition, we are learning the mechanisms whereby histologic and molecular remodeling drive stricture formation. Validated symptom tool for EoE assessment are under generation, but the alignment of symptoms and disease severity remain unclear.[125,126] Currently, there are no US Food and Drug Administration–approved EoE therapies and the role of combination therapies that spare chronic esophageal TCS or dietary elimination have not been explored.[84] Last, EoE phenotypes, including PPI-responsive esophageal eosinophilia and fibrostenotic EoE, need further elucidation both clinically and molecularly.

Despite these controversies, what is clear is that EoE is food antigen triggered, chronic disease of adults and children that is increasing in its prevalence. The diagnosis must be made using a clinicopathologic template that considers the symptoms, and endoscopic and clinical features. In addition, consideration must be given to the interventions that were utilized at the time of endoscopy, especially treatment with PPI and/or elimination diets. The pollen season in the context of aeroallergen sensitization should also be considered and patients should be treated to control inflammation and decrease the complications of food impactions and strictures.

REFERENCES

1. Liacouras CA, Furuta GT, Hirano I, et al. Eosinophilic esophagitis: updated consensus recommendations for children and adults. J Allergy Clin Immunol 2011;128(1):3–20.e6 [quiz: 21–2].
2. Straumann A, Spichtin HP, Grize L, et al. Natural history of primary eosinophilic esophagitis: a follow-up of 30 adult patients for up to 11.5 years. Gastroenterology 2003;125(6):1660–9.
3. Kagalwalla AF, Shah A, Ritz S, et al. Cow's milk protein-induced eosinophilic esophagitis in a child with gluten-sensitive enteropathy. J Pediatr Gastroenterol Nutr 2007;44(3):386–8.
4. Leslie C, Mews C, Charles A, et al. Celiac disease and eosinophilic esophagitis: a true association. J Pediatr Gastroenterol Nutr 2010;50(4):397–9.
5. Ooi CY, Day AS, Jackson R, et al. Eosinophilic esophagitis in children with celiac disease. J Gastroenterol Hepatol 2008;23(7 Pt 1):1144–8.
6. Thompson JS, Lebwohl B, Reilly NR, et al. Increased incidence of eosinophilic esophagitis in children and adults with celiac disease. J Clin Gastroenterol 2012;46(1):e6–11.
7. Balatsinou C, Milano A, Caldarella MP, et al. Eosinophilic esophagitis is a component of the anticonvulsant hypersensitivity syndrome: description of two cases. Dig Liver Dis 2008;40(2):145–8.
8. Schoepfer AM, Safroneeva E, Bussmann C, et al. Delay in diagnosis of eosinophilic esophagitis increases risk for stricture formation, in a time-dependent manner. Gastroenterology 2013;145(6):1230–6.e1-2.
9. Dellon ES, Kim HP, Sperry SL, et al. A phenotypic analysis shows that eosinophilic esophagitis is a progressive fibrostenotic disease. Gastrointest Endosc 2013;79(4):577–85.e4.
10. Nicodeme F, Hirano I, Chen J, et al. Esophageal distensibility as a measure of disease severity in patients with eosinophilic esophagitis. Clin Gastroenterol Hepatol 2013;11(9):1101–7.e1.
11. Kwiatek MA, Hirano I, Kahrilas PJ, et al. Mechanical properties of the esophagus in eosinophilic esophagitis. Gastroenterology 2011;140(1):82–90.
12. Noel RJ, Putnam PE, Collins MH, et al. Clinical and immunopathologic effects of swallowed fluticasone for eosinophilic esophagitis. Clin Gastroenterol Hepatol 2004;2(7):568–75.
13. Kagalwalla AF, Akhtar N, Woodruff SA, et al. Eosinophilic esophagitis: epithelial mesenchymal transition contributes to esophageal remodeling and reverses with treatment. J Allergy Clin Immunol 2012;129(5):1387–96.e7.
14. Aceves SS, Newbury RO, Dohil R, et al. Esophageal remodeling in pediatric eosinophilic esophagitis. J Allergy Clin Immunol 2007;119(1):206–12.
15. Rieder F, Nonevski I, Ma J, et al. T-helper 2 cytokines, transforming growth factor beta1, and eosinophil products induce fibrogenesis and alter muscle motility in patients with eosinophilic esophagitis. Gastroenterology 2014;146(5):1266–77.e1-9.
16. Persad R, Huynh HQ, Hao L, et al. Angiogenic remodeling in pediatric EoE is associated with increased levels of VEGF-A, angiogenin, IL-8, and activation of the TNF-alpha-NFkappaB pathway. J Pediatr Gastroenterol Nutr 2012;55(3):251–60.
17. Aceves SS, Chen D, Newbury RO, et al. Mast cells infiltrate the esophageal smooth muscle in patients with eosinophilic esophagitis, express TGF-beta1, and increase esophageal smooth muscle contraction. J Allergy Clin Immunol 2010;126(6):1198–204.e4.

18. Noel RJ, Putnam PE, Rothenberg ME. Eosinophilic esophagitis. N Engl J Med 2004;351(9):940–1.
19. Dellon ES. Epidemiology of eosinophilic esophagitis. Gastroenterol Clin North Am 2014;43(2):201–18.
20. Moawad FJ, Veerappan GR, Dias JA, et al. Race may play a role in the clinical presentation of eosinophilic esophagitis. Am J Gastroenterol 2012;107(8):1263.
21. Sperry SL, Woosley JT, Shaheen NJ, et al. Influence of race and gender on the presentation of eosinophilic esophagitis. Am J Gastroenterol 2012;107(2):215–21.
22. Weiler T, Mikhail I, Singal A, et al. Racial differences in the clinical presentation of pediatric eosinophilic esophagitis. J Allergy Clin Immunol Pract 2014;2(3): 320–5.
23. Prasad GA, Alexander JA, Schleck CD, et al. Epidemiology of eosinophilic esophagitis over three decades in Olmsted County, Minnesota. Clin Gastroenterol Hepatol 2009;7(10):1055–61.
24. Hruz P, Straumann A, Bussmann C, et al. Escalating incidence of eosinophilic esophagitis: a 20-year prospective, population-based study in Olten County, Switzerland. J Allergy Clin Immunol 2011;128(6):1349–50.e5.
25. Dellon ES, Jensen ET, Martin CF, et al. Prevalence of eosinophilic esophagitis in the United States. Clin Gastroenterol Hepatol 2014;12(4):589–96.e1.
26. Spergel JM, Book WM, Mays E, et al. Variation in prevalence, diagnostic criteria, and initial management options for eosinophilic gastrointestinal diseases in the United States. J Pediatr Gastroenterol Nutr 2011;52(3):300–6.
27. Almansa C, Krishna M, Buchner AM, et al. Seasonal distribution in newly diagnosed cases of eosinophilic esophagitis in adults. Am J Gastroenterol 2009; 104(4):828–33.
28. Elitsur Y, Aswani R, Lund V, et al. Seasonal distribution and eosinophilic esophagitis: the experience in children living in rural communities. J Clin Gastroenterol 2013;47(3):287–8.
29. Onbasi K, Sin AZ, Doganavsargil B, et al. Eosinophil infiltration of the oesophageal mucosa in patients with pollen allergy during the season. Clin Exp Allergy 2005;35(11):1423–31.
30. Wang FY, Gupta SK, Fitzgerald JF. Is there a seasonal variation in the incidence or intensity of allergic eosinophilic esophagitis in newly diagnosed children? J Clin Gastroenterol 2007;41(5):451–3.
31. Fogg MI, Ruchelli E, Spergel JM. Pollen and eosinophilic esophagitis. J Allergy Clin Immunol 2003;112(4):796–7.
32. Hurrell JM, Genta RM, Dellon ES. Prevalence of esophageal eosinophilia varies by climate zone in the United States. Am J Gastroenterol 2012;107(5):698–706.
33. Jensen ET, Kappelman MD, Kim H, et al. Early life exposures as risk factors for pediatric eosinophilic esophagitis. J Pediatr Gastroenterol Nutr 2013;57(1):67–71.
34. Dellon ES, Peery AF, Shaheen NJ, et al. Inverse association of esophageal eosinophilia with Helicobacter pylori based on analysis of a US pathology database. Gastroenterology 2011;141(5):1586–92.
35. Rothenberg ME, Spergel JM, Sherrill JD, et al. Common variants at 5q22 associate with pediatric eosinophilic esophagitis. Nat Genet 2010;42(4):289–91.
36. Sherrill JD, Gao PS, Stucke EM, et al. Variants of thymic stromal lymphopoietin and its receptor associate with eosinophilic esophagitis. J Allergy Clin Immunol 2010;126(1):160–5.e3.
37. Aceves SS, Newbury RO, Chen D, et al. Resolution of remodeling in eosinophilic esophagitis correlates with epithelial response to topical corticosteroids. Allergy 2010;65(1):109–16.

38. Rayapudi M, Mavi P, Zhu X, et al. Indoor insect allergens are potent inducers of experimental eosinophilic esophagitis in mice. J Leukoc Biol 2010;88(2):337–46.
39. Mishra A, Hogan SP, Brandt EB, et al. An etiological role for aeroallergens and eosinophils in experimental esophagitis. J Clin Invest 2001;107(1):83–90.
40. Cho JY, Doshi A, Rosenthal P, et al. Smad3 deficient mice have reduced esophageal fibrosis and angiogenesis in a mouse model of egg induced eosinophilic esophagitis. J Pediatr Gastroenterol Nutr 2014;59(1):10–6.
41. Cho JY, Rosenthal P, Miller M, et al. Targeting AMCase reduces esophageal eosinophilic inflammation and remodeling in a mouse model of egg induced eosinophilic esophagitis. Int Immunopharmacol 2014;18(1):35–42.
42. Rajavelu P, Rayapudi M, Moffitt M, et al. Significance of para-esophageal lymph nodes in food or aeroallergen-induced iNKT cell-mediated experimental eosinophilic esophagitis. Am J Physiol Gastrointest Liver Physiol 2012;302(7): G645–54.
43. Blanchard C, Stucke EM, Burwinkel K, et al. Coordinate interaction between IL-13 and epithelial differentiation cluster genes in eosinophilic esophagitis. J Immunol 2010;184(7):4033–41.
44. Zuo L, Fulkerson PC, Finkelman FD, et al. IL-13 induces esophageal remodeling and gene expression by an eosinophil-independent, IL-13R alpha 2-inhibited pathway. J Immunol 2010;185(1):660–9.
45. Blanchard C, Mingler MK, Vicario M, et al. IL-13 involvement in eosinophilic esophagitis: transcriptome analysis and reversibility with glucocorticoids. J Allergy Clin Immunol 2007;120(6):1292–300.
46. Straumann A, Bauer M, Fischer B, et al. Idiopathic eosinophilic esophagitis is associated with a T(H)2-type allergic inflammatory response. J Allergy Clin Immunol 2001;108(6):954–61.
47. Mishra A, Hogan SP, Brandt EB, et al. IL-5 promotes eosinophil trafficking to the esophagus. J Immunol 2002;168(5):2464–9.
48. Mishra A, Wang M, Pemmaraju VR, et al. Esophageal remodeling develops as a consequence of tissue specific IL-5-induced eosinophilia. Gastroenterology 2008;134(1):204–14.
49. Spergel JM, Rothenberg ME, Collins MH, et al. Reslizumab in children and adolescents with eosinophilic esophagitis: results of a double-blind, randomized, placebo-controlled trial. J Allergy Clin Immunol 2012;129(2):456–63, 463.e1–e3.
50. Assa'ad AH, Gupta SK, Collins MH, et al. An antibody against IL-5 reduces numbers of esophageal intraepithelial eosinophils in children with eosinophilic esophagitis. Gastroenterology 2011;141(5):1593–604.
51. Mavi P, Rajavelu P, Rayapudi M, et al. Esophageal functional impairments in experimental eosinophilic esophagitis. Am J Physiol Gastrointest Liver Physiol 2012;302(11):G1347–55.
52. Noti M, Wojno ED, Kim BS, et al. Thymic stromal lymphopoietin-elicited basophil responses promote eosinophilic esophagitis. Nat Med 2013;19(8):1005–13.
53. Konikoff MR, Noel RJ, Blanchard C, et al. A randomized, double-blind, placebo-controlled trial of fluticasone propionate for pediatric eosinophilic esophagitis. Gastroenterology 2006;131(5):1381–91.
54. Dellon ES, Chen X, Miller CR, et al. Tryptase staining of mast cells may differentiate eosinophilic esophagitis from gastroesophageal reflux disease. Am J Gastroenterol 2011;106(2):264–71.
55. Otani IM, Anilkumar AA, Newbury RO, et al. Anti-IL-5 therapy reduces mast cell and IL-9 cell numbers in pediatric patients with eosinophilic esophagitis. J Allergy Clin Immunol 2013;131(6):1576–82.

56. Hsu Blatman KS, Gonsalves N, Hirano I, et al. Expression of mast cell-associated genes is upregulated in adult eosinophilic esophagitis and responds to steroid or dietary therapy. J Allergy Clin Immunol 2011;127(5):1307–8.e3.

57. Abonia JP, Blanchard C, Butz BB, et al. Involvement of mast cells in eosinophilic esophagitis. J Allergy Clin Immunol 2010;126(1):140–9.

58. Nicholson AG, Li D, Pastorino U, et al. Full thickness eosinophilia in oesophageal leiomyomatosis and idiopathic eosinophilic oesophagitis. A common allergic inflammatory profile? J Pathol 1997;183(2):233–6.

59. Beppu LY, Anilkumar AA, Newbury R, et al. TGF-b1–induced phospholamban expression alters esophageal smooth muscle cell contraction in patients with eosinophilic esophagitis. J Allergy Clin Immunol 2014. [Epub ahead of print].

60. Lexmond WS, Neves JF, Nurko S, et al. Involvement of the iNKT cell pathway is associated with early-onset eosinophilic esophagitis and response to allergen avoidance therapy. Am J Gastroenterol 2014;109(5):646–57.

61. Jyonouchi S, Abraham V, Orange JS, et al. Invariant natural killer T cells from children with versus without food allergy exhibit differential responsiveness to milk-derived sphingomyelin. J Allergy Clin Immunol 2011;128(1):102–9.e13.

62. Rayapudi M, Rajavelu P, Zhu X, et al. Invariant natural killer T-cell neutralization is a possible novel therapy for human eosinophilic esophagitis. Clinical & Translational Immunology 2014;3:e9.

63. Zhu X, Wang M, Mavi P, et al. Interleukin-15 expression is increased in human eosinophilic esophagitis and mediates pathogenesis in mice. Gastroenterology 2010;139(1):182–93.e7.

64. Lucendo AJ, Navarro M, Comas C, et al. Immunophenotypic characterization and quantification of the epithelial inflammatory infiltrate in eosinophilic esophagitis through stereology: an analysis of the cellular mechanisms of the disease and the immunologic capacity of the esophagus. Am J Surg Pathol 2007; 31(4):598–606.

65. Dohil R, Newbury RO, Aceves S. Transient PPI responsive esophageal eosinophilia may be a clinical sub-phenotype of pediatric eosinophilic esophagitis. Dig Dis Sci 2012;57(5):1413–9.

66. Mishra A, Schlotman J, Wang M, et al. Critical role for adaptive T cell immunity in experimental eosinophilic esophagitis in mice. J Leukoc Biol 2007;81(4): 916–24.

67. Prussin C, Lee J, Foster B. Eosinophilic gastrointestinal disease and peanut allergy are alternatively associated with IL-5+ and IL-5(−) T(H)2 responses. J Allergy Clin Immunol 2009;124(6):1326–32.e6.

68. Upadhyaya B, Yin Y, Hill BJ, et al. Hierarchical IL-5 expression defines a subpopulation of highly differentiated human Th2 cells. J Immunol 2011;187(6): 3111–20.

69. Ridolo E, De Angelis GL, Dall'aglio P. Eosinophilic esophagitis after specific oral tolerance induction for egg protein. Ann Allergy Asthma Immunol 2011;106(1): 73–4.

70. Sanchez-Garcia S, Rodriguez Del Rio P, Escudero C, et al. Possible eosinophilic esophagitis induced by milk oral immunotherapy. J Allergy Clin Immunol 2012; 129(4):1155–7.

71. Spergel JM. Natural history of cow's milk allergy. J Allergy Clin Immunol 2013; 131(3):813–4.

72. Frischmeyer-Guerrerio PA, Guerrerio AL, Oswald G, et al. TGFbeta receptor mutations impose a strong predisposition for human allergic disease. Sci Transl Med 2013;5(195):195ra194.

73. Abonia JP, Wen T, Stucke EM, et al. High prevalence of eosinophilic esophagitis in patients with inherited connective tissue disorders. J Allergy Clin Immunol 2013;132(2):378–86.
74. Clayton F, Fang JC, Gleich GJ, et al. Eosinophilic esophagitis in adults is associated with IgG4 and not mediated by IgE. Gastroenterology 2014;147(3):602–9.
75. Yen EH, Hornick JL, Dehlink E, et al. Comparative analysis of FcepsilonRI expression patterns in patients with eosinophilic and reflux esophagitis. J Pediatr Gastroenterol Nutr 2010;51(5):584–92.
76. Vicario M, Blanchard C, Stringer KF, et al. Local B cells and IgE production in the oesophageal mucosa in eosinophilic oesophagitis. Gut 2010;59(1):12–20.
77. Simon D, Straumann A, Dahinden C, et al. Frequent sensitization to Candida albicans and profilins in adult eosinophilic esophagitis. Allergy 2013;68(7):945–8.
78. Blanchard C, Mingler MK, McBride M, et al. Periostin facilitates eosinophil tissue infiltration in allergic lung and esophageal responses. Mucosal Immunol 2008;1(4):289–96.
79. Lieberman JA, Morotti RA, Konstantinou GN, et al. Dietary therapy can reverse esophageal subepithelial fibrosis in patients with eosinophilic esophagitis: a historical cohort. Allergy 2012;67(10):1299–307.
80. Abu-Sultaneh SM, Durst P, Maynard V, et al. Fluticasone and food allergen elimination reverse sub-epithelial fibrosis in children with eosinophilic esophagitis. Dig Dis Sci 2011;56(1):97–102.
81. Lucendo AJ, Arias A, De Rezende LC, et al. Subepithelial collagen deposition, profibrogenic cytokine gene expression, and changes after prolonged fluticasone propionate treatment in adult eosinophilic esophagitis: a prospective study. J Allergy Clin Immunol 2011;128(5):1037–46.
82. Straumann A, Conus S, Degen L, et al. Budesonide is effective in adolescent and adult patients with active eosinophilic esophagitis. Gastroenterology 2010;139(5):1526–37, 1537.e1.
83. Islam SA, Ling MF, Leung J, et al. Identification of human CCR8 as a CCL18 receptor. J Exp Med 2013;210(10):1889–98.
84. Rothenberg ME, Aceves S, Bonis PA, et al. Working with the US Food and Drug Administration: progress and timelines in understanding and treating patients with eosinophilic esophagitis. J Allergy Clin Immunol 2012;130(3):617–9.
85. Molina-Infante J, Zamorano J. Distinguishing eosinophilic esophagitis from gastroesophageal reflux disease upon PPI refractoriness: what about PPI-responsive esophageal eosinophilia? Digestion 2012;85(3):210.
86. Schroeder S, Capocelli KE, Masterson JC, et al. Effect of proton pump inhibitor on esophageal eosinophilia. J Pediatr Gastroenterol Nutr 2013;56(2):166–72.
87. Ramirez RM, Jacobs RL. Eosinophilic esophagitis treated with immunotherapy to dust mites. J Allergy Clin Immunol 2013;132(2):503–4.
88. Butz BK, Wen T, Gleich GJ, et al. Efficacy, dose reduction, and resistance to high-dose fluticasone in patients with eosinophilic esophagitis. Gastroenterology 2014;147(2):324–33.e5.
89. Dohil R, Newbury R, Fox L, et al. Oral viscous budesonide is effective in children with eosinophilic esophagitis in a randomized, placebo-controlled trial. Gastroenterology 2010;139(2):418–29.
90. Gupta SK, Vitanza JM, Collins MH. Efficacy and safety of oral budesonide suspension in pediatric patients with eosinophilic esophagitis. Clin Gastroenterol Hepatol 2014. [Epub ahead of print].

91. Dellon ES, Sheikh A, Speck O, et al. Viscous topical is more effective than nebulized steroid therapy for patients with eosinophilic esophagitis. Gastroenterology 2012;143(2):321–4.e1.
92. Markowitz JE, Spergel JM, Ruchelli E, et al. Elemental diet is an effective treatment for eosinophilic esophagitis in children and adolescents. Am J Gastroenterol 2003;98(4):777–82.
93. Spergel JM, Brown-Whitehorn TF, Cianferoni A, et al. Identification of causative foods in children with eosinophilic esophagitis treated with an elimination diet. J Allergy Clin Immunol 2012;130(2):461–7.e5.
94. Henderson CJ, Abonia JP, King EC, et al. Comparative dietary therapy effectiveness in remission of pediatric eosinophilic esophagitis. J Allergy Clin Immunol 2012;129(6):1570–8.
95. Peterson KA, Byrne KR, Vinson LA, et al. Elemental diet induces histologic response in adult eosinophilic esophagitis. Am J Gastroenterol 2013;108(5):759–66.
96. Kagalwalla AF, Sentongo TA, Ritz S, et al. Effect of six-food elimination diet on clinical and histologic outcomes in eosinophilic esophagitis. Clin Gastroenterol Hepatol 2006;4(9):1097–102.
97. Kagalwalla AF, Amsden K, Shah A, et al. Cow's milk elimination: a novel dietary approach to treat eosinophilic esophagitis. J Pediatr Gastroenterol Nutr 2012;55(6):711–6.
98. Kagalwalla AF, Shah A, Li BU, et al. Identification of specific foods responsible for inflammation in children with eosinophilic esophagitis successfully treated with empiric elimination diet. J Pediatr Gastroenterol Nutr 2011;53(2):145–9.
99. Gonsalves N, Yang GY, Doerfler B, et al. Elimination diet effectively treats eosinophilic esophagitis in adults; food reintroduction identifies causative factors. Gastroenterology 2012;142(7):1451–9.e1.
100. Lucendo AJ, Arias A, Gonzalez-Cervera J, et al. Empiric 6-food elimination diet induced and maintained prolonged remission in patients with adult eosinophilic esophagitis: a prospective study on the food cause of the disease. J Allergy Clin Immunol 2013;131(3):797–804.
101. Molina-Infante J, Martin-Noguerol E, Alvarado-Arenas M, et al. Selective elimination diet based on skin testing has suboptimal efficacy for adult eosinophilic esophagitis. J Allergy Clin Immunol 2012;130(5):1200–2.
102. Paquet B, Begin P, Paradis L, et al. Variable yield of allergy patch testing in children with eosinophilic esophagitis. J Allergy Clin Immunol 2013;131(2):613.
103. Leung J, Hundal NV, Katz AJ, et al. Tolerance of baked milk in patients with cow's milk-mediated eosinophilic esophagitis. J Allergy Clin Immunol 2013;132(5):1215–6.e1.
104. Lucendo AJ, Arias A, Gonzalez-Cervera J, et al. Tolerance of a cow's milk-based hydrolyzed formula in patients with eosinophilic esophagitis triggered by milk. Allergy 2013;68(8):1065–72.
105. Sperry SL, Crockett SD, Miller CB, et al. Esophageal foreign-body impactions: epidemiology, time trends, and the impact of the increasing prevalence of eosinophilic esophagitis. Gastrointest Endosc 2011;74(5):985–91.
106. Straumann A, Bussmann C, Zuber M, et al. Eosinophilic esophagitis: analysis of food impaction and perforation in 251 adolescent and adult patients. Clin Gastroenterol Hepatol 2008;6(5):598–600.
107. Ally MR, Dias J, Veerappan GR, et al. Safety of dilation in adults with eosinophilic esophagitis. Dis Esophagus 2013;26(3):241–5.

108. Dellon ES, Gibbs WB, Rubinas TC, et al. Esophageal dilation in eosinophilic esophagitis: safety and predictors of clinical response and complications. Gastrointest Endosc 2010;71(4):706–12.
109. Assa'ad AH, Putnam PE, Collins MH, et al. Pediatric patients with eosinophilic esophagitis: an 8-year follow-up. J Allergy Clin Immunol 2007;119(3):731–8.
110. Straumann A, Conus S, Degen L, et al. Long-term budesonide maintenance treatment is partially effective for patients with eosinophilic esophagitis. Clin Gastroenterol Hepatol 2011;9(5):400–9.e1.
111. Kuchen T, Straumann A, Safroneeva E, et al. Swallowed topical corticosteroids reduce the risk for long-lasting bolus impactions in eosinophilic esophagitis. Allergy 2014;69(9):1248–54.
112. Spergel JM, Brown-Whitehorn TF, Beausoleil JL, et al. 14 years of eosinophilic esophagitis: clinical features and prognosis. J Pediatr Gastroenterol Nutr 2009;48(1):30–6.
113. Wolthers OD, Heuck C. Assessment of the relation between short and intermediate term growth in children with asthma treated with inhaled glucocorticoids. Allergy 2004;59(11):1193–7.
114. Wolthers OD, Pedersen S. Controlled study of linear growth in asthmatic children during treatment with inhaled glucocorticosteroids. Pediatrics 1992;89(5 Pt 1):839–42.
115. Gray SL, LaCroix AZ, Larson J, et al. Proton pump inhibitor use, hip fracture, and change in bone mineral density in postmenopausal women: results from the Women's Health Initiative. Arch Intern Med 2010;170(9):765–71.
116. Ngamruengphong S, Leontiadis GI, Radhi S, et al. Proton pump inhibitors and risk of fracture: a systematic review and meta-analysis of observational studies. Am J Gastroenterol 2011;106(7):1209–18 [quiz: 1219].
117. Dilger K, Lopez-Lazaro L, Marx C, et al. Active eosinophilic esophagitis is associated with impaired elimination of budesonide by cytochrome P450 3A enzymes. Digestion 2013;87(2):110–7.
118. Sugnanam KK, Collins JT, Smith PK, et al. Dichotomy of food and inhalant allergen sensitization in eosinophilic esophagitis. Allergy 2007;62(11):1257–60.
119. Barbi E, Gerarduzzi T, Longo G, et al. Fatal allergy as a possible consequence of long-term elimination diet. Allergy 2004;59(6):668–9.
120. David TJ. Anaphylactic shock during elimination diets for severe atopic eczema. Arch Dis Child 1984;59(10):983–6.
121. Flinterman AE, Knulst AC, Meijer Y, et al. Acute allergic reactions in children with AEDS after prolonged cow's milk elimination diets. Allergy 2006;61(3):370–4.
122. Flick RP, Katusic SK, Colligan RC, et al. Cognitive and behavioral outcomes after early exposure to anesthesia and surgery. Pediatrics 2011;128(5):e1053–61.
123. Furuta GT, Kagalwalla AF, Lee JJ, et al. The oesophageal string test: a novel, minimally invasive method measures mucosal inflammation in eosinophilic oesophagitis. Gut 2013;62(10):1395–405.
124. Acevos SS. Unmet therapeutic needs in eosinophilic esophagitis. Dig Dis 2014; 32(1–2):143–8.
125. Dellon ES, Irani AM, Hill MR, et al. Development and field testing of a novel patient-reported outcome measure of dysphagia in patients with eosinophilic esophagitis. Aliment Pharmacol Ther 2013;38(6):634–42.
126. Franciosi JP, Hommel KA, Greenberg AB, et al. Development of the pediatric quality of life inventory eosinophilic esophagitis module items: qualitative methods. BMC Gastroenterol 2012;12(1):135.

Atopic Dermatitis in Children

Clinical Features, Pathophysiology, and Treatment

Jonathan J. Lyons, MD, Joshua D. Milner, MD,
Kelly D. Stone, MD, PhD*

KEYWORDS

- Atopic dermatitis • Eczema • Allergy • Netherton syndrome • Hyper-IgE syndrome

KEY POINTS

- Atopic dermatitis is a complex disorder resulting from gene-environment interactions.
- Defective skin barrier function and immune dysregulation are paramount to disease pathogenesis.
- Pruritus is universal, is a major comorbidity, and is poorly responsive to antihistamines.
- Effective treatment requires therapies targeted to restore both barrier function and to control inflammation.
- Education of patients regarding the principal defects and provision of a comprehensive skin care plan is essential.

INTRODUCTION

Atopic dermatitis (AD) is a chronic, relapsing, and highly pruritic dermatitis that generally develops in early childhood, and has a characteristic age-dependent distribution. AD is relatively common, affecting 10% to 20% of children in developed countries.[1] Patients with AD frequently have elevated total immunoglobulin E (IgE) levels, sometimes markedly elevated, the level of which appears to correlate with disease severity.[2] Patients with AD also can have elevated allergen-specific IgE levels, indicating sensitization, but not necessarily clinical allergy, an area of great confusion for patient management, particularly with regard to food allergy.[3] The major medical comorbidities associated with AD are infections, including *Staphylococcus aureus*

This research was supported by the Intramural Research Program of the National Institutes of Health, National Institute of Allergy and Infectious Diseases.

Genetics and Pathophysiology of Allergy Section, Laboratory of Allergic Diseases, National Institute of Allergy and Infectious Diseases, National Institutes of Health, Bethesda, MD, USA
* Corresponding author. Laboratory of Allergic Diseases, National Institute of Allergy and Infectious Diseases, 10 Center Drive, Building 10, Room 12C103, Bethesda, MD 20892-1899.
E-mail address: stonek@niaid.nih.gov

superinfection and eczema herpeticum; however, chronic pruritus and sleep loss, as well as the time and expense associated with treatment, are often most distressing for patients and families. AD has been associated with poor school performance, poor self-esteem, and family dysfunction.[4–7]

The causes of AD are still poorly understood, although genetic predisposition in the setting of inciting environmental factors appears critical. Similar to asthma and other complex chronic disorders, AD should be viewed as a common end manifestation of many different genetic defects, resulting in impaired epidermal barrier function and immune dysregulation. Additional identification and characterization of genetic defects among patients with AD is needed; this may lead to better characterization of the disease and development of more effective therapies.

For now, management is based on targeting the known defects in AD, namely skin barrier dysfunction and cutaneous inflammation, along with treatment (in some cases prophylactically) of associated infections. The pruritus associated with AD is often the most distressing symptom and is treated with skin hydration and topical anti-inflammatories, but is poorly responsive to antihistamines in most patients. Behavioral interventions, such as biofeedback and relaxation techniques, also can be helpful in controlling scratching. Although a comprehensive treatment plan with extensive education is effective is controlling AD in most patients, better treatments are needed, particularly disease-modifying therapies that can be initiated in early childhood.

CLINICAL FEATURES

AD is characterized by a chronic, relapsing dermatitis that is pruritic, begins in the first 5 years of life in 90% of patients (but not in the first weeks of life, as seen in the autosomal dominant hyper-IgE syndrome), and usually presents in a characteristic age-dependent distribution with facial, scalp, and extensor involvement in infants and young children, and predominant flexural involvement in older children and adults. Pruritus is universal and xerosis is a common feature in children with AD. Acute lesions are characterized by pruritic papules with erythema, excoriations, and serous exudate, whereas chronic AD is characterized by areas of lichenification and fibrotic nodules, often accompanied by acute lesions (**Fig. 1**).

Because pathognomonic lesions are not present to definitively diagnose AD, diagnostic criteria have been described; the most widely cited being the "Hanifin and Rajka" criteria[8] and subsequent modifications, including the UK Working Party's Diagnostic Criteria for Atopic Dermatitis (**Box 1**).[9] Five major clinical features based

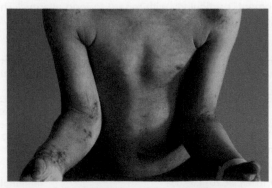

Fig. 1. Typical distribution of skin lesions in a child with AD.

Box 1
Clinical features of atopic dermatitis

Major features:

Pruritus

Characteristic morphology and distribution:

  Facial and extensor involvement in infants and children; flexural involvement with lichenification in adults

Chronic or chronic, relapsing course

Personal or family history of atopy, including asthma, allergic rhinitis, atopic dermatitis

Minor features:

Early age of onset

Xerosis

Palmar hyperlinearity, ichthyosis, keratosis pilaris

Immediate skin test reactivity, elevated serum immunoglobulin E

Cutaneous infection, including *Staphylococcus aureus* and Herpes simplex virus

Nipple eczema

Cheilitis

Pityriasis alba

White dermatographism, delayed blanching

Perifollicular accentuation

Anterior subcapsular cataracts

Itch when sweating

Nonspecific hand or foot dermatitis

Recurrent conjunctivitis

Dennie-Morgan folds

Keratoconus

Facial erythema or pallor

Adapted from Hanifin JM, Rajka G. Diagnostic features of atopic dermatitis. Acta Dermatovener Suppl (Stockholm) 1980;92:44–7.

---

upon these criteria are (1) pruritus; (2) a chronic, relapsing course; (3) typical distribution; (4) family or personal history of atopy; and (5) onset before 2 years of age. In addition, associated minor criteria are frequently observed in patients with AD and aid in diagnosis.

Common triggers for flares include heat, sweating, anxiety, frustration, and infections. Additionally, in a subset of patients with moderate to severe disease refractory to standard therapy, food allergy may play a role in exacerbations, particularly in younger children.[10] Testing for food allergy in children should be limited because of the low positive predictive value of both skin testing and *in vitro* serum assays for allergen-specific IgE.[11] Food allergy appears to be greatly overdiagnosed in children with AD, so elimination diets should be approached cautiously to avoid unnecessary restrictions.[3] Likewise, blind panel food allergy testing or avoidance of foods in the absence of a history suggestive of a food-specific IgE-mediated reaction is not recommended.

Infectious Complications

Staphylococcus aureus colonization is common in patients with AD, affecting more than 90%, and the density of *S. aureus* on the skin correlates directly with AD severity.[12,13] Even in the absence of clear signs of infection patients with severe AD may improve with antibiotics.[14,15] Clinical signs of *S. aureus* infection requiring treatment with topical or systemic antibiotics include honey-colored crusting, pustules, and folliculitis. Colonization of the nares with *S. aureus* and transmission with hands may be an important reservoir for cutaneous colonization.[16] In addition, *S. aureus* strains isolated from children with AD and their parents are identical based on pulse field electrophoresis, suggesting intrafamilial transmission is a source of recolonization after antibiotic treatment.[17] Increased colonization rates in children with AD have been observed and may be related to skin barrier disruption; exposed binding sites for the bacteria in the extracellular matrix, disruptions in innate immunity, and cellular immune dysfunction with predominant Th2 responses likely contribute.[18,19] Specific IgE to staphylococcal enterotoxin also has been found in sera of patients with AD and is associated with disease severity in children.[20,21]

Viral infections that occur in patients with AD include eczema herpeticum (EH), eczema coxsackium, eczema vaccinatum, and molluscum contagiosum. EH results from dissemination of herpes simplex virus (HSV-1 or HSV-2) in patients with AD, commonly with the first exposure, and is characterized by punched-out erosions and vesicles, occasionally complicated by secondary infection with staphylococcal or streptococcal species. Fever, lymphadenopathy, and malaise are common with EH. EH can be severe with keratoconjunctivitis and multiorgan involvement leading to fatality, and requires prompt diagnosis and initiation of antiviral medication. Risk factors for EH include early-onset and severe AD, marked elevations in total IgE, elevated allergen-specific IgE levels, peripheral eosinophilia, and the presence of filaggrin (*FLG*) mutations.[22] Disseminated coxsackie A6 viral infections with eruptions at sites of AD lesions have recently been described and termed "eczema coxsackium," but data on this infectious complication are limited.[23] For patients with AD, even with quiescent disease, smallpox vaccination or contact with persons vaccinated with smallpox can result in the potentially fatal complication of eczema vaccinatum from dissemination and poor immune control of the virus.[24]

DIFFERENTIAL DIAGNOSIS

A number of diseases may present with eczematous rashes and can be misdiagnosed as AD (**Box 2**). Several primary immunodeficiency diseases exist with prominent allergic inflammation, elevated total IgE levels, eosinophilia, and an eczematous rash that can be mistaken for typical AD. The autosomal-dominant hyper-IgE syndrome presents with an eczematous rash in the first weeks of life, which is atypical for AD.[25] *DOCK8* deficiency, which is a combined immunodeficiency with prominent cutaneous viral susceptibility, is associated with rash that is usually more dramatic than that seen in typical AD.[26] *PGM3* deficiency, a congenital disorder of glycosylation resulting in a hyper-IgE phenotype with unusual features, including neurologic and skeletal anomalies and increased circulating Th17 cells, also can present with an eczematous rash.[27] Wiskott-Aldrich syndrome, in which the dermatitis is variable, is characterized by thrombocytopenia with small platelets.[28] Immunodysregulation polyendocrinopathy enteropathy X-linked (IPEX) syndrome presents in the first weeks of

---

Box 2
Differential diagnosis for atopic dermatitis

Contact dermatitis

Seborrheic dermatitis

Drug reactions

Infantile psoriasis

Scabies

Nutritional deficiencies: zinc/biotin

Acrodermatitis enteropathica

Netherton syndrome

Ichthyosis vulgaris

Peeling skin disorder, type B

Severe dermatitis, multiple allergies and metabolic wasting (SAM) syndrome

Primary immunodeficiency diseases and Omenn syndrome

Lymphocytic-variant hypereosinophilic syndrome (HES)

Cutaneous T-cell lymphoma

---

life with prominent allergic inflammation and dermatitis, and later with autoimmune disease.[29] Netherton syndrome is a genetic disease affecting primarily the barrier function of the skin and is characterized by ichthyosis, diffuse erythroderma, severe atopy with elevated total IgE levels, eosinophilia, and trichorrhexis invaginatum.[30] Finally, genetic defects in corneodesmosin (*CDSN*) and desmoglein-1 (*DSG1*) also have been reported and are associated with eczematous dermatitis, elevated IgE levels, and clinical allergic disease.[31,32]

With all of these disorders, although diffuse eczematous dermatitis, elevated IgE levels, eosinophilia, and allergic diseases are present, there are distinguishing "syndromic" features characteristic of each disease that may aid in diagnosis (see **Box 2**). Severe and extensive skin involvement, particularly beginning near or at birth, may suggest the presence of a genetic cause for disease. Salient associated features usually necessitating additional clinical investigation include recurrent or severe infections, particularly recurrent abscesses, lymphadenitis, or pneumonia. Late onset of disease (after second decade of life), absence of concomitant allergic disease, and persistent blood eosinophilia (absolute eosinophil count >1000 cells/μL), particularly in the setting of appropriate skin care should also prompt further work-up for an alternate underlying diagnosis.

Clonal diseases, including cutaneous T-cell lymphoma and lymphocytic variant hypereosinophilic syndrome, should be considered in patients presenting with diffuse eczematous rashes after 5 years of age, but these are uncommon in children. Other considerations in the differential diagnosis include contact dermatitis, particularly in older children presenting with eczematous rashes that begin in late childhood and adolescence; nutritional deficiencies; scabies, which can be distinguished by a characteristic distribution; seborrheic dermatitis; and psoriasis.

PATHOPHYSIOLOGY

AD is associated with both disruption of the epithelial barrier of the skin and allergic inflammation in the skin of hosts whose genetic background results in a predisposition to atopy. AD and food allergy present in the first years of life and are the initial steps in the "atopic march." Broad environmental modifiers that are poorly characterized appear to be critical for the development of AD in genetically susceptible children. The following sections review defects in pathways that are fundamental to AD development in humans, including barrier disruption and immune dysregulation. The focus is to reveal patterns in the early pathogenesis of AD that guide treatment strategies and suggest targets for novel therapeutics.

Genetics

Twin concordance studies demonstrate that genetic factors are the primary determinant for the development of AD, with estimates for genetic contribution to disease being approximately 80%.[33,34] Despite these findings, a common defective pathway that gives rise to the clinical phenotype of AD in the human host has not been identified. Genome-wide association studies have identified a number of genetic susceptibility loci in patients with AD. Many susceptibility loci enriched within the AD population are within or near genes critical to innate immunity, Th2-mediated inflammation, and skin barrier function, highlighting the importance of these pathways in AD pathogenesis.[34]

A small number of heritable genetic atopic syndromes, which are included in the differential diagnosis of common AD, have been characterized that have shed additional light on the pathogenesis of the disease (**Table 1**). Loss of skin barrier integrity appears essential for the development of AD; several genetic diseases affecting skin barrier function have been described, including Netherton syndrome and peeling skin syndrome, type b, all of which have features of allergic inflammation. In concert with barrier dysfunction, virtually every lineage of immune cell has an implicated role in the immunopathogenesis of AD, with certain populations, such as CD4[+] T cells, clearly being necessary for disease development.

BARRIER DEFECTS IN THE SKIN

A number of proteins contribute to the structure and primary function of the skin as a barrier, preventing water loss and impeding the penetration of irritants, immunogens, and pathogens, most notably *S. aureus*. Damaging mutations in genes critical to normal barrier function of the skin have been shown to strongly segregate with early and severe forms of AD and ichthyosis, usually associated with elevations in total serum IgE levels. Among these are mutations in *FLG*, *DSG1*, *CDSN*, and serine protease inhibitor Kazal-type 5 (*SPINK5*) (see **Box 2**).

Skin Barrier Function and Filaggrin

Filaggrin (*FLG*) is a polyfunctional protein, present in the epidermis, which undergoes complex proteolytic processing during normal desquamation. This processing contributes to the numerous roles *FLG* has in skin barrier maintenance during its life cycle, and terminates in the release of Natural Moisturizing Factor (NMF), which contributes to water retention and skin hydration.[35] In the past decade, several loss-of-function mutations in *FLG* have been shown to result in deficiency of the protein, reduced levels of NMF, and severe early-onset AD and ichthyosis, with marked elevations of total IgE.[36,37] In addition to its effects on the structure and function of skin, *FLG* haploinsufficiency may contribute to AD pathogenesis in additional ways, including effects on skin pH, promotion of proinflammatory cytokine expression, and unimpeded growth of *S. aureus*.[38–40] *FLG* mutations also convey a major risk for development of peanut

Table 1
Heritable genetic syndromes resulting in atopic dermatitis

	Syndrome	Gene	Primary Defect	Common Distinguishing Features
Immune pathway defects	Autosomal dominant hyper-IgE syndrome	STAT3	Abnormal cytokine signaling	Bacterial pneumonias; lung bullae/bronchiectasis; absent T_H17
	Autosomal recessive hyper-IgE syndromes	DOCK8	Cytoskeletal dysfunction	Cutaneous viral susceptibility; progressive combined immunodeficiency
		PGM3	Abnormal glycosylation	Marked neurologic impairment; reduced branching glycans; leukopenia; increased T_H17
	Wiskott-Aldrich syndrome	WAS	Cytoskeletal dysfunction	X-linked; thrombocytopenia; progressive combined immunodeficiency
	IPEX syndrome	FOXP3	Absent Tregs	Endocrine abnormalities; chronic diarrhea
	Omenn syndrome	RAG1/2[a]	Lymphopenia; oligoclonal T cells	"Leaky" SCID; oligoclonal T-cell expansion; thymus present
Skin barrier defects	Atypical complete DiGeorge[b]	del22q11.2	Lymphopenia; oligoclonal T cells	"Leaky" SCID; velo-cardio-facial abnormalities; oligoclonal T-cell expansion; absent thymus
	Ichthyosis vulgaris	FLG	Impaired skin hydration and barrier maintenance	Palmar hyperlinearity; keratosis pilaris
	Netherton syndrome	SPINK5	Inappropriate protease activation	Erythroderma; ichthyosis; trichorrhexis invaginatum ("bamboo hair")
	Peeling skin syndrome type B	CDSN	Impaired intercellular adhesion	Erythroderma; ichthyosis; thin/fine hair
	SAM syndrome	DSG1	Impaired intercellular adhesion	Erythroderma; hypotrichosis; growth retardation due to metabolic disturbance

Abbreviations: IPEX, immune dysregulation, polyendocrinopathy, enteropathy, X linked; SAM, severe dermatitis, multiple allergies and metabolic wasting; SCID, severe combined immunodeficiency.

[a] Multiple other hypomorphic mutations leading to a "leaky" (presence of a few T cells) SCID phenotype may result in Omenn syndrome.

[b] Atypical complete DiGeorge is due to a chromosomal deletion, not a single genetic mutation; it also has a "leaky" phenotype.

allergy and asthma, with the latter occurring only among patients with comorbid AD, supporting a role for epicutaneous sensitization in systemic atopic disease.[41]

The Corneodesmosome: Corneodesmosin and Desmoglein-1 Deficiencies

Skin barrier integrity is dependent on intact cell-cell adhesion and resistance of shearing forces. The desmosome is a junctional protein complex in skin that acts as an anchor for the keratin cytoskeleton and facilitates cell-cell adhesion, resisting mechanical stress.[42,43] Mutations in 2 desmosome proteins in human skin, *DSG1* and *CDSN*, have been found to cause severe AD. Complete loss of *CDSN* expression due to damaging mutations results in peeling skin syndrome, type B, a diffusely ichthyotic and erythrodermic skin condition with associated severe pruritus and atopy.[31] Genetic deficiency of *DSG1* results in severe dermatitis, multiple allergies, and metabolic wasting (SAM) syndrome, associated with elevated IgE levels.[32] Of note, autoantibodies directed at *DSG1* in skin result in the bullous disease pemphigus foliaceous (PF). Remarkably, despite a similar skin defect, atopy is not reported as a common feature of PF.[44]

Protease Activity in the Skin and Netherton Syndrome

During normal desquamation, desmosomes must be processed and degraded by proteases in a regulated manner near the skin surface. Lympho-epithelial Kazal-type–related inhibitor (LEKTI) encoded by the serine protease inhibitor Kazal-type 5 (*SPINK5*) gene is a major inhibitor of endogenous skin proteases, and under low pH, releases kallikrein family proteases (KLK5, KLK7, KLK14) to facilitate normal exfoliation.[45] In this way, the epidermal pH gradient is able to limit extensive proteolysis to the outermost layers of epidermis (**Fig. 2**B). Damaging autosomal recessive mutations in *SPINK5* lead to loss of LEKTI and enhanced serine protease activity deep in the epidermis resulting in increased desmosomal destruction and increased skin permeability. This is clinically manifest as Netherton syndrome, characterized by generalized erythroderma, ichthyosis, trichorrhexis invaginatum (bamboo hair), elevated IgE, and atopy.[30] Genetic variants in *KLK7* also have been reported in association with AD.[46]

INNATE IMMUNE CONTRIBUTIONS TO ATOPIC DERMATITIS

Innate immune cells play a major role in the immunopathogenesis of AD (see **Fig. 2**A). Once a defect in the skin barrier is established, dendritic cells (DCs) and denuded epithelium are exposed to exogenous irritants, danger signals, and pathogens. This leads to DC and keratinocyte activation via innate immune receptor ligation by damage-associated molecular patterns (DAMPs) and pathogen-associated molecular patterns (PAMPs). In the genetically susceptible host, activated epithelial cells prime DCs to promote Th2 programs through elaboration of thymic stromal lymphopoietin (TSLP), interleukin (IL)-33, and IL-25.[47] Intense pruritus associated with AD lesions may lead to further activation through mechanical epithelial disruption by vigorous scratching, and promote disease progression. Numerous inherited immunodeficiency diseases exist that are caused by innate immune defects. However, atopy has not been well characterized among these syndromes. Despite this, multiple susceptibility loci have been identified within innate immune receptors that are overrepresented among atopic individuals, some segregating with more severe AD phenotypes.[34] For example, single nucleotide polymorphisms (SNPs) have been reported in toll-like receptor-2, which appear to result in loss of function and impaired sensing of *Staphylococcus*. One missense SNP, R753Q, is believed to have a functional consequence, impairing host defense and increase staphylococcal colonization; it is found

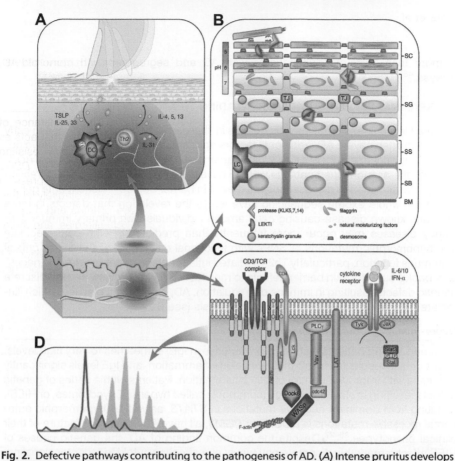

Fig. 2. Defective pathways contributing to the pathogenesis of AD. (*A*) Intense pruritus develops in lesional skin; defective barrier function leads to immune activation by irritants and microbes, with IL-25, IL-33, and TSLP contributing to Th2-mediated inflammation. IL-4 and IL-13 induce class switching to IgE, and further impair skin barrier function by reducing both *FLG* and antimicrobial peptide expression. Highly pruritogenic IL-31 is also elaborated leading to additional excoriation, further skin barrier degradation, and immune activation, thus potentiating disease. (*B*) Mutations in several proteins expressed in the epidermis result in severe AD; these include *FLG*, lympho-epithelial Kazal-type-related inhibitor (LEKTI), as well as *CDSN* and *DSG1* (components of desmo-somes). FLG is critical to skin barrier integrity and hydration. Inactive profilaggrin polymers exist inside keratohyalin granules within the stratum granulosum (SG) layer. As epithelial cells transition into the stratum corneum (SC), adjacent proteases (eg, KLK5) are released by LEKTI in a pH-dependent manner, acting on these granules to yield FLG monomers that contribute to skin barrier function, as well as on desmosomes to facilitate normal exfoliation. Loss of LEKTI function results in inappropriate protease activity deep within the SG resulting in the severe skin barrier defect characteristic of Netherton syndrome. Similar disease results from absence of proteins necessary for desmosome function. Further proteolysis of FLG releases small hygroscopic mole-cules and free amino acids that comprise natural moisturizing factor (NMF). Decreased FLG results from null mutations or Th2-mediated inflammation, and leads to impaired skin hydration, dysre-gulated pH, and barrier dysfunction. BM, basement membrane; LC, Langerhans cell; SB, stratum basale; SS, stratum spinosum; TJ, tight junction. (*C*) Multiple heritable immune defects lead to AD; defective proteins or pathways are colored in red. Genetic defects leading to severe limitation of CD3/TCR diversity may result in AD. Loss of TCR diversity may also contribute to the prominent AD phenotypes observed in Wiskott-Aldrich syndrome protein (WASp) defects. Defects in STAT3 and DOCK8 pathways lead to the autosomal dominant and recessive forms of HIES characterized by allergy and eczema. (*D*) Representative spectratype of a patient with oligoclonal T-cell expansion (*red*) compared with a normal polyclonal TCR repertoire (*shaded*); typical of abnormality seen in Omenn syndrome or atypical complete DiGeorge.

in more than 10% of adult patients with AD and segregates with more severe disease.[48]

DISCRETE IMMUNE PATHWAY DEFECTS LEADING TO ATOPIC DERMATITIS

Despite clear evidence that intrinsic defects in skin barrier function predispose to early onset and often severe AD, additional factors appear to be necessary for AD development. A significant number of individuals carrying null *FLG* alleles fail to develop AD.[49] Additionally, as mentioned patients with PF have not been reported to have increased allergic sensitization or disease, despite their skin barrier defect.[44] Recent data generated from whole exome sequencing have led to the revelation that defects in more than one known disease-causing gene among individuals with primary immunodeficiency diseases may occur more frequently than predicted.[50] One can speculate that hypomorphic mutations or SNPs with functional consequences in genes critical to immune function, particularly Th2-mediated inflammation, might provide the necessary background for skin barrier defects to manifest as AD. We review several discrete genetic defects resulting in immune dysregulation, AD, and allergic disease, which illuminate mechanisms relevant to AD pathogenesis (see **Box 2**).

Hyper-Immunoglobulin E Syndromes

Common among patients with AD is an increase in IgE, sometimes to very high levels. This increase results from Th2-mediated skin inflammation, and IgE levels significantly decrease with improved control of skin inflammation. Patients with a series of genetic defects resulting in elevations of IgE (commonly called hyper-IgE syndromes, or HIES), resulting from dominant negative mutations in *STAT3*, as well as hypomorphic autosomal recessive mutations in *DOCK8* or *PGM3*, all have AD as a major feature of their clinical phenotypes.[25–27] Despite the common finding of AD, the genetic causes of HIES affect remarkably disparate pathways; one affecting cytokine receptor signaling, one cellular cytoskeletal rearrangement, and one global cellular glycosylation patterns. Mechanisms underlying allergic phenotypes among forms of HIES remain an area of active investigation; however, immune dysregulation resulting in enhanced Th2-mediated inflammation appears common.

EFFECT OF TH2 INFLAMMATION ON SKIN BARRIER FUNCTION

Although barrier defects appear to require immunologic factors to manifest as AD, exuberant Th2 inflammation may itself cause defective skin barrier integrity. *FLG* can be directly modulated by the Th2 cytokines, IL-13 and IL-4.[51] Additionally, IL-10, IL-4, and IL-13 have been shown to reduce antimicrobial peptide (AMP) expression in keratinocytes, and patients with AD have been shown to have a relative deficiency in AMP production.[19,52,53] This may contribute to staphylococcal colonization, increased risk for viral and bacterial superinfections, and increased disease severity.

IMPAIRED CD4+ T-CELL REPERTOIRE AND REGULATORY T CELLS

CD4+ T cells are essential to development of AD. Diversity of T-cell receptors (TCRs) has been estimated at 2.5×10^7 and represents the repertoire human CD4+ T cells have to recognize non-self and inform adaptive immune responses.[54] When this diversity is limited, such as is seen in pediatric patients with HIV following immune reconstitution, an increased incidence of AD is observed.[55] More severe repertoire deficits may result from hypomorphic genetic mutations in genes, such as *IL2RG*, *JAK3*, or *RAG*, in which patients have a "leaky" phenotype; so-called because a few T cells are present.[56] In this setting, massive expansion of one or a few clonal populations may occur, leading to the striking phenotype of Omenn syndrome characterized by erythroderma, severe eczema, high IgE, and eosinophilia, frequently from birth.[57] Atypical complete DiGeorge represents a similar "leaky" process and shares many clinical features with Omenn syndrome, including severe AD.[58] A reduction in TCR diversity also can be seen in progressive combined immunodeficiencies, such as *DOCK8* deficiency and Wiskott-Aldrich syndrome, which are both associated with moderate to severe AD (see **Fig. 2**C, D).[59,60]

How Impaired TCR diversity may result in AD remains unproven. However, evidence suggests that a loss of $CD25^{bright}CD127^{neg}FoxP3^{+}CD4^{+}$ regulatory T-cell (Treg) diversity may contribute to immunopathogenesis.[28] Primary support for this hypothesis comes from IPEX syndrome due to FoxP3 deficiency, in which patients have a selective loss of Tregs.[29] Affected individuals present with severe AD, high IgE, and eosinophilia, in addition to diarrhea and autoimmunity. Patients with Wiscott-Aldrich syndrome also have been shown to have specific Treg functional defects that likely contribute to their clinical phenotype, which includes AD and allergic disease.[61] Last, eczematous dermatitis and high IgE are both prominent features of acute graft-versus-host disease (aGvHD).[62] Although the pathogenesis of aGvHD is complex and results from inappropriate and deleterious alloreactivity of donor T cells, reduced TCR diversity and oligoclonality are observed, with a specific loss of Tregs.[63,64] Remarkably, donor Treg infusion has been shown to prevent development of eczema and other clinical features of aGvHD.[65]

PHYSIOLOGY OF PRURITUS AND INTERLEUKIN-31 RECEPTOR ALPHA/ONCOSTATIN M RECEPTOR BETA COMPLEX MUTATIONS

Intense pruritus is a hallmark of AD lesions. Although complete discussion of the neurologic, physical, and immunologic contributions to itch are beyond the scope of this review, skin excoriation due to chronic and severe pruritus contributes to progression of skin lesions and promotes superinfection. Unlike in allergic rhinitis or urticaria, histamine receptors 1 and 2 do not appear to be significant mediators of pruritus in AD.[66]

IL-31 is a cytokine expressed by Th2 cells and is a strong pruritogen (see **Fig. 2**A).[67] IL-31 signals through a cognate heterodimeric receptor complex consisting of IL-31 receptor alpha (IL31RA) and oncostatin M receptor beta (OSMR). Increased IL-31 expression has been observed in AD lesions, and injection of IL-31 causes intense pruritus.[67,68] Mutations in both *OSMR* and *IL31RA* result in familial primary localized cutaneous amyloidosis, a syndrome characterized by severe cutaneous pruritus.[69,70] Despite chronic excoriation resulting in some features consistent with chronic AD lesions, there is no report of increased IgE or atopy within this population.

Hyperalgesia via nociceptive pathways also has been implicated in multiple animal models of pruritus. Recently, human sensory neurons have been shown to express IL-31RA and signal after exposure to IL-31 *in vivo* and *in vitro*; this process appears to be transient receptor channel potential cation channel ankyrin subtype 1 (TRPA1)-dependent in murine models.[71] Interestingly, TRPA1 is necessary for both histamine-independent itch mediated by bradykinin and sensing of noxious environmental irritants.[72,73]

CHRONIC MANAGEMENT
General Approach

The goals of AD management are to improve quality of life and prevent infectious complications, while minimizing potential medication side effects. Optimal control of all aspects of AD morbidity, including pruritus, is best achieved through *skin hydration, restoration of the skin barrier*, and *control of skin inflammation*. Because AD is a chronic, relapsing disorder with flares occurring at variable intervals, a comprehensive home treatment plan is critical to successful management, including steps to manage an acute flare. Chronic management of AD requires extensive patient education on the clinical features and associations of the disorder, its natural history, review of potential triggers for disease flares, discussion of medications and potential side effects, and provision of an individualized and comprehensive treatment plan that is based on the underlying pathophysiology (**Fig. 3**). Treatment plans should be directed at underlying defects: skin hydration and emollients to address barrier dysfunction and topical (or rarely systemic immunosuppressants) to quell skin inflammation. Antimicrobials also should be included in patients with recurrent infection, and methods to reduce exposure to potential triggers should be addressed. Compulsive attention to the details of the treatment plan, regular follow-up for adjustment of treatment plans for moderate to severe cases, and extensive education at each visit are critical for successful management. Multidisciplinary treatment teams are helpful in managing moderate to severe cases.[74]

Hydration and Use of Occlusive Topical Moisturizers

As has been discussed, disruption of the skin barrier is a central feature of AD, leading to transepidermal water loss and xerosis.[75] Diminished levels of ceramide observed in AD skin reduce water-binding capacity and potentiate this problem.[76,77] Treatment guidelines recommend regular skin hydration with soaking baths and use of occlusive topical ointments and creams for optimal control. This strategy has demonstrated efficacy in reducing the requirement for topical and systemic immunosuppressants (corticosteroid-sparing effect).[10,78,79] Although increased use of topical occlusive treatments is associated with improved AD control,[80] the optimal regimen for use of topical occlusives has not been extensively studied.[81] In our experience, regular, daily soaking baths of 15 minutes in lukewarm plain water, with immediate application of occlusive ointments (soak-and-seal),[82] and application of occlusive treatments through the day, are the most important aspects of treatment. For facial and neck involvement, a towel gently draped over the head and neck can be used in the bath to assist with hydration. Frequency of baths can be increased to 2 or 3 times daily during severe flares. Showers are not as effective at hydrating the skin and are not a satisfactory alternative to soaking baths in moderate to severe cases.

Application of emollients to dry skin immediately after soaking baths functions to create a barrier impeding water loss, thereby restoring the stratum corneum, reducing the requirement for topical corticosteroids to control flares, and reducing pruritus.[81,83,84] Occlusion is the primary desired function of emollients, with ointments being more effective than creams. Lotions are not effective in AD; high water content leads to evaporative drying, and irritants such as fragrances and preservatives, may irritate or inflame non-intact skin. Although ointments, such as petroleum jelly or hydrated petrolatum, are more occlusive than creams and generally more effective, ointments may be poorly tolerated in some patients and can lead to occlusive folliculitis. Creams are frequently better tolerated during hot, humid days and during school, thus promoting compliance. There is no clear evidence that the newer ceramide-containing creams improve patient outcomes. In general, we provide both an ointment and a cream and educate patients on the relative benefits of each.

Topical Corticosteroids

To address the inflammatory component of AD, topical corticosteroids are the most effective treatment, used on an as-needed basis to treat acute flares, and in more

Eczema Management Plan

Putting your ducks in a row to prevent and treat eczema flares and maintain healthy skin

	Green Duck Routine: Daily Skin Maintenance Symptoms: none	Yellow Duck Routine: Mild Eczema Flares Symptoms: itchiness, red patches on the skin, open sores, or broken skin	Red Duck Routine: Severe Eczema Flares Symptoms: skin flares that have not responded to treatments for mild eczema
Bath	Soak in a bath of lukewarm (not hot) water for 15 minutes. Cleanse with a non-drying, fragrance-free soap only when needed. Gently pat skin dry and apply moisturizer within 3 minutes after bathing.	Soak in lukewarm bath once or twice per day for 15 minutes. Add ¼ cup bleach to the bath every other day. Gently pat skin dry and apply topical medicine and moisturizer as below within 3 minutes after bathing (Remember: Do not mix topical medications and moisturizers).	Soak in a lukewarm bath at least twice per day for 15 minutes. Add ¼ cup bleach to the bath every other day. Gently pat skin dry and apply topical medicine and moisturizer as below within 3 minutes after bathing (Remember: Do not mix topical medications and moisturizers).
Apply Medicine	None	**To the face (and groin and underarms):** Apply hydrocortizone 2.5% ointment only to affected areas 2 times per day, for a maximum of 14 days, including immediately after baths. **To the eyelids:** Apply protopic 0.03% ointment to eyelids 2 times a day for up to 10 days for eyelid eczema. **To the body:** Apply triamcinolone 0.1% ointment only to affected areas 2 times per day, for a maximum of 21 days, including immediately after baths.	**To the face (and groin and underarms):** Apply topical desonide 0.05% ointment only to affected areas 2 times per day for a maximum of 14 days, including immediately after baths. **To the eyelids:** Apply protopic 0.03% ointment to eyelids 2 times a day for up to 10 days for eyelid eczema. **To the body:** Apply mometasone 0.1% ointment only to affected areas 1 time per day, for a maximum of 10 days, including immediately after baths.
Moisturize	Apply moisturizer (Hydrolatum® or Vanicream®) immediately after baths and at least 2 additional times per day. **Do not use lotions (lotions dry skin) or scented moisturizers.**	Apply moisturizer (Hydrolatum® or Vanicream®) to all healed and unaffected areas of the body immediately after baths (do not apply over topical medicines), and at least 2 additional times per day. Apply cool compresses to affected areas at night as needed for nighttime itching.	Apply moisturizer (Hydrolatum® or Vanicream® 10 to all healed and unaffected areas of the body immediately after baths (do not apply over topical medicines), and several additional time(s) per day. Apply cool compresses to affected areas at night as needed for nighttime itching.
Antibiotics	Apply mupirocin to open areas of the skin 2 times per day, until healed, to prevent infection. Apply mupirocin inside each nostril 2 times per day for 5 days. Repeat monthly.	Apply mupirocin to open areas of the skin 2 times per day, until healed, to prevent infection. Apply mupirocin inside each nostril 2 times per day for 5 days. Repeat monthly.	Apply mupirocin to open areas of the skin 2 times per day, until healed, to prevent infection. Apply mupirocin inside each nostril 2 times per day for 5 days. Repeat monthly.
Next Steps		When skin is healed, follow the green duck routine for daily skin maintenance. If skin worsens or doesn't improve after several days of yellow duck routine treatment, follow the red duck routine for severe eczema flares.	When skin starts to improve, follow the yellow duck routine for mild eczema flares.

Name: _____ Follow-up Appointment: _____ To schedule an appointment and for questions, call: ( ) -

Fig. 3. Example of eczema management plan. (*Courtesy of* Laboratory of Allergic Diseases, National Institute of Allergy and Infectious Diseases, National Institutes of Health.)

severe cases, to maintain control. Topical corticosteroids diminish inflammation, pruritus, and *S. aureus* colonization of the skin. Particularly in children, great care must be taken to balance use of the lowest-potency topical corticosteroid necessary to achieve control so as to minimize potential side effects, while not under-treating the inflammation. For moderate to severe AD, instruction for stepwise adjustments in the topical corticosteroid potency to be used, based on severity of flare and the area of the body involved, should be included in the comprehensive eczema action plan (see **Fig. 3**). When mid-potency to high-potency corticosteroids are used for flares, stepwise decreases in potency are necessary to prevent rebound exacerbations. Education of patients and their families on the relative strengths of topical corticosteroids prescribed, potential systemic and local side effects, and strategies for dose adjustments is critical to treatment success. Any concerns of "steroid phobia" that may limit compliance should be openly discussed. As previously noted, aggressive skin hydration and use of emollients is steroid-sparing and should be emphasized in discussions with families.

Topical corticosteroids are available in a wide range of potencies, from the least-potent group 1 preparations (eg, hydrocortisone 1% ointment), to the most-potent group 7 preparations (eg, clobetasol propionate 0.05% ointment). The greater the potency of topical corticosteroid used, the greater the risk of systemic and local side effects, particularly when used on large areas of the body over extended periods. For each corticosteroid, there are multiple vehicles, including ointments, creams, and lotions. Due to differences in level of occlusion, the vehicle affects potency through degree of absorption; for a given topical corticosteroid, ointments are more potent than creams, which are more potent than lotions. In general, ointments are preferred because they provide a more occlusive barrier for maintaining skin hydration and promote better absorption of the corticosteroid. Ointments also contain fewer preservatives.

Lower-potency topical corticosteroids should be used for areas on the body with thinner skin, greater chance for absorption, and higher risk for local side effects. These include the face, eyelids, genitalia, and intertriginous areas. For other areas of the body, short courses of higher-potency corticosteroids may be needed to achieve control of flares. Choice of topical corticosteroid is based on the severity of disease, distribution, and age of patient. For infants and toddlers, lower-potency corticosteroids should be used for all areas of the skin. Of note, fluticasone 0.05% cream is approved for short-term use in children 3 months or older and mometasone cream and ointment are approved for children 2 years or older; both can be used once daily as needed for flares.

Discussion of the details of application of topical corticosteroids and emollients is key to successful outcomes. The topical corticosteroid should be applied as a thin layer to areas of flare first. Topical emollient should be applied second in a thick layer to all unaffected areas of skin, avoiding application over areas already treated with topical steroid. Application of emollient over topical corticosteroid dilutes the corticosteroid and unnecessarily spreads it to unaffected areas of skin. Particularly in young children, there is a tendency to vigorously rub in both the topical steroid and emollient; this should be avoided. Provision of sufficient amounts of topical corticosteroids is also important, with attention to the severity and extent of disease.

Local side effects include atrophy, striae, acne, telangiectasias, and secondary infections. The major systemic side effect is adrenal suppression, the risk of which is greater with higher-potency topical corticosteroids and with use of occlusive dressings.

Systemic corticosteroids should be avoided in the treatment of AD, even with severe disease. Although systemic corticosteroids provide rapid improvement in AD flares, discontinuation generally results in a significant rebound inflammatory response resulting in another, often more severe, disease flare. Given the chronic relapsing course of AD and significant side effects from prolonged systemic corticosteroid treatment, there is rarely a role for these medications in the treatment of AD. Although systemic corticosteroids are sometimes perceived to be more potent, topical corticosteroids likely achieve higher concentrations at the site of inflammation within the superficial layers of the skin.[85] For children with AD and persistent asthma requiring systemic corticosteroids for asthma exacerbations, we recommend anticipatory treatment of the AD with higher-potency topical corticosteroids as the systemic corticosteroids are weaned or stopped, so as to blunt the rebound inflammatory response.

Topical Calcineurin Inhibitors

The anti-inflammatory effects of topical calcineurin inhibitors result from selective blocking of cytokine transcription in activated T cells. Use of topical calcineurin inhibitors does not result in skin atrophy, making this class of medication effective particularly in controlling eyelid and facial dermatitis. Calcineurin inhibitors also may be useful as a steroid-sparing agent for patients requiring long-term anti-inflammatory treatment. Efficacy as a maintenance medication when applied to areas of frequent flares 3 times weekly also has been demonstrated, although these medicines are not approved by the Food and Drug Administration for this use.[86] Two topical calcineurin inhibitors are available:

- Pimecrolimus (Elidel) is available as a 1% cream and is approved for use in children 2 years and older.
- Tacrolimus (Protopic) is available as a 0.03% or 0.1% ointment. The 0.03% ointment is approved for children 2 years and older, whereas the 0.1% ointment is approved for children 16 years and older.

The major side effect of both calcineurin inhibitors is transient burning that generally subsides after a few days of use. A black box warning was added to this class of medications in 2005 because of concerns of association with specific cancers. A review of the data by the Topical Calcineurin Inhibitor Task Force of the American Academy of Allergy, Asthma and Immunology (AAAAI) and American College of Allergy, Asthma and Immunology (ACAAI), however, did not identify a clear association.[87]

Antimicrobial Treatments

S. aureus colonization is common in patients with AD. Treatment of infection should be guided by antimicrobial sensitivities to ensure coverage of potentially antibiotic-resistant organisms. Use of bleach baths has been reported in the treatment of dermatitis associated with hyper-IgE syndromes and is included in pediatric treatment guidelines for AD, but there are few data supporting efficacy in widespread use.[89–90] However, among children 6 months to 17 years of age with moderate-severe AD and evidence of secondary *S. aureus* infection, use of dilute bleach baths twice weekly and application of intranasal mupirocin twice daily for 5 days, then repeated monthly, over a 3-month period, resulted in significant improvement of AD severity compared with placebo,[91] and should be considered for any patient who has required more than one course of systemic antibiotics for *S. aureus* skin infections. Mupirocin also can be applied to excoriated areas of skin twice daily to further prevent infection. Due to evidence for intra-familial transmission of *Staphylococcus*, treatment of family members with intranasal mupirocin also should be considered.

Antihistamines Are Generally Ineffective in the Treatment of Pruritus Associated with Atopic Dermatitis

Pruritus is the most common feature of AD and the most detrimental for quality of life. Scratching perpetuates cutaneous inflammation through release of TSLP and other mediators, feeding the cycle of continued inflammation and pruritus. As already discussed, the pruritus in AD results from a number of mediators, including neuropeptides and cytokines, namely IL-31. As a result, antihistamines are generally ineffective in controlling the pruritus of AD. Double-blind randomized cross-over trials have demonstrated a lack of efficacy in treating itch by oral antihistamine,[92] and histamine stimulation failed to evoke pruritus in skin of patients with AD.[93] Although some sleep benefit may be derived from first-generation sedating oral antihistamines, this may be largely negated by the resulting "hangover" effect and impairment in cognitive performance, particularly among children.[94] Until more effective therapies are developed, treatment of pruritus should be focused on addressing skin inflammation and barrier dysfunction.

Wet Wrap Therapy

Wet wrap therapy was initially described more than 20 years ago and consists of application of dilute topical corticosteroids and emollients after a soaking bath, followed by a layer of wet dressing or cloths, then dry clothes.[95] Wet wraps can be used in patients with moderate to severe disease that responds poorly to standard skin care. Wet wraps soothe the skin, promote hydration, prevent scratching, and increase absorption of topical corticosteroids. Wet wraps with dilute topical corticosteroids are effective in clinical trials for controlling flares and maintaining control over short periods of several weeks.[96–98] In patients with severe AD, we have found that wet wraps result in remission of AD, when followed by a routine skin care regimen, over a period of 1 year (Stone and colleagues, in preparation). Wet wraps can result in maceration of skin, folliculitis, and enhanced absorption of topical corticosteroids, and thus should be used only with close medical supervision. Routine skin care is critical between wet wrap treatments, particularly liberal use of emollients.

Systemic Immunosuppressants

For patients with severe AD that is refractory to standard therapies, with careful attention to compliance, systemic immunosuppressants are a treatment option. Systemic immunosuppressants that have been reported include cyclosporine, mycophenolate mofetil, azathioprine, and methotrexate.[99,100] None of these therapies has a direct effect on restoring barrier function. In our experience, systemic immunosuppressants are not optimally effective unless careful attention to hydration and aggressive use of emollients is also promoted.

SUMMARY

AD is a complex disorder that requires both a genetic predisposition and exposure to poorly defined environmental factors. Disease results from a defective skin barrier and immune dysregulation. Effective treatment requires targeted therapies to both restore barrier function and control inflammation. Treating both defects is crucial to optimal outcomes for patients with moderate to severe disease. Education of patients regarding the underlying defects and provision of a comprehensive skin care plan is essential.

ACKNOWLEDGMENTS

We thank Krista T. Townsend for her contributions to **Fig. 2**.

REFERENCES

1. Williams H, Robertson C, Stewart A, et al. Worldwide variations in the prevalence of symptoms of atopic eczema in the International Study of Asthma and Allergies in Childhood. J Allergy Clin Immunol 1999;103(1 Pt 1):125–38 PubMed PMID: 9893196.
2. Flohr C, Johansson SG, Wahlgren CF, et al. How atopic is atopic dermatitis? J Allergy Clin Immunol 2004;114(1):150–8 PubMed PMID: 15241359.
3. Fleischer DM, Bock SA, Spears GC, et al. Oral food challenges in children with a diagnosis of food allergy. J Pediatr 2011;158(4):578–83.e1 PubMed PMID: 21030035.
4. Su JC, Kemp AS, Varigos GA, et al. Atopic eczema: its impact on the family and financial cost. Arch Dis Child 1997;76(2):159–62 PubMed PMID: 9068310. Pubmed Central PMCID: 1717083.
5. Paller AS, McAlister RO, Doyle JJ, et al. Perceptions of physicians and pediatric patients about atopic dermatitis, its impact, and its treatment. Clin Pediatr 2002; 41(5):323–32 PubMed PMID: 12086198.
6. Chamlin SL, Frieden IJ, Williams ML, et al. Effects of atopic dermatitis on young American children and their families. Pediatrics 2004;114(3):607–11 PubMed PMID: 15342828.
7. Beattie PE, Lewis-Jones MS. An audit of the impact of a consultation with a paediatric dermatology team on quality of life in infants with atopic eczema and their families: further validation of the infants' dermatitis quality of life index and dermatitis family impact score. Br J Dermatol 2006;155(6):1249–55 PubMed PMID: 17107397.
8. Hanifin JM, Rajka G. Diagnostic features of atopic dermatitis. Acta Derm Venereol Suppl (Stockh) 1980;92:44–7.
9. Williams HC, Burney PG, Hay RJ, et al. The U.K. Working Party's diagnostic criteria for atopic dermatitis. I. Derivation of a minimum set of discriminators for atopic dermatitis. Br J Dermatol 1994;131(3):383–96 PubMed PMID: 7918015.
10. Schneider L, Tilles S, Lio P, et al. Atopic dermatitis: a practice parameter update 2012. J Allergy Clin Immunol 2013;131(2):295–9.e1-27 PubMed PMID: 23374261.
11. Boyce JA, Assa'ad A, Burks AW, et al. Guidelines for the diagnosis and management of food allergy in the United States: summary of the NIAID-Sponsored expert panel report. J Allergy Clin Immunol 2010;126(6):1105–18 PubMed PMID: 21134568.
12. Leyden JJ, Marples RR, Kligman AM. *Staphylococcus aureus* in the lesions of atopic dermatitis. Br J Dermatol 1974;90(5):525–30 PubMed PMID: 4601016.
13. Williams RE, Gibson AG, Aitchison TC, et al. Assessment of a contact-plate sampling technique and subsequent quantitative bacterial studies in atopic dermatitis. Br J Dermatol 1990;123(4):493–501 PubMed PMID: 2095181.
14. Leyden JJ, Kligman AM. The case for steroid–antibiotic combinations. Br J Dermatol 1977;96(2):179–87 PubMed PMID: 843453.
15. Boguniewicz M, Sampson H, Leung SB, et al. Effects of cefuroxime axetil on *Staphylococcus aureus* colonization and superantigen production in atopic dermatitis. J Allergy Clin Immunol 2001;108(4):651–2 PubMed PMID: 11590398.
16. Williams JV, Vowels BR, Honig PJ, et al. *S. aureus* isolation from the lesions, the hands, and the anterior nares of patients with atopic dermatitis. Pediatr Dermatol 1998;15(3):194–8 PubMed PMID: 9655314.

17. Bonness S, Szekat C, Novak N, et al. Pulsed-field gel electrophoresis of *Staphylococcus aureus* isolates from atopic patients revealing presence of similar strains in isolates from children and their parents. J Clin Microbiol 2008;46(2):456–61 PubMed PMID: 18077648. Pubmed Central PMCID: 2238135.

18. Cho SH, Strickland I, Boguniewicz M, et al. Fibronectin and fibrinogen contribute to the enhanced binding of *Staphylococcus aureus* to atopic skin. J Allergy Clin Immunol 2001;108(2):269–74 PubMed PMID: 11496245.

19. Ong PY, Ohtake T, Brandt C, et al. Endogenous antimicrobial peptides and skin infections in atopic dermatitis. N Engl J Med 2002;347(15):1151–60 PubMed PMID: 12374875.

20. Bunikowski R, Mielke M, Skarabis H, et al. Prevalence and role of serum IgE antibodies to the *Staphylococcus aureus*-derived superantigens SEA and SEB in children with atopic dermatitis. J Allergy Clin Immunol 1999;103(1 Pt 1): 119–24 PubMed PMID: 9893195.

21. Lin YT, Shau WY, Wang LF, et al. Comparison of serum specific IgE antibodies to staphylococcal enterotoxins between atopic children with and without atopic dermatitis. Allergy 2000;55(7):641–6 PubMed PMID: 10921463.

22. Leung DY. Why is eczema herpeticum unexpectedly rare? Antiviral Res 2013; 98(2):153–7 PubMed PMID: 23439082. Pubmed Central PMCID: 3773952.

23. Mathes EF, Oza V, Frieden IJ, et al. "Eczema coxsackium" and unusual cutaneous findings in an enterovirus outbreak. Pediatrics 2013;132(1):e149–57 PubMed PMID: 23776120.

24. Vora S, Damon I, Fulginiti V, et al. Severe eczema vaccinatum in a household contact of a smallpox vaccinee. Clin Infect Dis 2008;46(10):1555–61 PubMed PMID: 18419490.

25. Holland SM, DeLeo FR, Elloumi HZ, et al. STAT3 mutations in the hyper-IgE syndrome. N Engl J Med 2007;357(16):1608–19 PubMed PMID: 17881745.

26. Zhang Q, Davis JC, Lamborn IT, et al. Combined immunodeficiency associated with DOCK8 mutations. N Engl J Med 2009;361(21):2046–55 PubMed PMID: 19776401. Pubmed Central PMCID: 2965730.

27. Zhang Y, Yu X, Ichikawa M, et al. Autosomal recessive phosphoglucomutase 3 (PGM3) mutations link glycosylation defects to atopy, immune deficiency, autoimmunity, and neurocognitive impairment. J Allergy Clin Immunol 2014; 133(5):1400–9 PubMed PMID: 24589341. Pubmed Central PMCID: 4016982.

28. Ozcan E, Notarangelo LD, Geha RS. Primary immune deficiencies with aberrant IgE production. J Allergy Clin Immunol 2008;122(6):1054–62 [quiz: 1063–4]. PubMed PMID: 19084106.

29. d'Hennezel E, Bin Dhuban K, Torgerson T, et al. The immunogenetics of immune dysregulation, polyendocrinopathy, enteropathy, X linked (IPEX) syndrome. J Med Genet 2012;49(5):291–302 PubMed PMID: 22581967.

30. Chavanas S, Bodemer C, Rochat A, et al. Mutations in SPINK5, encoding a serine protease inhibitor, cause Netherton syndrome. Nat Genet 2000;25(2): 141–2 PubMed PMID: 10835624.

31. Oji V, Eckl KM, Aufenvenne K, et al. Loss of corneodesmosin leads to severe skin barrier defect, pruritus, and atopy: unraveling the peeling skin disease. Am J Hum Genet 2010;87(2):274–81 PubMed PMID: 20691404. Pubmed Central PMCID: 2917721.

32. Samuelov L, Sarig O, Harmon RM, et al. Desmoglein 1 deficiency results in severe dermatitis, multiple allergies and metabolic wasting. Nat Genet 2013; 45(10):1244–8 PubMed PMID: 23974871. Pubmed Central PMCID: 3791825.

33. Thomsen SF, Ulrik CS, Kyvik KO, et al. Importance of genetic factors in the etiology of atopic dermatitis: a twin study. Allergy Asthma Proc 2007;28(5): 535–9 PubMed PMID: 18034971.
34. Morar N, Willis-Owen SA, Moffatt MF, et al. The genetics of atopic dermatitis. J Allergy Clin Immunol 2006;118(1):24–34 [quiz: 35–6]. PubMed PMID: 16815134.
35. Sandilands A, Sutherland C, Irvine AD, et al. Filaggrin in the frontline: role in skin barrier function and disease. J Cell Sci 2009;122(Pt 9):1285–94 PubMed PMID: 19386895. Pubmed Central PMCID: 2721001.
36. Smith FJ, Irvine AD, Terron-Kwiatkowski A, et al. Loss-of-function mutations in the gene encoding filaggrin cause ichthyosis vulgaris. Nat Genet 2006;38(3): 337–42 PubMed PMID: 16444271.
37. Sandilands A, Terron-Kwiatkowski A, Hull PR, et al. Comprehensive analysis of the gene encoding filaggrin uncovers prevalent and rare mutations in ichthyosis vulgaris and atopic eczema. Nat Genet 2007;39(5):650–4 PubMed PMID: 17417636.
38. Jungersted JM, Scheer H, Mempel M, et al. Stratum corneum lipids, skin barrier function and filaggrin mutations in patients with atopic eczema. Allergy 2010; 65(7):911–8 PubMed PMID: 20132155.
39. Kezic S, O'Regan GM, Lutter R, et al. Filaggrin loss-of-function mutations are associated with enhanced expression of IL-1 cytokines in the stratum corneum of patients with atopic dermatitis and in a murine model of filaggrin deficiency. J Allergy Clin Immunol 2012;129(4):1031–9.e1 PubMed PMID: 22322004. Pubmed Central PMCID: 3627959.
40. Miajlovic H, Fallon PG, Irvine AD, et al. Effect of filaggrin breakdown products on growth of and protein expression by Staphylococcus aureus. J Allergy Clin Immunol 2010;126(6):1184–90.e3 PubMed PMID: 21036388. Pubmed Central PMCID: 3627960.
41. Irvine AD, McLean WH, Leung DY. Filaggrin mutations associated with skin and allergic diseases. N Engl J Med 2011;365(14):1315–27 PubMed PMID: 21991953.
42. Kottke MD, Delva E, Kowalczyk AP. The desmosome: cell science lessons from human diseases. J Cell Sci 2006;119(Pt 5):797–806 PubMed PMID: 16495480.
43. Jonca N, Leclerc EA, Caubet C, et al. Corneodesmosomes and corneodesmosin: from the stratum corneum cohesion to the pathophysiology of genodermatoses. Eur J Dermatol 2011;21(Suppl 2):35–42 PubMed PMID: 21628128.
44. James KA, Culton DA, Diaz LA. Diagnosis and clinical features of pemphigus foliaceus. Dermatol Clin 2011;29(3):405–12 viii. PubMed PMID: 21605805. Pubmed Central PMCID: 3108573.
45. Deraison C, Bonnart C, Lopez F, et al. LEKTI fragments specifically inhibit KLK5, KLK7, and KLK14 and control desquamation through a pH-dependent interaction. Mol Biol Cell 2007;18(9):3607–19 PubMed PMID: 17596512. Pubmed Central PMCID: 1951746.
46. Vasilopoulos Y, Cork MJ, Murphy R, et al. Genetic association between an AACC insertion in the 3'UTR of the stratum corneum chymotryptic enzyme gene and atopic dermatitis. J Invest Dermatol 2004;123(1):62–6 PubMed PMID: 15191543.
47. Kuo IH, Yoshida T, De Benedetto A, et al. The cutaneous innate immune response in patients with atopic dermatitis. J Allergy Clin Immunol 2013; 131(2):266–78 PubMed PMID: 23374259.
48. Niebuhr M, Langnickel J, Draing C, et al. Dysregulation of toll-like receptor-2 (TLR-2)-induced effects in monocytes from patients with atopic dermatitis: impact of the TLR-2 R753Q polymorphism. Allergy 2008;63(6):728–34 PubMed PMID: 18445187.

49. Henderson J, Northstone K, Lee SP, et al. The burden of disease associated with filaggrin mutations: a population-based, longitudinal birth cohort study. J Allergy Clin Immunol 2008;121(4):872–7.e9 PubMed PMID: 18325573.

50. Dinwiddie DL, Kingsmore SF, Caracciolo S, et al. Combined DOCK8 and CLEC7A mutations causing immunodeficiency in 3 brothers with diarrhea, eczema, and infections. J Allergy Clin Immunol 2013;131(2):594–7.e1-3 PubMed PMID: 23374272. Pubmed Central PMCID: 3570814.

51. Howell MD, Kim BE, Gao P, et al. Cytokine modulation of atopic dermatitis filaggrin skin expression. J Allergy Clin Immunol 2007;120(1):150–5 PubMed PMID: 17512043. Pubmed Central PMCID: 2669594.

52. Howell MD, Boguniewicz M, Pastore S, et al. Mechanism of HBD-3 deficiency in atopic dermatitis. Clin Immunol 2006;121(3):332–8 PubMed PMID: 17015038.

53. Howell MD, Novak N, Bieber T, et al. Interleukin-10 downregulates anti-microbial peptide expression in atopic dermatitis. J Invest Dermatol 2005;125(4):738–45 PubMed PMID: 16185274.

54. Arstila TP, Casrouge A, Baron V, et al. A direct estimate of the human alphabeta T cell receptor diversity. Science 1999;286(5441):958–61 PubMed PMID: 10542151.

55. Siberry GK, Leister E, Jacobson DL, et al. Increased risk of asthma and atopic dermatitis in perinatally HIV-infected children and adolescents. Clin Immunol 2012;142(2):201–8 PubMed PMID: 22094294. Pubmed Central PMCID: 3273595.

56. Shearer WT, Dunn E, Notarangelo LD, et al. Establishing diagnostic criteria for severe combined immunodeficiency disease (SCID), leaky SCID, and Omenn syndrome: the Primary Immune Deficiency Treatment Consortium experience. J Allergy Clin Immunol 2014;133(4):1092–8 PubMed PMID: 24290292. Pubmed Central PMCID: 3972266.

57. Villa A, Notarangelo LD, Roifman CM. Omenn syndrome: inflammation in leaky severe combined immunodeficiency. J Allergy Clin Immunol 2008;122(6): 1082–6 PubMed PMID: 18992930.

58. Markert ML, Alexieff MJ, Li J, et al. Complete DiGeorge syndrome: development of rash, lymphadenopathy, and oligoclonal T cells in 5 cases. J Allergy Clin Immunol 2004;113(4):734–41 PubMed PMID: 15100681.

59. Wada T, Schurman SH, Garabedian EK, et al. Analysis of T-cell repertoire diversity in Wiskott-Aldrich syndrome. Blood 2005;106(12):3895–7 PubMed PMID: 16091449. Pubmed Central PMCID: 1895101.

60. Dasouki M, Okonkwo KC, Ray A, et al. Deficient T cell receptor excision circles (TRECs) in autosomal recessive hyper IgE syndrome caused by DOCK8 mutation: implications for pathogenesis and potential detection by newborn screening. Clin Immunol 2011;141(2):128–32 PubMed PMID: 21763205.

61. Humblet-Baron S, Sather B, Anover S, et al. Wiskott-Aldrich syndrome protein is required for regulatory T cell homeostasis. J Clin Invest 2007;117(2):407–18 PubMed PMID: 17218989. Pubmed Central PMCID: 1764857.

62. Heyd J, Donnenberg AD, Burns WH, et al. Immunoglobulin E levels following allogeneic, autologous, and syngeneic bone marrow transplantation: an indirect association between hyperproduction and acute graft-v-host disease in allogeneic BMT. Blood 1988;72(2):442–6 PubMed PMID: 3042039.

63. Dong S, Maiella S, Xhaard A, et al. Multiparameter single-cell profiling of human CD4+FOXP3+ regulatory T-cell populations in homeostatic conditions and during graft-versus-host disease. Blood 2013;122(10):1802–12 PubMed PMID: 23818545.

64. Clave E, Busson M, Douay C, et al. Acute graft-versus-host disease transiently impairs thymic output in young patients after allogeneic hematopoietic stem cell transplantation. Blood 2009;113(25):6477–84 PubMed PMID: 19258596.
65. Di Ianni M, Falzetti F, Carotti A, et al. Tregs prevent GVHD and promote immune reconstitution in HLA-haploidentical transplantation. Blood 2011;117(14): 3921–8 PubMed PMID: 21292771.
66. Darsow U, Pfab F, Valet M, et al. Pruritus and atopic dermatitis. Clin Rev Allergy Immunol 2011;41(3):237–44 PubMed PMID: 21207193.
67. Dillon SR, Sprecher C, Hammond A, et al. Interleukin 31, a cytokine produced by activated T cells, induces dermatitis in mice. Nat Immunol 2004;5(7): 752–60 PubMed PMID: 15184896.
68. Sonkoly E, Muller A, Lauerma AI, et al. IL-31: a new link between T cells and pruritus in atopic skin inflammation. J Allergy Clin Immunol 2006;117(2):411–7 PubMed PMID: 16461142.
69. Arita K, South AP, Hans-Filho G, et al. Oncostatin M receptor-beta mutations underlie familial primary localized cutaneous amyloidosis. Am J Hum Genet 2008;82(1):73–80 PubMed PMID: 18179886. Pubmed Central PMCID: 2253984.
70. Lin MW, Lee DD, Liu TT, et al. Novel IL31RA gene mutation and ancestral OSMR mutant allele in familial primary cutaneous amyloidosis. Eur J Hum Genet 2010;18(1):26–32 PubMed PMID: 19690585. Pubmed Central PMCID: 2987153.
71. Cevikbas F, Wang X, Akiyama T, et al. A sensory neuron-expressed IL-31 receptor mediates T helper cell-dependent itch: involvement of TRPV1 and TRPA1. J Allergy Clin Immunol 2014;133(2):448–60 PubMed PMID: 24373353. Pubmed Central PMCID: 3960328.
72. Wilson SR, Gerhold KA, Bifolck-Fisher A, et al. TRPA1 is required for histamine-independent, Mas-related G protein-coupled receptor-mediated itch. Nat Neurosci 2011;14(5):595–602 PubMed PMID: 21460831. Pubmed Central PMCID: 3181150.
73. Bautista DM, Jordt SE, Nikai T, et al. TRPA1 mediates the inflammatory actions of environmental irritants and proalgesic agents. Cell 2006;124(6):1269–82 PubMed PMID: 16564016.
74. Boguniewicz M, Nicol N, Kelsay K, et al. A multidisciplinary approach to evaluation and treatment of atopic dermatitis. Semin Cutan Med Surg 2008;27(2): 115–27 PubMed PMID: 18620133.
75. De Benedetto A, Kubo A, Beck LA. Skin barrier disruption: a requirement for allergen sensitization? J Invest Dermatol 2012;132(3 Pt 2):949–63 PubMed PMID: 22217737. Pubmed Central PMCID: 3279586.
76. Imokawa G, Abe A, Jin K, et al. Decreased level of ceramides in stratum corneum of atopic dermatitis: an etiologic factor in atopic dry skin? J Invest Dermatol 1991;96(4):523–6 PubMed PMID: 2007790.
77. Hara J, Higuchi K, Okamoto R, et al. High-expression of sphingomyelin deacylase is an important determinant of ceramide deficiency leading to barrier disruption in atopic dermatitis. J Invest Dermatol 2000;115(3):406–13 PubMed PMID: 10951276.
78. Lucky AW, Leach AD, Laskarzewski P, et al. Use of an emollient as a steroid-sparing agent in the treatment of mild to moderate atopic dermatitis in children. Pediatr Dermatol 1997;14(4):321–4 PubMed PMID: 9263319.
79. Grimalt R, Mengeaud V, Cambazard F, et al. The steroid-sparing effect of an emollient therapy in infants with atopic dermatitis: a randomized controlled study. Dermatology 2007;214(1):61–7 PubMed PMID: 17191050.

80. Cork MJ, Britton J, Butler L, et al. Comparison of parent knowledge, therapy utilization and severity of atopic eczema before and after explanation and demonstration of topical therapies by a specialist dermatology nurse. Br J Dermatol 2003;149(3):582–9 PubMed PMID: 14510993.
81. Chiang C, Eichenfield LF. Quantitative assessment of combination bathing and moisturizing regimens on skin hydration in atopic dermatitis. Pediatr Dermatol 2009;26(3):273–8 PubMed PMID: 19706087. Pubmed Central PMCID: 2762386.
82. Gutman AB, Kligman AM, Sciacca J, et al. Soak and smear: a standard technique revisited. Arch Dermatol 2005;141(12):1556–9 PubMed PMID: 16365257.
83. Loden M. Effect of moisturizers on epidermal barrier function. Clin Dermatol 2012;30(3):286–96 PubMed PMID: 22507043.
84. Lee CH, Chuang HY, Shih CC, et al. Transepidermal water loss, serum IgE and beta-endorphin as important and independent biological markers for development of itch intensity in atopic dermatitis. Br J Dermatol 2006;154(6):1100–7 PubMed PMID: 16704640.
85. McClain RW, Yentzer BA, Feldman SR. Comparison of skin concentrations following topical versus oral corticosteroid treatment: reconsidering the treatment of common inflammatory dermatoses. J Drugs Dermatol 2009;8(12): 1076–9 PubMed PMID: 20027934.
86. Paller AS, Eichenfield LF, Kirsner RS, et al. Three times weekly tacrolimus ointment reduces relapse in stabilized atopic dermatitis: a new paradigm for use. Pediatrics 2008;122(6):e1210–8 PubMed PMID: 19015204.
87. Fonacier L, Spergel J, Charlesworth EN, et al. Report of the topical calcineurin inhibitor task force of the American College of Allergy, Asthma and Immunology and the American Academy of Allergy, Asthma and Immunology. J Allergy Clin Immunol 2005;115(6):1249–53 PubMed PMID: 15940142.
88. Eberting CL, Davis J, Puck JM, et al. Dermatitis and the newborn rash of hyper-IgE syndrome. Arch Dermatol 2004;140(9):1119–25 PubMed PMID: 15381553.
89. Krakowski AC, Eichenfield LF, Dohil MA. Management of atopic dermatitis in the pediatric population. Pediatrics 2008;122(4):812–24 PubMed PMID: 18829806.
90. Birnie AJ, Bath-Hextall FJ, Ravenscroft JC, et al. Interventions to reduce *Staphylococcus aureus* in the management of atopic eczema. Cochrane Database Syst Rev 2008;(3):CD003871. PubMed PMID: 18646096.
91. Huang JT, Abrams M, Tlougan B, et al. Treatment of *Staphylococcus aureus* colonization in atopic dermatitis decreases disease severity. Pediatrics 2009; 123(5):e808–14 PubMed PMID: 19403473.
92. Wahlgren CF, Hagermark O, Bergstrom R. The antipruritic effect of a sedative and a non-sedative antihistamine in atopic dermatitis. Br J Dermatol 1990; 122(4):545–51 PubMed PMID: 2110817.
93. Rukwied R, Lischetzki G, McGlone F, et al. Mast cell mediators other than histamine induce pruritus in atopic dermatitis patients: a dermal microdialysis study. Br J Dermatol 2000;142(6):1114–20 PubMed PMID: 10848733.
94. Kay GG. The effects of antihistamines on cognition and performance. J Allergy Clin Immunol 2000;105(6 Pt 2):S622–7 PubMed PMID: 10856168.
95. Goodyear HM, Spowart K, Harper JI. 'Wet-wrap' dressings for the treatment of atopic eczema in children. Br J Dermatol 1991;125(6):604 PubMed PMID: 1760370.
96. Devillers AC, Oranje AP. Efficacy and safety of 'wet-wrap' dressings as an intervention treatment in children with severe and/or refractory atopic dermatitis: a

critical review of the literature. Br J Dermatol 2006;154(4):579–85 PubMed PMID: 16536797.

97. Lee JH, Lee SJ, Kim D, et al. The effect of wet-wrap dressing on epidermal barrier in patients with atopic dermatitis. J Eur Acad Dermatol Venereol 2007; 21(10):1360–8 PubMed PMID: 17958842.

98. Schnopp C, Holtmann C, Stock S, et al. Topical steroids under wet-wrap dressings in atopic dermatitis–a vehicle-controlled trial. Dermatology 2002;204(1): 56–9 PubMed PMID: 11834851.

99. Denby KS, Beck LA. Update on systemic therapies for atopic dermatitis. Curr Opin Allergy Clin Immunol 2012;12(4):421–6 PubMed PMID: 22622476.

100. Arkwright PD, Motala C, Subramanian H, et al. Management of difficult-to-treat atopic dermatitis. J Allergy Clin Immunol Pract 2013;1(2):142–51 PubMed PMID: 24565453.

Pediatric Allergic Rhinitis

Chet A. Tharpe, MD, Stephen F. Kemp, MD*

KEYWORDS

- Allergic rhinitis • Conjunctivitis • Concurrent conditions • Avoidance
- Pharmacotherapy • Immunomodulation

KEY POINTS

- Allergic rhinitis significantly affects sleep, cognition, performance, and quality of life.
- Allergic rhinitis is diagnosed clinically based on compatible history and risk factors, characteristic signs and symptoms, and the confirmed presence of allergen-specific immunoglobulin E (if clinically indicated).
- For most patients, allergic rhinitis is a persistent condition that requires years of ongoing management, which combines allergen avoidance strategies and pharmacotherapy, with consideration of allergen immunotherapy for severe or refractory cases.
- Treatment of allergic rhinitis improves concurrent asthma, and allergen immunotherapy might potentially prevent asthma in some children with allergic rhinitis.
- Optimized partnership between patient, caregiver, and health care professional helps to maximize response to allergic rhinitis treatment, while reducing/allaying concerns about safety or therapeutic complications.

INTRODUCTION

Allergic rhinitis (AR) is a chronic immunoglobulin (Ig)E–dependent respiratory disease of the upper airway characterized by rhinorrhea, sneezing, congestion, and/or naso-ocular pruritus.[1] Estimates for its prevalence vary regionally and by age group. Several risk factors have been proposed or identified (**Box 1**). The International Study of Asthma and Allergies in Childhood systematically evaluated the prevalence of asthma, allergic rhinoconjunctivitis, and eczema in approximately 1.2 million children in 98 countries and determined the overall prevalence of AR in children aged 6 to 7 years and 13 to 14 years was 8.5% and 14.6%, respectively.[2]

CLINICAL MANIFESTATIONS

AR characteristically presents with paroxysms of rhinorrhea, sneezing, and congestion, often accompanied by pruritus of the eyes, nose, and palate. Postnasal drainage,

Disclosures: The authors have nothing to disclose.
Division of Clinical Immunology and Allergy, Department of Medicine, The University of Mississippi Medical Center, 768 Lakeland Drive, Building LJ, Jackson, MS 39216, USA
* Corresponding author.
E-mail address: skemp@umc.edu

Immunol Allergy Clin N Am 35 (2015) 185–198
http://dx.doi.org/10.1016/j.iac.2014.09.003
0889-8561/15/$ – see front matter © 2015 Elsevier Inc. All rights reserved.

immunology.theclinics.com

> **Box 1**
> **Risk factors for pediatric allergic rhinitis**
>
> Family history
>
> Male gender
>
> Firstborn status
>
> Early systemic use of antibiotics
>
> Maternal smoking
>
> Exposure to indoor aeroallergens
>
> Serum IgE greater than 100 IU/mL before age 6 years
>
> Presence of allergen-specific IgE
>
> *Data from* Wallace DV, Dykewicz MS, Bernstein DI, et al. The diagnosis and management of rhinitis: an updated practice parameter. J Allergy Clin Immunol 2008;122:S1–84; Matheson MC, Dharmage SC, Abramson MJ, et al. Early-life risk factors and incidence of rhinitis: results from the European Community Respiratory Health Study—an international population-based cohort study. J Allergy Clin Immunol 2011;128:816–23; Saulyte J, Regueira C, Montes-Martinez A, et al. Active or passive exposure to tobacco smoking and allergic rhinitis, allergic dermatitis, and food allergy in adults and children: a systematic review and meta-analysis. PLoS Med 2014;11:e1001611.

cough, fatigue, and irritability are other common symptoms.[1,3,4] Of these, nasal congestion is the most common.[5] Young children, however, typically do not blow their noses, but they may instead exhibit repeated sniffing, snorting, throat-clearing, and coughing. Additionally, a palatal click can sometimes be audible if children use their tongues to scratch their itchy palates. Chronic mouth breathing owing to nasal obstruction in children with AR has been linked to facial abnormalities and an increased incidence of dental malocclusions and snoring.[6,7]

COGNITIVE FUNCTION AND QUALITY OF LIFE

Sleep-disordered breathing, fatigue, and generalized malaise are important sequelae of undertreated AR.[5,8,9] Irritability and behavioral issues are often seen as a result of AR in children.[9,10] Children with AR are more likely to have emotional and social complications.[5]

AR can also impair cognitive functioning and academic performance.[5,11,12] Sedating antihistamines can be unintentional cofactors.[13] Complications of AR such as sleep disorders and eustachian tube dysfunction with associated conductive hearing loss likely contribute to learning impairment.[14]

CONCURRENT CONDITIONS

AR occurs in association with several other diseases, including asthma, allergic conjunctivitis, and sinusitis.

Asthma

Asthma and rhinitis often coexist and are believed to represent a spectrum of the same disease entity. Rhinitis is correlated with and is a risk factor for the occurrence and severity of asthma. Up to 50% of individuals with chronic rhinitis have asthma. Conversely, most individuals with asthma also have chronic rhinitis.[15] Accordingly, expert panels recommend that patients with AR should be evaluated for asthma and vice versa, and, if identified, the 2 conditions should be treated concurrently.[15,16]

Allergic Conjunctivitis

Up to 60% of patients with AR have concurrent conjunctivitis.[17] Pediatric data are similar. For example, Ibáñez and colleagues[18] reported 53.6% of children with AR had ocular symptoms and found a correlation between severity and duration of AR and the likelihood of concurrent conjunctivitis. Allergic conjunctivitis characteristically presents with bilateral pruritus, an urge to rub the eyes, tearing (watery discharge), hyperemia and chemosis, and conjunctival edema. Eyelid edema is also common.

Sinusitis

Nasal inflammation from AR can obstruct the sinus ostiomeatal complex, contributing to acute or chronic sinusitis. Symptoms of bacterial sinusitis include nasal congestion, mucopurulent drainage, facial/dental discomfort, and cough. Mucopurulent drainage and cough are the most useful predictors of bacterial sinusitis in children, but no single symptom has high predictive value for discriminating between bacterial sinusitis and rhinitis.[19]

Oral Allergy Syndrome (Pollen-Food Allergy Syndrome)

Oral allergy syndrome (OAS) is a localized form of food allergy that develops in some pollen-allergic individuals who ingest immunologically related, uncooked fruits (eg, apples, peaches, cucumbers, melons) or raw vegetables during the pertinent pollen season. Characteristic symptoms include pruritus, tingling, redness, and swelling of the lips, tongue, and soft palate. OAS symptoms have been reported in 25% of children with AR.[20] Sensitization to birch, the most common pollen sensitization reported with OAS, was found in 31% of children with AR who ingested fruits (eg, apples) sharing birch pollen-related proteins.[20]

Other Conditions

AR probably contributes to eustachian tube dysfunction, causing concurrent otitis media with effusion, which can be associated with conductive hearing loss and language delay.[21,22] Nasal obstruction caused by severe AR can also cause sleep-disordered breathing and anosmia.[23,24]

PATTERNS OF SYMPTOMS

AR has traditionally been classified as either seasonal or perennial, depending on whether symptoms occur at a particular time of year or are present throughout the year. The US Food and Drug Administration continues to use this classification in its approval process for AR therapeutics. The Allergic Rhinitis in Asthma guidelines developed in collaboration with the World Health Organization classify AR according to temporal pattern (intermittent or persistent) and symptomatic severity (mild or moderate/severe) (**Box 2**).

DIAGNOSIS

AR is diagnosed clinically based on compatible history and risk factors, characteristic signs and symptoms, and the confirmed presence of allergen-specific IgE (if clinically indicated).

HISTORY

Seasonal/intermittent AR is often diagnosed by history alone, because each recurring pollen season produces symptoms. For example, symptoms caused by tree and

---

Box 2
Allergic Rhinitis in Asthma classification of allergic rhinitis

Intermittent means that the symptoms are present:

• Less than 4 d/wk

• Or for less than 4 weeks

Persistent means that the symptoms are present:

• More than 4 d/wk

• And for more than 4 weeks

Mild means that none of the following items are present:

• Sleep disturbance

• Impairment of daily activities, leisure, and/or sport

• Impairment of school or work

• Troublesome symptoms

Moderate-severe means that one or more of the following items are present:

• Sleep disturbance

• Impairment of daily activities, leisure, and/or sport

• Impairment of school or work

• Troublesome symptoms

From Bousquet J, Van Cauwenberge P, Khaltaev N, et al. Allergic rhinitis and its impact on asthma. J Allergy Clin Immunol 2001;108:S147–334; with permission.

---

grass pollen allergy typically occur in the spring, whereas those caused by ragweed pollen occur in the fall, although exposures may vary regionally. Clinical history alone might also permit the diagnosis of episodic AR if there is an obvious, consistent association between exposure and symptom onset (eg, sneezing commences within minutes of visiting with an individual who has indoor cats). In contrast, the culprit allergens (eg, dust mites or animal emanations) in perennial/persistent AR might not be evident by history alone.

PHYSICAL FINDINGS

The nose, oropharynx, tympanic membranes, and eyes should each be examined for findings of AR or concurrent conditions. The nasal mucosa in active disease often has mucosal edema accompanied by pallor or a pale bluish hue. Clear drainage may be visible anteriorly or posteriorly. Posterior drainage is often observed with hyperplastic lymphoid tissue lining the posterior pharynx (cobblestoning). An effusion of serous fluid may accumulate behind the tympanic membrane when significant nasal mucosal edema and eustachian tube dysfunction are present.

Certain facial features, when present, also suggest AR.[25] A transverse nasal crease can be caused by a child's repeated vertical rubbing of the tip of the nose (allergic salute). Infraorbital edema and discoloration caused by venous stasis is often described as allergic shiners. Dennie-Morgan lines are accentuated folds below the lower eyelids that suggest allergic conjunctivitis. Allergic facies, observed in some young children, consist of chronic mouth breathing, dental malocclusion, and high-arched palate.

NATURAL HISTORY

AR is uncommon in children younger than 2 years, because it typically requires a few years of allergen exposure to develop.[26] If a very young child has persistent nasal symptoms, another diagnosis should be considered (see Differential Diagnosis in later discussion). In children, sensitization (presence of allergen-specific IgE) precedes the appearance of clinical allergy, which develop first to allergens continuously present in the respirable environment (eg, dust mites, animal emanations) and then to pollens and other seasonal aeroallergens.[20] In a prospective study of 2024 children, AR prevalence increased from 5% at age 4 years to 14% at age 8 years.[20] Up to 80% of patients with AR have symptoms before age 20 years.[27]

DIAGNOSTIC TESTING

Diagnostic testing is not necessary before making the presumptive diagnosis of AR and initiating empiric treatment. However, allergen-specific IgE testing can confirm the diagnosis and facilitate individualized AR management. Care should be taken to select for testing only those allergens considered clinically relevant based on the history, clinical manifestations, and local aerobiology, as clinically irrelevant results can occur.[28] Skin prick testing (SPT) and in vitro specific-IgE (sIgE) testing are sensitive diagnostic methods. Properly performed SPT is generally preferred because it is less expensive than sIgE testing and provides rapid results, which the patient/caregiver can observe.[1] SPT is usually performed by allergy/immunology specialists because rare systemic reactions during testing are possible. Conversely, sIgE testing might be preferable for children with extensive dermatitis, persistent need for medication that interferes with the SPT wheal-and-flare response, or a relative contraindication to SPT (eg, uncontrolled asthma).[1]

DIFFERENTIAL DIAGNOSIS

Various disorders can mimic AR or coexist with it. **Box 3** provides an age-based differential diagnosis for pediatric AR.

PATHOPHYSIOLOGY

Sensitized individuals respond to allergen exposure by producing allergen-specific IgE. IgE antibodies bind to IgE receptors on mast cells throughout the respiratory mucosa and to circulating basophils. When the same allergen is subsequently inhaled, it binds to IgE molecules, which cross-link on the mast cell surface, resulting in activation and release of inflammatory mediators. Nasal mast cells release histamine, leukotrienes, prostaglandins, bradykinin, and platelet-activating factor, among other mediators, which produce the clinical stigmata of AR. Tissue eosinophilia is also a feature of AR, and eosinophilic mediators augment nasal inflammation. The allergic nasal response consists of an immediate phase, which peaks 15 to 30 minutes after allergen exposure and corresponds to mast cell mediator release, followed in approximately 60% to 70% of individuals by a late phase, which peaks 6 to 12 hours after exposure and corresponds to infiltration of nasal mucosa with inflammatory cells (eg, eosinophils, basophils, T lymphocytes).[29,30]

MANAGEMENT STRATEGIES

Optimized partnership between patient, caregiver, and health care professional helps to maximize response to AR treatment while reducing/allaying concerns about safety

Box 3
Age-based differential diagnosis for pediatric allergic rhinitis

Infants (0–1 y)

Infectious rhinitis: viral URI, sinusitis, chlamydia, syphilis

Allergic rhinitis: indoor and food allergens

Nonallergic, noninfectious rhinitis

- Irritant rhinitis

Obstruction

- Anatomic abnormality: trisomy 21
- Partial or unilateral choanal atresia
- Tumor: encephalocele, meningocele

Toddlers (1–3 y)

Allergic rhinitis: indoor and food allergens

Infectious rhinitis: recurrent URI, sinusitis (CF, primary ciliary dyskinesia, immunodeficiency[a])

Nonallergic, noninfectious rhinitis

- Irritant rhinitis

Obstruction

- Adenoidal or turbinate hypertrophy
- Foreign body

Children (3–12 y)

Allergic rhinitis: indoor and outdoor allergens

Infectious rhinitis: recurrent URI, sinusitis (CF, primary ciliary dyskinesia, immunodeficiency[a])

Nonallergic, noninfectious rhinitis

- Physical rhinitis (gustatory, cold, sunlight)
- Irritant rhinitis
- NARES
- Rhinitis medicamentosa: topical decongestants

Obstruction

- Adenoidal or turbinate hypertrophy
- Foreign body
- Nasal polyp
- Tumor

Adolescents (12–18 y)

Allergic rhinitis: indoor and outdoor allergens

Infectious rhinitis: viral URI, sinusitis (immunodeficiency[a])

Nonallergic, noninfectious rhinitis

- Physical rhinitis (gustatory, cold, sunlight)
- NARES
- Rhinitis medicamentosa: topical decongestants, cocaine
- Idiopathic (vasomotor)

Obstruction

- Adenoidal or turbinate hypertrophy
- Nasal polyps, septal deviation
- Tumor: angiofibroma

Abbreviations: CF, cystic fibrosis; NARES, nonallergic rhinitis with eosinophilia syndrome; URI, upper respiratory infection.
[a] IgA deficiency, hypogammaglobulinemia, human immunodeficiency virus infection.

Adapted from Zacharisen MC. Rhinitis in children, adolescents, the elderly, and pregnant women: special considerations. Immunol Allergy Clin North Am 2000;20:428; with permission.

or therapeutic complications. The 4 key components of AR management are patient/caregiver education, environmental control measures, pharmacotherapy, and immunomodulation.

Environmental Control Measures

Environmental control by avoidance of relevant allergens and symptomatic triggers is a key initial step in the management of AR. However, complete avoidance is rarely possible. Evidence on pet allergen avoidance is lacking, and recent reviews have found minimal to no evidence to support dust mite avoidance measures, the most common of which are impermeable pillow and mattress covers.[31,32] Avoidance of respiratory irritants, such as tobacco smoke and strong perfumes, seems reasonable.

Pharmacotherapy

Because of the limited effectiveness of environmental control measures, pharmacotherapeutics are often needed for children with moderate/severe or persistent AR symptoms. **Fig. 1** summarizes guideline-directed therapy, which may involve more than one agent.[1,7,15] Treatment of AR with intranasal corticosteroids, antihistamines, or leukotriene modifiers is also effective in reducing or controlling asthma symptoms.[15]

Corticosteroids

Systemic corticosteroids should rarely be used in children with AR because safer, effective alternatives are available.[1,7,15] Intranasal corticosteroids (INCS) are the most effective therapy for AR in children.[1,15,33] INCSs treat the inflammatory clinical manifestations of AR and have also shown great benefit in improving the comorbidities of asthma and bronchial hyperresponsiveness, conjunctivitis, sleep disorders, and quality-of-life impairment.[34–38]

There is no evidence to indicate that any INCS is clinically superior if used correctly at the recommended dose.[39] Symptomatic improvement has been reported within 12 hours of use.[40] In the Pediatric Allergies in America survey, 19% of parents reported that INCSs provided relief for their child in less than 1 hour and 31% in 1 hour.[5] However, full benefit may not be achieved for days to weeks after starting therapy.

The potential for systemic absorption of INCSs to have effects on the hypothalamic-pituitary-adrenal axis and on growth has been evaluated in many studies, most of which showed limited or no hypothalamic-pituitary-adrenal effects at recommended doses.[41–45] Second-generation INCSs have markedly lower bioavailability compared with first-generation agents, resulting in a lower risk of side effects (**Table 1**). Longer-term studies of the growth effects caused by inhaled corticosteroids administered for asthma are also reassuring. Caution is needed, however, if corticosteroids are used for concurrent conditions, as the adverse effects of topical corticosteroid preparations can be additive. Appropriate recommendations for children prescribed INCSs include (1) lowest effective dose, (2) regular height measurements, and (3) periodic re-evaluation of need for INCS.

Oral and Intranasal Antihistamines

Second-generation oral and intranasal antihistamines (**Table 2**) are effective for AR and are generally well tolerated.[1,15] Metabolites of second-generation antihistamines, such as fexofenadine (the metabolite of terfenadine) or levocetirizine (a purified isomer of cetirizine), were designed to have fewer central nervous system effects, although

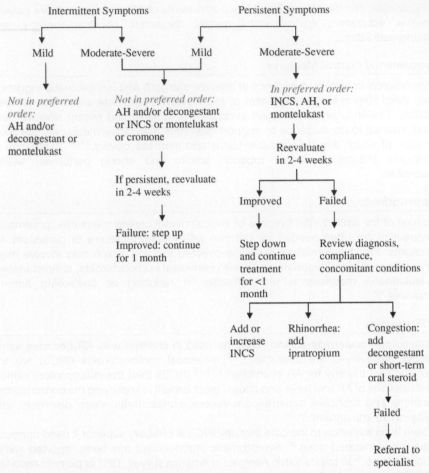

Fig. 1. Suggested treatment algorithm for pediatric allergic rhinitis. Consider allergen avoidance measures, intranasal antihistamines, and immunomodulatory therapy where appropriate. AH, antihistamines. (*From* Gentile D, Bartholow A, Valovirta E, et al. Current and future directions in pediatric allergic rhinitis. J Allergy Clin Immunol: In Practice 2013;1:218; with permission.)

this has not been confirmed.[46] Antihistamine sprays have a rapid onset of action (less than 15 minutes after use).[40] Dual azelastine-fluticasone therapy is also available.

First-generation antihistamines should no longer be used in children because of their risk of sedation and other unfavorable effects.[13]

Leukotriene Modifiers

Montelukast has been effective in seasonal and perennial AR pediatric studies.[47,48] It is the only leukotriene modifier approved in the United States for the treatment of pediatric AR. Adverse neuropsychiatric changes have been reported in some individuals, but studies have shown no significant difference when compared with placebo.[49,50] Pending further information, professional societies have advised that patients might continue montelukast unless mood disturbance develops.[51]

Table 1
Intranasal preparations used in pediatric AR

Generic Name	Brand Name(s)	Aqueous/Aerosol	MOA	RX/OTC	Dosing
Azelastine	Astelin	Aqueous	AH	RX	5–11 y: 1 SEN BID; ≥12 y: 2 SEN BID (137 μg/spray)
Azelastine	Astepro	Aqueous	AH	RX	6–11 y: 1 SEN BID; ≥12 y: 1–2 SEN BID (205.5 μg/spray)
Azelastine/Fluticasone propionate	Dymista	Aqueous	AH/CS	RX	≥12 y: 1 SEN BID (137 μg/50 μg/spray)
Beclomethasone dipropionate	Beconase AQ	Aqueous	CS	RX	≥6 y: 1–2 SEN BID (42 μg/spray)
Beclomethasone dipropionate	Qnasl	Aerosol	CS	RX	≥12 y: 2 SEN daily (80 μg/spray)
Budesonide	Rhinocort Aqua	Aqueous	CS	RX	≥6 y: 1–2 SEN daily (32 μg/spray)
Ciclesonide	Omnaris	Aqueous	CS	RX	≥6 y: 2 SEN daily (50 μg/spray)
Ciclesonide	Zetonna	Aerosol	CS	RX	≥12 y: 1 SEN daily (37 mcg/spray)
Flunisolide	(Brand name product no longer available in US)	Aqueous	CS	RX	6–14 y: 2 SEN B D; ≥15 y: 2 SEN BID-TID (max 8 SEN per day) (25,29 μg/spray)
Cromolyn	NasalCrom	Aqueous	Chromone	OTC	≥2 y: 1 SEN TID-QID (max 6 SEN per day)
Fluticasone furoate	Veramyst	Aqueous	CS	RX	≥2 y: 1–2 SEN daily (27.5 μg/spray)
Fluticasone propionate	Flonase	Aqueous	CS	RX	≥4 y: 1–2 SEN daily (50 μg/spray)
Ipratropium bromide	Atrovent	Aqueous	AC	RX	≥6 y: 2 SEN BID-TID (42 μg; 0.03% spray)
Mometasone furoate	Nasonex	Aqueous	CS	RX	2–11 y: 1 SEN daily; ≥12 y: 2 SEN daily (50 μg/spray)
Olopatadine	Patanase	Aqueous	AH	RX	6–11 y: 1 SEN BID; ≥12 y: 2 SEN BID (665 μg/spray)
Oxymetazoline	Afrin	Aqueous	Topical Vasoconstrictor	OTC	≥6 y: 1–2 SEN BID for up to 3 d
Triamcinolone	Nasacort AQ	Aqueous	CS	OTC	2–5 y: 1 SEN daily; ≥6 y: 1–2 SEN daily (55 μg/spray)

Fluticasone propionate, fluticasone furoate, mometasone furoate, and ciclesonide are second-generation intranasal CS with undetectable to less than 2% systemic bioavailability. The remaining intranasal CS are first-generation agents, which have 10%–50% bioavailability.

Abbreviations: AC, anticholinergic; AH, antihistamine; BID, twice daily; CS, corticosteroid; MOA, mechanism of action; OTC, over the counter; QD, once daily; QID, four times daily; RX, prescription; SEN, spray each nostril; TID, three times daily.

Data from deShazo RD, Kemp SF. Pharmacotherapy of allergic rhinitis. In: Post TW, editor. UpToDate. Waltham (MA): UpToDate. Accessed May 10, 2014.

Table 2
Oral preparations used in pediatric AR

Generic Name	Brand Name	MOA	RX/OTC	Dosing
Cetirizine	Zyrtec	AH	OTC	6 mo–1 y: 2.5 mg daily; 1–2 y: 2.5 mg daily or BID; 2–5 y: 2.5–5 mg daily; ≥6 y: 5–10 mg daily
Desloratadine	Clarinex	AH	RX	6–11 mo: 1 mg daily; 1–5 y: 1.25 mg daily; 6–11 y: 2.5 mg daily; ≥12 y: 5 mg daily
Fexofenadine	Allegra	AH	OTC	2–11 y: 30 mg BID; ≥12 y: 60 mg BID or 180 mg daily
Levocetirizine	Xyzal	AH	RX	6 mo-5 y: 1.25 mg QPM; 6–11 y: 2.5 mg QPM; ≥12 y: 2.5–5 mg QPM
Loratadine	Alavert; Claritin	AH	OTC	2–6 y: 5 mg daily; ≥6 y: 10 mg daily
Montelukast	Singulair	LTRA	RX	6–23 mo: 4 mg (oral granules) daily; 2–5 y: 4 mg (tablet or granules) daily; 6–14 y: 5 mg daily; ≥15 y: 10 mg daily

Abbreviations: AH, antihistamine; BID, twice daily; LTRA, leukotriene receptor antagonist; MOA, mechanism of action; OTC, over the counter; QPM, once nightly; RX, prescription; SEN, spray each nostril; TID, three times daily.

Intranasal Cromolyn

Cromolyn sodium is a weakly effective topical mast cell stabilizer that is well tolerated but needs to be administered 4 times daily for efficacy.[15] It can also be used prophylactically for episodic rhinitis before allergen exposure.

Intranasal Anticholinergics

Ipratropium nasal spray can limit nasal drainage but offers no relief for pruritus or congestion. It is sometimes useful in children with profuse rhinorrhea uncontrolled by INCS use.[1]

Intranasal Decongestants

Vasoconstrictor decongestant sprays, such as oxymetazoline, can be used briefly in children to relieve severe nasal congestion, but prolonged use can lead to rhinitis medicamentosa characterized by rebound nasal congestion.[1] In contrast, the combination of intranasal decongestant and INCS in adults may effectively treat nasal congestion without rhinitis medicamentosa,[52] but this approach has not been evaluated in children.

Saline Irrigation

As adjunctive therapy, nasal irrigation with saline prepared from distilled or sterilized water may assist AR management by clearing secretions, allergens, and irritants.[53,54] Irrigation devices should be cleaned as directed and replaced regularly.

IMMUNOMODULATION
Allergen Immunotherapy

Allergen immunotherapy (AIT) encompasses both subcutaneous immunotherapy (SCIT) and sublingual immunotherapy. SCIT involves the supervised administration of gradually increasing doses of therapeutic vaccines of aeroallergens to which an individual has shown allergen-specific IgE. Over time, an optimal maintenance dose is attained that effectively modulates the immune response to the aeroallergen(s), resulting in fewer symptoms on exposure. Multiple immunomodulatory mechanisms are probably involved.[55] AIT is unique among therapeutic modalities in its ability to provide sustained immunomodulation of allergic respiratory disease, including the reduced incidence of asthma in children with AR.[56,57]

Sublingual immunotherapy involves the application of allergen (typically one allergen only) to the sublingual tissues or oral mucosa either as oral solutions or rapidly disintegrating tablets. Compared with SCIT, it has significantly lower risk and little difference in overall efficacy based on meta-analyses.[58,59] Two grass preparations and one ragweed preparation received US Food and Drug Administration approval for use in the United States in 2014.

Anti-immunoglobulin E Therapy

Omalizumab is a recombinant human monoclonal IgG anti-IgE antibody that binds to circulating IgE to prevent its binding to the surface receptors of mast cells and basophils. For patients 12 years and older, anti-IgE is effective for moderate-to-severe persistent asthma and for concurrent AR.[7,15]

REFERRAL

An allergist/immunologist can be particularly helpful for children with any of the following:

- Severe or prolonged symptoms despite avoidance measures and pharmacotherapy; AIT has been found to alter the progression of allergic respiratory disease, including the prevention of subsequent asthma development.
- Comorbid conditions
- Intolerance of pharmacotherapy
- Interest in immunomodulation as a therapeutic option

SUMMARY

AR presents both challenges and opportunities for the pediatric patient, caregiver, and health care professional. Proper diagnosis facilitates patient/caregiver education and permits consideration of multiple therapeutic modalities tailored to the individual patient. AR management in a specific child is age dependent and influenced by the severity and frequency of the symptoms and the presence of any concurrent conditions. Current strategies permit symptomatic control and improved quality of life for most patients.

REFERENCES

1. Wallace DV, Dykewicz MS, Bernstein DI, et al. The diagnosis and management of rhinitis: an updated practice parameter. J Allergy Clin Immunol 2008;122:S1–84.
2. Mallol J, Crane J, von Mutius E, et al. The International Study of Asthma and Allergies in Childhood (ISAAC) Phase Three: a global synthesis. Allergol Immunopathol (Madr) 2013;41:73–85.
3. Ng ML, Warlow RS, Chrishanthan N, et al. Preliminary criteria for the definition of allergic rhinitis: a systematic evaluation of clinical parameters in a disease cohort (I). Clin Exp Allergy 2000;30:1314–31.
4. Ng ML, Warlow RS, Chrishanthan N, et al. Preliminary criteria for the definition of allergic rhinitis: a systematic evaluation of clinical parameters in a disease cohort (II). Clin Exp Allergy 2000;30:1417–22.

5. Meltzer EO, Blaiss MS, Derebery J, et al. Burden of allergic rhinitis: results from the Pediatric Allergies in America survey. J Allergy Clin Immunol 2009;124(Suppl 3):S43–70.

6. Chng SY, Goh DY, Wang XS. Snoring and atopic disease: a strong association. Pediatr Pulmonol 2004;38:210–6.

7. Gentile D, Bartholow A, Valovirta E, et al. Current and future directions in pediatric allergic rhinitis. J Allergy Clin Immunol: In Practice 2013;1:214–26.

8. Thompson A, Sardana N, Craig TC. Sleep impairment and daytime sleepiness in patients with allergic rhinitis: the role of congestion and inflammation. Ann Allergy Asthma Immunol 2013;111:446–51.

9. Blaiss MS. Pediatric allergic rhinitis: physical and mental complications. Allergy Asthma Proc 2008;29:1–6.

10. Brawley A, Silverman B, Kearney S, et al. Allergic rhinitis in children with attention-deficit/hyperactivity disorder. Ann Allergy Asthma Immunol 2004;92:663–7.

11. Walker S, Khan-Wasti S, Fletcher M, et al. Seasonal allergic rhinitis is associated with a detrimental effect on examination performance in United Kingdom teenagers: case-control study. J Allergy Clin Immunol 2007;120:381–7.

12. Marshall PS, O'Hara C, Steinberg P. Effects of seasonal allergic rhinitis on selected cognitive abilities. Ann Allergy Asthma Immunol 2000;84:403–10.

13. Church MK, Maurer M, Simons FE, et al. Risk of first-generation H(1)-antihistamines: a GA(2)LEN position paper. Allergy 2010;65:459–66.

14. Jáuregui I, Mullol J, Dávila I, et al. Allergic rhinitis and school performance. J Investig Allergol Clin Immunol 2009;19(Suppl 1):32–9.

15. Brozek JL, Bousquet J, Baena-Cagnani CE, et al. Allergic Rhinitis and its Impact on Asthma (ARIA) guidelines: 2010 revision. J Allergy Clin Immunol 2010;126:466–76.

16. Bachert C, Vignola AM, Gevaert P, et al. Allergic rhinitis, rhinosinusitis and asthma: one airway disease. Immunol Allergy Clin North Am 2004;24:19–43.

17. Barney NP, Cook EB, Stahl JL. Allergic and immunologic diseases of the eye. In: Adkinson NF Jr, Bochner BS, Busse WW, et al, editors. Middleton's allergy: principles and practice. 8th edition. , St Louis (MO): Elsevier; 2014. p. 618–37.

18. Ibáñez MD, Valero AL, Montoro J, et al. Analysis of comorbidities and therapeutic approach for allergic rhinitis in a pediatric population in Spain. Pediatr Allergy Immunol 2013;24:678–84.

19. Slavin RG, Spector SL, Bernstein IL, et al. The diagnosis and management of sinusitis: a practice parameter update. J Allergy Clin Immunol 2005;116:S13–47.

20. Westman M, Stjärne P, Asarnoj A, et al. Natural course and comorbidities of allergic and nonallergic rhinitis in children. J Allergy Clin Immunol 2012;129:403–8.

21. Bernstein JM. The role of IgE-mediated hypersensitivity in the development of otitis media with effusion. Otolaryngol Clin North Am 1992;25:197–211.

22. Nguyen LH, Manoukian JJ, Sobol SE, et al. Similar allergic inflammation in the middle ear and upper airway: evidence linking otitis media with effusion to the united airways concept. J Allergy Clin Immunol 2004;114:1110–5.

23. Rappai M, Collop N, Kemp S, et al. The nose and sleep-disordered breathing: what we know and what we do not know. Chest 2003;124:2309–23.

24. Alkhalil M, Lockey R. Pediatric obstructive sleep apnea syndrome (OSAS) for the allergist: update on the assessment and management. Ann Allergy Asthma Immunol 2011;107:104–9.

25. Howarth PH. Allergic and nonallergic rhinitis. In: Adkinson NF Jr, Yuninger JW, Busse WW, et al, editors. Middleton's allergy: principles and practice. 6th edition. St Louis (MO): Mosby; 2003. p. 1391–410.

26. Kulig M, Klettke U, Wahn V, et al. Development of seasonal allergic rhinitis during the first 7 years of life. J Allergy Clin Immunol 2000;106:832–9.
27. Skoner DP. Allergic rhinitis: definition, epidemiology, pathophysiology, detection, and diagnosis. J Allergy Clin Immunol 2001;108(Suppl 1):S2–8.
28. Sicherer SH, Wood RA. American Academy of Pediatrics Section on Allergy and Immunology. Allergy testing in childhood: using allergen-specific IgE tests. Pediatrics 2012;129:193–7.
29. Orban NT, Saleh H, Durham SR. Allergic and non-allergic rhinitis. In: Adkinson NF Jr, Bochner BS, Busse WW, et al, editors. Middleton's allergy: principles and practice. 7th edition. St Louis (MO): Elsevier; 2009. p. 973–90.
30. Broide DH. Allergic rhinitis: pathophysiology. Allergy Asthma Proc 2010;31:370–4.
31. Nurmatov U, van Schayck CP, Hurwitz B, et al. House dust mite avoidance measures for perennial allergic rhinitis: an updated Cochrane systematic review. Allergy 2012;67:158–65.
32. Arroyave WD, Rabito FA, Carlson JC, et al. Impermeable dust mite covers in primary and tertiary prevention of allergic disease: a meta-analysis. Ann Allergy Asthma Immunol 2014;112:237–48.
33. Rachelefsky G, Farrar JR. A control model to evaluate pharmacotherapy for allergic rhinitis in children. JAMA Pediatr 2013;167:380–6.
34. Bielory L. Ocular symptom reduction in patients with seasonal allergic rhinitis treated with the intranasal corticosteroid mometasone furoate. Ann Allergy Asthma Immunol 2008;100:272–9.
35. Corren J, Manning BE, Thompson SF, et al. Rhinitis therapy and the prevention of hospital care for asthma: a case-control study. J Allergy Clin Immunol 2004;113:415–9.
36. Crystal-Peters J, Neslusan C, Crown WH, et al. Treating allergic rhinitis in patients with comorbid asthma: the risk of asthma-related hospitalizations and emergency department visits. J Allergy Clin Immunol 2002;109:57–62.
37. Bender BG, Milgrom H. Comparison of the effects of fluticasone propionate aqueous nasal spray and loratadine on daytime alertness and performance in children with seasonal allergic rhinitis. Ann Allergy Asthma Immunol 2004;92:344–9.
38. Mansfield LE, Diaz G, Posey CR, et al. Sleep disordered breathing and daytime quality of life in children with allergic rhinitis during treatment with intranasal budesonide. Ann Allergy Asthma Immunol 2004;92:240–4.
39. Luskin AT, Blaiss MS, Farrar JR, et al. Is there a role for aerosol nasal sprays in the treatment of allergic rhinitis: a white paper. Allergy Asthma Proc 2011;32:168–77.
40. van Cauwenberge P, Bachert C, Passalacqua G, et al. Consensus statement on the treatment of allergic rhinitis. European Academy of Allergology and Clinical Immunology. Allergy 2000;55:116–34.
41. Schenkel EJ, Skoner DP, Bronsky EA, et al. Absence of growth retardation in children with perennial allergic rhinitis after one year of treatment with mometasone furoate aqueous nasal spray. Pediatrics 2000;105:E22.
42. Allen DB, Meltzer EO, Lemanske RF, et al. No growth suppression in children treated with the maximum recommended dose of fluticasone propionate aqueous nasal spray for one year. Allergy Asthma Proc 2002;23:407–13.
43. Skoner DP, Gentile D, Angelini B, et al. The effects of intranasal triamcinolone acetonide and intranasal fluticasone propionate on short-term bone growth and HPA axis in children with allergic rhinitis. Ann Allergy Asthma Immunol 2003;90:56–62.

44. Möller C, Ahlström H, Henricson KA, et al. Safety of nasal budesonide in the long-term treatment of children with perennial rhinitis. Clin Exp Allergy 2003;33:816–22.
45. Galant SP, Melamed IR, Nayak AS, et al. Lack of effect of fluticasone propionate aqueous nasal spray on the hypothalamic-pituitary-adrenal axis in 2- and 3-year-old patients. Pediatrics 2003;112:96–100.
46. Verster JC, Volkerts ER. Antihistamines and driving ability: evidence from on-the-road driving studies during normal traffic. Ann Allergy Asthma Immunol 2004;92: 294–303.
47. Li AM, Abdullah VJ, Tsen CS, et al. Leukotriene receptor antagonist in the treatment of childhood allergic rhinitis—a randomized placebo-controlled study. Pediatr Pulmonol 2009;44:1085–92.
48. Razi C, Bakirtas A, Harmanci K, et al. Effect of montelukast on symptoms and exhaled nitric oxide levels in 7- to 14-year-old children with seasonal allergic rhinitis. Ann Allergy Asthma Immunol 2006;97:767–74.
49. Philip G, Hustad C, Noonan G, et al. Reports of suicidality in clinical trials of montelukast. J Allergy Clin Immunol 2009;124:691–6.e6.
50. Philip G, Hustad CM, Malice MP, et al. Analysis of behavior-related adverse experiences in clinical trials of montelukast. J Allergy Clin Immunol 2009;124: 699–706.e8.
51. Joint statement on FDA investigation of Singulair from the AAAAI and ACAAI. In: Peters-Golden M. Agents affecting the 5-lipoxygenase pathway in the treatment of asthma. In: Post TW, editor, Waltham, MA.
52. Baroody FM, Brown D, Gavanescu L, et al. Oxymetazoline adds to the effectiveness of fluticasone furoate in the treatment of perennial allergic rhinitis. J Allergy Clin Immunol 2011;127:927–34.
53. Li H, Sha Q, Zuo K, et al. Nasal saline irrigation facilitates control of allergic rhinitis by topical steroid in children. ORL J Otorhinolaryngol Relat Spec 2009;71:50–5.
54. Wang YH, Yang CP, Ku MS, et al. Efficacy in the treatment of acute sinusitis in children. Int J Pediatr Otorhinolaryngol 2009;73:1696–701.
55. Akdis M, Akdis CA. Mechanisms of allergen-specific immunotherapy: multiple suppressor factors at work in immune tolerance to allergens. J Allergy Clin Immunol 2014;133:621–31.
56. Niggemann B, Jacobsen L, Dreborg S, et al. Five-year follow-up on the PAT study: specific immunotherapy and long-term prevention of asthma in children. Allergy 2006;61:855–9.
57. Passalacqua G, Durham SR, Global Allergy and Asthma European Network. Allergic rhinitis and its impact on asthma update: allergen immunotherapy. J Allergy Clin Immunol 2007;119:881–91.
58. Radulovic S, Wilson D, Calderon M, et al. Systematic reviews of sublingual immunotherapy (SLIT). Allergy 2011;66:740–52.
59. Kim JM, Lin SY, Suarez-Cuervo C, et al. Allergen-specific immunotherapy for pediatric asthma and rhinoconjunctivitis: a systematic review. Pediatrics 2013; 131:1155–67.

Anaphylaxis and Urticaria

Kelli W. Williams, MD, MPH[a], Hemant P. Sharma, MD, MHS[b,*]

KEYWORDS

- Anaphylaxis • Urticaria • Treatment • Prevention

KEY POINTS

- Anaphylaxis is a serious, life-threatening allergic reaction that affects approximately 2% of the population.
- Urticaria is a rash of transient, erythematous, pruritic wheals that affects up to 25% of the population.
- All cases of anaphylaxis warrant thorough clinical evaluation by the allergist–immunologist, although most cases of urticaria are self-limited and do not require specialist referral.

INTRODUCTION

Anaphylaxis is an acute, severe systemic allergic reaction that can ultimately lead to death if not recognized early and treated properly. Resulting from the rapid release of mast cell–derived and basophil-derived mediators, an anaphylactic reaction can begin quickly and be difficult to control. Fortunately, if recognized early, anaphylaxis can be easily treatable.

Although often a component of anaphylaxis, urticaria is a common allergic complaint that can occur as an isolated incident or as a recurring problem. Urticaria is a rash that consists of transient, erythematous, pruritic, and usually blanching wheals. They can be found on any part of the body and can be triggered by a multitude of eliciting factors. Often, urticaria is quite bothersome and can last from minutes to months.

This article summarizes our current knowledge on the epidemiology, pathogenesis, associated triggers, diagnosis, and treatment of both anaphylaxis and urticaria. Preventative strategies are also discussed.

Disclosures: Nothing to disclose (K.W. Williams); Spokesperson for unbranded anaphylaxis education campaign sponsored by Mylan Specialty; Consultant, Nutricia NA (H.P. Sharma).
[a] Laboratory of Clinical Infectious Diseases, National Institute of Allergy and Infectious Diseases, National Institutes of Health, 9000 Rockville Pike, Bethesda, MD 20892, USA; [b] Division of Allergy and Immunology, Children's National Medical Center, Children's National Health System, 111 Michigan Avenue NW, Washington, DC 20010, USA
* Corresponding author.
E-mail address: HSharma@childrensnational.org

ANAPHYLAXIS
Epidemiology

Anaphylaxis is an acute, life-threatening systemic allergic reaction that affects up to 2% of the population.[1,2] The majority of cases of anaphylaxis are in children, where the prevalence of food allergy has been estimated as high as 8%.[2–4] The exact proportion of cases resulting in fatality is unknown, but is rare overall.[5]

Recently a nationwide, cross-sectional, random digital dial telephone survey of 1000 adults was completed. In this population, nearly 8% of participants reported a prior anaphylactic reaction, but, when symptoms were evaluated, the lifetime prevalence of anaphylaxis was 1.6%.[6]

Previously, anaphylaxis was characterized as an allergic reaction that involved 2 or more organ systems or hypotension.[7] However, in the last 10 years, formal clinical diagnostic criteria for anaphylaxis have been developed by the National Institute of Allergy and Infectious Diseases and the Food Allergy and Anaphylaxis Network (now known as Food Allergy Research and Education; **Box 1**).[8] Despite these criteria,

---

Box 1
Diagnostic criteria for anaphylaxis

Anaphylaxis is diagnosed when 1 of the following criteria is met:

1. Development of acute illness within minutes to hours after exposure causing skin and/or mucosal tissue involvement (eg, rash, generalized urticaria, pruritus, flushing, angioedema, laryngeal edema).

    And at least 1 of the following are present:

    - Evidence of respiratory compromise (eg, dyspnea, cough, difficulty breathing, wheezing, stridor);

    - Hypotension (defined in point 3) or evidence of end organ dysfunction (eg, syncope, hypotonia, urinary incontinence).

2. Development of 2 or more of the following within minutes to hours after exposure to a likely allergen for that patient:

    - Skin or mucosal tissue involvement, including rash, generalized urticaria, pruritus, flushing, angioedema, laryngeal edema;

    - Respiratory compromise, including dyspnea, cough, difficulty breathing, wheezing, stridor, and hypoxia;

    - Hypotension or symptoms concerning for hypotension, including syncope, hypotonia, and urinary incontinence; and

    - Gastrointestinal symptoms, including nausea, vomiting, diarrhea, and crampy abdominal pain.

3. Development of hypotension within minutes to hours after exposure to a known allergen for that patient:

    - Infants and children age less than 1 year: SBP less than 70; children ages 1 to 10 years: SBP < (70 mm Hg + [2 × age in years]); children ages 11 to 17 years: SBP less than 90 mm Hg; or for all children: A greater than 30% decrease from that person's baseline.

    - Adults: SBP less than 90 mm Hg or greater than 30% decrease from that person's baseline.

Abbreviation: SBP, systolic blood pressure.
Adapted from Sampson HA, Muñoz-Furlong A, Campbell RL, et al. Second symposium on the definition and management of anaphylaxis: summary report–second National Institute of Allergy and Infectious Disease/Food Allergy and Anaphylaxis Network symposium. Ann Emerg Med 2006;47(4):374; with permission.

several retrospective chart analyses of emergency department visits have confirmed the underdiagnosis of anaphylaxis, with reports of 25% to 57% of anaphylaxis cases not properly diagnosed as anaphylaxis.[7,9,10] The true prevalence of anaphylaxis is likely underreported owing to underdiagnosis.[11] Several studies have reported increasing prevalence over the last few decades.[12–15]

Pathophysiology

Murine studies have revealed both immunoglobulin (Ig)E-dependent and IgE-independent mechanisms of anaphylaxis.[16–18] IgE-mediated reactions result after allergen sensitization has occurred. During sensitization, allergen-specific IgE antibodies bind with high affinity to FcεRI receptors on both tissue mast cells and circulating basophils. Upon exposure to the sensitized allergen, IgE cross-linking promotes the immediate release of several mediators and cytokines, including histamine, tryptase, chymase, platelet-activating factor, prostaglandin D2, cysteinyl leukotrienes, interleukin-6, and tumor necrosis factor-α.[19,20] Rapid degranulation of these substances into the systemic circulation contributes to the multiorgan dysfunction seen in anaphylaxis and ultimately can result in death.[21]

In an IgE-independent mechanism initiated by allergen exposure, IgG can bind to form IgG–antigen immune complexes.[16] These immune complexes cross-link with FcεRIII receptors found on macrophages and induce the release of additional platelet-activating factor, but not histamine or tryptase.[22,23]

By inducing smooth muscle constriction and augmenting vascular permeability, histamine is responsible for the flushing, pruritus, rhinorrhea, tachycardia, and bronchospasm seen in anaphylaxis. The release of tryptase from mast cells allows for the amplification of the allergic response by stimulating further mast cell degranulation. Additionally, tryptase activates downstream pathways, including the complement cascade, coagulation pathway, and the kallikrein–kinin system. These pathways contribute to the hypotension and angioedema seen in many cases of anaphylaxis. Like histamine, platelet-activating factor enhances vascular permeability and contributes to the clinical manifestations, notably the hypotension, seen in anaphylaxis.[19,21,22,24] Recently, platelet-activating factor levels were found to correlate directly and significantly with severity scores of anaphylaxis, and this clinical correlation was not observed with tryptase and histamine levels.[25]

Triggers

Immunoglobulin E–mediated triggers

The most commonly identified cause of anaphylaxis is food allergy, contributing up to 50% of all cases of anaphylaxis (**Box 2**).[26] Affecting up to 8% of American children, food allergy is the major cause of anaphylaxis in children.[1,3,27] Although any food can cause anaphylaxis, the most commonly implicated foods are peanuts, tree nuts, and shellfish, with peanuts being the most common cause in children and shellfish the most common cause in adults.[28,29] Although the prevalence of tree nut allergy is lower than peanut allergy, a higher rate of fatal anaphylaxis has been reported with tree nut allergy.[30] Milk, soy, eggs, wheat, fish, food additives, and spices have also been associated with severe reactions.[31]

Delayed anaphylaxis occurring 4 to 6 hours after ingestion of mammalian meat, particularly beef, has recently been described. These patients were found to have sensitization to the carbohydrate galactose-α-1,3-galactose, which is found in select mammalian meats.[32] Sensitization to galactose-α-1,3-galactose has been described after bites of *Ixodes* ticks.[33]

Box 2
Common triggers of anaphylaxis and urticaria

Allergic triggers: Reaction owing to immunoglobulin E-mediated response to allergen

   Foods, such as peanut, shellfish, tree nuts, milk, soy, wheat, egg, and fish

   Drugs, such as β-lactam antibiotics and nonsteroidal anti-inflammatory drugs

   Insect venom, such as from honey bee, wasps, yellow jackets, hornets, and fire ants

   Biologics, such as allergen immunotherapy, vaccine additives, monoclonal antibodies

   Latex

   Food additives, such as carmine, gelatin, and spices

Nonimmunologic triggers: Reaction owing to direct activation of mast cells and basophils

   Physical factors, such as exercise, cold, and heat

   Medications, such as opioids

   Radiocontrast media

Other systemic triggers

   Systemic mastocytosis or a clonal mast cell disorder

   Idiopathic anaphylaxis

Data from Refs.[2,8,21]

Drug allergy is also a common cause of anaphylaxis, particularly in adults.[1,2,6] Of the countless drugs that have been implicated in anaphylaxis, most reactions are secondary to antibiotic exposure. Anaphylaxis owing to β-lactam antibiotics have been reported for over 50 years.[21,34] The incidence of penicillin-associated anaphylaxis has been reported as high as 1 to 5 per 10,000 patient courses of treatment.[35] Nonsteroidal anti-inflammatory drugs are identified frequently as common triggers of anaphylaxis, with ibuprofen and naproxen being implicated most often.[1,36] Webb and Lieberman[27] identified aspirin-associated anaphylaxis in 35% of drug allergy anaphylaxis. Although any medication can cause anaphylaxis, frequent reports have been described after treatment with insulin, heparin, erythromycin, and cancer chemotherapeutics.[27,37]

Biologic agents have also been associated frequently with anaphylaxis. Commonly implicated biologic agents include allergen immunotherapy, vaccinations, adjuvants, immune-modulating agents, and monoclonal antibodies.[8,38,39]

Anaphylaxis has been reported with latex exposure, especially among health care workers, patients with frequent procedures or genitourinary abnormalities, and workers with frequent occupational exposure to latex.[40,41] In patients without a known latex exposure, latex allergy has also been associated with atopy and family history of latex allergy.[42]

Anaphylaxis owing to Hymenoptera venom allergy can occur in up to 3% of insect stings in adults and 1% in children. In particular, honey bee, wasps, yellow jackets, white-faced hornets, yellow hornets, and fire ants have been associated with anaphylaxis, and first-time sting reactions can be fatal.[8,43,44] Bites from the deer fly and *Triatoma* have been reported in rare cases of anaphylaxis.[27]

Non–Immunoglobulin E–mediated triggers

Although diagnostic testing and clinical history aid substantially in our ability to identify a cause of anaphylaxis, up to 60% of anaphylaxis cases have no discernible basis.[27,45]

Idiopathic anaphylaxis is a diagnosis of exclusion that results when there are no identifiable triggers and other systemic disorders, such as mastocytosis, have been ruled out. Most cases of idiopathic anaphylaxis occur in adult women.[27,46] Idiopathic anaphylaxis is more prevalent among atopic individuals, with nearly 50% having associated atopy in 1 large cohort of patients with idiopathic anaphylaxis.[46]

Anaphylaxis has been reported to occur through non–IgE-mediated mechanisms. In particular, immediate mast cell and basophil degranulation can be triggered after exposure to radiocontrast media, opioid medications, and vancomycin.[47–50] Antigen–antibody immune complexes can also form after the administration of blood products and intravenous immunoglobulins. The immune complexes activate the complement system, which allows for the circulation of C3a, C4a, and C5a. These anaphylatoxins can trigger systemic mast cell and basophil degranulation leading to anaphylaxis.[51]

Physical stimuli, such as exercise, have also been reported to induce anaphylaxis. Exercise-induced anaphylaxis is most commonly reported in young adults, but can occur at any age.[52–54] Most cases of exercise-induced anaphylaxis present with symptoms during exercise or shortly afterward (<15 minutes). The pathophysiology of exercise-induced anaphylaxis remains unclear, but proposed mechanisms include release of endorphins and neuropeptides, such as gastrin, during exercise that trigger mast cell degranulation.[52,55,56]

Food-dependent, exercise-induced anaphylaxis has also been widely reported, usually with exposure to a specific food within minutes to hours before exercise and anaphylaxis with or immediately after activity. Foods that have been commonly implicated include wheat, soy, and nuts, although it can occur with others foods.[52,54,57–59] Taking aspirin or other nonsteroidal anti-inflammatory drugs before exercise has also been associated with anaphylaxis.[60,61]

Opioid medications, such as morphine, codeine, and meperidine, have been reported to elicit clinical anaphylaxis. Opioids can directly stimulate mast cell degranulation, releasing histamine and tryptase into circulation and contributing to the symptoms of anaphylaxis.[62,63]

Mastocytosis is a rare, heterogenous group of disorders characterized by clonal proliferation of mast cells in 1 or more organ systems. Systemic disease, in which there is significant bone marrow involvement, often presents with anaphylaxis.[64,65] This is owing to the propensity of the abundant and disruptive mast cells to degranulate. As a result, patients often have elevated baseline tryptase levels (>20 ng/mL).[66] Systemic mastocytosis is associated with c-KIT point mutations.[67] Other common symptoms of systemic mastocytosis include flushing, pruritus, syncope, urticaria, abdominal pain, tachycardia, and hypotension.

Diagnosis

The diagnosis of anaphylaxis relies heavily on the clinician obtaining a thorough history and physical examination, while paying particular attention to any possible or known allergen exposures. Because anaphylaxis is a systemic allergic reaction, the signs and symptoms can affect multiple organ systems (**Box 3**). The skin and mucosal tissues are most commonly involved, with urticaria and/or angioedema reported in nearly 90% of anaphylactic reactions.[27]

In 2005, the National Institute of Allergy and Infectious Diseases and Food Allergy and Anaphylaxis Network developed clinical diagnostic criteria to define anaphylaxis (see **Box 1**). In 2012, Campbell and colleagues[68] evaluated the validity of the National Institute of Allergy and Infectious Diseases/Food Allergy and Anaphylaxis Network diagnostic criteria for anaphylaxis and results yielded a sensitivity of 96.7% and a specificity of 82.4%.

Box 3
Common signs and symptoms of anaphylaxis

Skin or mucosal tissue
Rash
Generalized urticaria
Flushing
Pruritus
Angioedema
Piloerection
Oral pruritus or tingling
Conjunctival erythema
Laryngeal edema
Respiratory
Dyspnea
Cough
Difficulty breathing
Wheezing
Stridor
Chest tightness
Rhinorrhea
Nasal congestion
Sneezing
Nasal pruritus
Dysphonia
Hoarseness
Cardiovascular
Syncope
Feeling faint or dizzy
Confusion
Altered mental state
Chest pain
Heart palpitations
Tachycardia
Bradycardia
Urinary incontinence
Cardiac arrest
Gastrointestinal
Nausea
Vomiting
Diarrhea

Crampy abdominal pain

Difficulty swallowing

Neurologic

Anxiety

Feeling of impending doom

Seizures

Headache

Irritability

Confusion

Data from Joint Task Force on Practice Parameters, American Academy of Allergy, Asthma and Immunology, American College of Allergy, Asthma and Immunology, et al. The diagnosis and management of anaphylaxis: an updated practice parameter. J Allergy Clin Immunol 2005;115(3 Suppl 2):S483–523; and Lieberman P. Middleton's allergy: principles and practice. Seventh edition. In: Adkinson NF, et al, editors. Anaphylaxis, Chapter 59. vol. 2. Philadelphia: Elsevier Inc; 2010. p. 1027–50.

Although anaphylaxis is a clinical diagnosis, laboratory testing may aid in confirming the severe systemic reaction. Because tryptase is among the early mediators released by mast cells during an acute allergic reaction, serum tryptase levels are often elevated (>11.5 ng/mL) in anaphylaxis. Serum tryptase levels peak 1 to 2 hours after symptom onset and normalize after 5 to 6 hours. It is crucial to obtain the serum tryptase level during its narrow window in circulation, usually within 3 hours of symptom onset.[69,70] Mast cells in the gastrointestinal and respiratory tracts may contain less tryptase per cell, contributing to inconsistently elevated tryptase levels in food-induced anaphylaxis.[5] Because of this variation, it is important to understand that an elevated tryptase level with a concerning clinical history is highly suggestive of anaphylaxis, although a normal tryptase level does not rule out anaphylaxis. Histamine is the first mediator released by mast cells; however, it normalizes within 45 minutes so is often of little diagnostic value.[71]

All patients who experience anaphylaxis should be referred for allergy–immunology evaluation. Depending on the clinical history, assessment of IgE-mediated sensitization to allergens of interest may be warranted. In vivo and in vitro tests to evaluate for IgE-mediated allergy are available for most foods, latex, and a few medications. Skin prick testing with extracts from suspected foods have a high negative predictive value and high sensitivity in predicting clinical allergy.[72–74] IgE antibody directed at specific allergens can also be measured in the blood. Patients with a clinical history concerning for allergy and evidence of IgE-directed sensitization, either by skin prick test or allergen-specific IgE antibody, are viewed to have clinical allergy. False-positive results can occur; therefore, the clinical history is most important.

Although anaphylaxis most commonly presents as an acute systemic reaction, secondary and delayed reactions have also been reported. Occurring up to 72 hours after an exposure to an allergen, biphasic reactions can occur in up to 25% of fatal or near-fatal anaphylactic reactions.[75]

Treatment and Prevention

The most crucial step in treating anaphylaxis is quickly recognizing the signs and symptoms so that therapy can be started immediately. Delayed treatment is associated with death.[5,30,74,76,77] As with any medical emergency, the clinician should first ensure that the patient's airway is protected and preserved. If there is evidence of respiratory compromise, the patient may need intubation and/or oxygen. Vital signs should be quickly assessed, and if there is evidence of circulatory compromise the patient should be placed in the recumbent position with legs elevated.

Intramuscular epinephrine is the first-line therapy for anaphylaxis.[78,79] Epinephrine should be injected into the front–lateral thigh, because studies have shown this location produces a rapid rise in plasma and tissue epinephrine levels.[80,81] The recommended adult dose is 0.3 mg of 1:1000 solution (1 mg/mL). Children should receive 0.01 mg/kg of 1:1000 solution with a maximum single dose of 0.3 mg. For ease of administration during anaphylaxis, there are several epinephrine autoinjectors available commercially. These autoinjectors come in standard adult doses (0.3 mg) and pediatric doses (0.15 mg) for children less than 25 kg. Additional doses of epinephrine may be given every 5 to 15 minutes if clinical symptoms do not improve. It is crucial for all patients and their families to be educated on proper technique of autoinjector administration. Because of the risk for a biphasic reaction, every patient who receives epinephrine should seek medical care for continuous monitoring of vital signs and clinical symptoms.

Although not the preferred route of administration, epinephrine can slowly be given intravenously (usually over 5 minutes) at a dose of 0.1 mg of 1:10,000 solution (0.1 mg/mL). Usually, intravenous epinephrine is reserved for patients who do not respond to repeated intramuscular injections.[82]

As adjuncts to epinephrine, but not in place of it, nebulized short-acting bronchodilators and antihistamines are used to reduce symptoms associated with anaphylaxis. In particular, H1 and H2 antagonists are commonly used to halt the progression of hives, flushing, and pruritus. Additionally, using a combination of both has shown superior effect in anaphylaxis than using an H1 antagonist alone.[83]

The use of corticosteroids in the acute management of IgE-mediated anaphylaxis is unclear. Although the Cochrane Database Systemic Review on corticosteroid use in anaphylaxis was unable to identify benefits in the acute management in anaphylaxis, Tole and Lieberman[75] demonstrated potential efficacy in reducing the frequency of biphasic anaphylactic reactions.[84]

Although rare, death from anaphylaxis results from cardiovascular collapse or respiratory failure. The most common triggers in anaphylaxis-related death have been insect stings, food allergy, drug allergy, and radiocontrast media.[30,85] Several studies have shown that a delay in epinephrine administration is a risk factor for anaphylaxis-related death and biphasic anaphylactic reactions.[5,30,75,77]

The crucial step in preventing anaphylaxis is identifying the trigger. Once identified, avoidance of this trigger is essential. This may mean avoiding particular foods, medications, outdoor areas where insects may habitate, or reducing exercise. Venom immunotherapy has proven successful in preventing stinging insect anaphylaxis in up to 98% of patients who previously had anaphylaxis from a sting.[44] For patients who have had anaphylaxis to a medication but require future doses, an induction of tolerance procedure may be performed under an allergist's care to safely administer the medication. Formerly known as drug desensitization, induction of tolerance is temporary and achieved by administering small but gradually increasing doses of the medication.[37] Patients who have been diagnosed with anaphylaxis should carry a medical alert identifying the allergy and an epinephrine autoinjector at all times.

URTICARIA
Epidemiology

Urticaria is an allergic rash that affects up to 25% of the population at some point in their lifetime.[86–89] The rash usually consists of transient, erythematous, pruritic, and circumscribed wheals, or hives (**Fig. 1**). There are 2 main categories of urticaria depending on the time course of the rash: Acute and chronic. Although each urticarial lesion may last minutes to hours, acute urticaria is an episode of hives that lasts less than 6 weeks. Chronic urticaria is hives that persist or recur, usually multiple days in a week, for longer than 6 weeks' duration.[86,90] Acute urticaria occurs more frequently in children than adults. Similar to anaphylaxis, acute urticaria is more prevalent in adult females than males.[87,91–95]

Affecting up to 1% of the population, chronic urticaria is more common in adults than children. Chronic urticaria often begins in the third to fifth decade of life and is most prevalent among women.[87,96–98] Although both acute and chronic urticaria usually resolve on their own, chronic urticaria may persist for years. Autoantibody-associated urticaria is responsible for 30% to 50% of all cases of chronic urticaria and is now considered a subset of chronic idiopathic urticaria.[90] As in anaphylaxis, physical activity can trigger urticaria. Physical urticaria represents 20% to 30% of all cases of chronic urticaria.[99] Another subtype of chronic urticaria is cholinergic urticaria, which accounts for 5% of all cases.[100,101]

Pathophysiology

As seen in anaphylaxis, urticaria results from the activation and degranulation of mast cells, which are abundant in the skin. Mast cell degranulation incites the rapid release

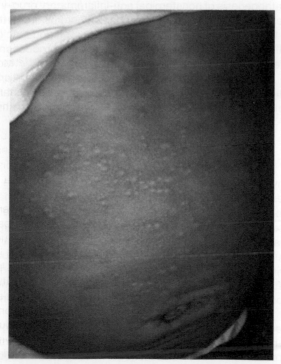

Fig. 1. Classic urticaria with scattered erythematous, pruritic, and usually blanching wheals.

of mediators and cytokines, including histamine, substance P, platelet-activating factor, tumor necrosis factor-α, interleukin-1, prostaglandin D2, and leukotrienes C4 and D4. Each of these contributes to the vasodilation, increased vascular permeability, and acute inflammation that leads to urticaria.[102,103]

Although urticaria can occur as a result of direct mast cell activation and degranulation, most urticaria results from immune-mediated hypersensitivity reactions.[102] The most common immunologic pathway in acute urticaria is IgE mediated, similar to that seen in anaphylaxis.

IgG antibodies to both IgE and/or the FcER1 α-subunit have been described to be pathogenic in patients with chronic urticaria. Through this autoimmune mechanism, histamine release theoretically can be triggered. Because these autoantibodies have also been reported in healthy subjects, there is controversy over the clinical pathogenicity.[102–104] In patients with autoantibody-associated urticaria, there is significant prevalence of other autoimmune conditions, including autoimmune thyroid disorders, celiac disease, systemic lupus erythematosus, rheumatoid arthritis, and type 1 diabetes.[90,105]

Both immune complex–mediated and cytotoxic hypersensitivity are thought to be involved with urticaria owing to infectious processes.[106–108] Additionally, cytotoxic reactions have been reported after blood product transfusions.[102]

Most physical urticarias result from the direct mast cell degranulation initiated by the specific physical stimulus, such as with heat, water, or vibration.[99] The pathogenesis of cholinergic urticaria is not well understood. Because cholinergic urticaria has been associated with hypohidrosis, the urticaria could result from leakage of the sweat into the dermis. Other theories include a muscarinic-mediated mechanism and a neurogenic reflex.[87,109–111]

Although the pathogenesis of nonsteroidal anti-inflammatory drug–induced urticaria is not well understood, the suggested mechanism stems from the inhibition of cyclooxygenase-1, which shunts the metabolism of arachidonic acid toward the 5-lipoxygenase pathway. This ultimately leads to increased production and release of cysteinyl leukotrienes, thus contributing to urticaria formation.[112] Molecular genetic mechanisms are also being sought in patients with nonsteroidal anti-inflammatory drug–induced urticaria. Although several target genes related to histamine and leukotriene metabolism have been suggested to be involved, research on the pathogenesis is ongoing.[113]

Triggers

Acute urticaria

Similar to anaphylaxis, 30% to 50% of acute urticaria cases are idiopathic (see **Box 2**).[114–116] Despite this, an allergy and immunology evaluation may be warranted in some cases because identifying the trigger may prevent future reactions. IgE-mediated hypersensitivity reactions to foods, medications, latex, and insect stings can trigger urticaria and anaphylaxis (see **Box 2**). Nonsteroidal anti-inflammatory drugs are particularly prone to inducing urticaria.[112] Additionally, patients who are sensitized to environmental aeroallergens, such as grass or pet dander, can develop acute urticaria after contact with the allergen.[87] A similar postinflammatory reaction can occur after bites from mosquitos, fleas, and bedbugs, and is known as papular urticaria.[117]

In children, infections are a major cause of acute urticaria. Although the pathogenesis of infection-related urticaria is unclear, the development of urticaria during an acute infectious process has been well described. Among the infectious agents, upper respiratory tract viruses, *Mycoplasma pneumoniae*, and parasitic infections have been commonly reported in children.[88,118,119] In adults, infectious hepatitis and mononucleosis have been implicated in acute urticaria.[120,121]

Chronic urticaria

Thirty percent to 60% of patients with chronic urticaria have positive autoantibodies directed at IgE, the FcER1 α-subunit, or positive autologous serum skin tests.[87,90,105] Chronic urticaria has also been associated with infection. Microbes that have been commonly associated with chronic urticaria include *Helicobacter pylori*, Group A *Streptococci*, hepatitis B and C, Epstein–Barr virus, and parasitic infection.[90,119,122–125]

The physical urticarias and their known triggers have been well described. Dermatographism results from friction applied to the skin, such as by stroking with a smooth, blunt object. Cold and heat urticaria presents minutes after contact or exposure to cold or hot objects, liquids, or air. Aquagenic urticaria results from direct skin contact with water, and can result from exposure to any water source and regardless of the water temperature. Cholinergic urticaria is precipitated by an increase in core body temperature and most often associated with exercise. Clinically, cholinergic urticaria is distinct from typical urticaria because they are smaller (usually 1–3 mm in diameter), punctate, and usually found in primarily on the chest and back. Delayed pressure urticaria results from sustained pressure. Vibratory urticaria is elicited after direct exposure to vibration. Solar urticaria is triggered by direct skin exposure to sunlight. Removal of these physical stimuli usually results in quick resolution of the urticaria.[99,126]

Chronic urticaria has also been associated with a variety of systemic disorders, including malignancy (eg, B-cell lymphoma, Hodgkin lymphoma), connective tissue disorders, Schnitzler syndrome, mastocytosis, hypereosinophilic syndrome, and Muckle–Wells syndrome.[105] Those patients with chronic urticaria and no identifiable trigger are ultimately diagnosed with chronic idiopathic urticaria.

Diagnosis

As with anaphylaxis, the diagnosis of urticaria relies greatly on the clinician conducting a thorough history and physical examination. Classically, urticaria are raised erythematous wheals that are pruritic. They are usually well-circumscribed or coalescing, and often migrate around the body. Any 1 lesion should last no more than 24 hours, and lesions that last longer or are associated with bruising may suggest urticarial vasculitis. Because urticaria are often transient, photographs of the lesions may be helpful in making the diagnosis when the rash has resolved. The history alone may suggest likely triggers. Typically, urticaria caused by an allergic reaction is distinguished by appearance of symptoms shortly (usually within 2 hours) after a new exposure and a time-limited course of symptoms (resolving within 1 day). Urticaria that lasts days is very unlikely to be caused by an allergic process. The differential diagnosis is broad, but includes erythema multiforme, allergic or irritant contact dermatitis, cellulitis, urticarial vasculitis, systemic lupus erythematosus, cryoglobulinemia, mastocytosis, and malignancy.[105,127]

If IgE-mediated hypersensitivity reaction is suspected, skin prick testing and/or serum IgE testing directed at the allergen may be available. This is often the case with food allergy, latex allergy, and rarely medication allergy. When no test is available and/or clinical suspicion is low, an allergen challenge may be done under close medical supervision.

Although blood work is not usually necessary in an initial evaluation for urticaria, a complete blood count with differential white blood cell, blood culture, C-reactive protein, and/or erythrocyte sedimentation rate may be helpful if infection is suspected. Microbial-specific antibodies can also be done. If suspicion is high for an inflammatory or systemic cause of the urticaria, a more thorough laboratory evaluation should be pursued.

Some patients with chronic urticaria may warrant further autoantibody studies, when clinically relevant. In particular, antithyroglobulin and antimicrosomal antibodies are often checked. Some clinicians may find testing for autoantibodies directed at IgE and the FcER1 α-subunit helpful, although this does not usually change clinical management.[86,87] Autologous serum skin tests, autologous plasma skin tests, and basophil histamine release assays have also been performed in patients with chronic urticaria. These tests are not confirmatory and routine performance of these tests is not recommended in patients with chronic urticaria.[90,103]

A punch skin biopsy should be performed when there is refractory urticaria or a concern for urticarial vasculitis. Skin biopsy typically reveals perivascular leukocytic infiltration with eosinophilis, neutrophils, and/or basophils. With urticarial vasculitis, skin biopsies should have evidence of leukocytoclasia and deposition of fibrinogen, complement, and/or immunoglobulins.[86,105]

Because physical and cholinergic urticaria are inducible by stimuli, there are a variety of diagnostic tests available to confirm these diagnoses. Provocative testing should be done in the office setting on an area of skin that has not been recently affected by urticaria. The most common form of physical urticaria is symptomatic dermatographism, which is confirmed by the development of wheal formation and pruritus after moderate stroking of the skin by a smooth, blunt object. The ice cube test is used to confirm cold urticaria. The clinician should place an ice cube (placed in a glass object or Ziplock bag to avoid water from touching the skin), cool pack, or cold water bath on the volar aspect of the forearm for up to 5 minutes. The arm should be evaluated for urticaria formation 10 minutes after removing the ice cube. Similarly, heat urticaria can be provoked by applying a hot stimulus to the skin (eg, glass or metal container with hot water, hot pack, or hot water bath). The heated device should be at a temperature of approximately 45°C. Aquagenic urticaria is diagnosed after the application of tap or distilled water to the skin and observation for urticarial emergence.[87,128]

Delayed pressure urticaria is evaluated by placing metal rods of various weights on the volar aspect of the forearm for 15 minutes. If urticaria appear 6 hours later, the diagnosis is confirmed. Vibratory urticaria can be diagnosed after the arm is placed on a vortex mixer for 10 minutes. The arm should be read for urticaria 10 minutes after provocation is complete. Solar urticaria can be provoked by exposing the buttocks separately to ultraviolet A, ultraviolet B, and visible light. Solar urticaria typically appears within 10 minutes after completed exposure. Cholinergic urticaria can be confirmed by following 2 steps. First, the patient should conduct moderate exercise for 15 minutes beyond the point of sweating. Ten minutes after completion, the skin should be evaluated for urticarial rash. If this test is positive, the patient should then undergo a passive warming study at least 24 hours after the exercise test. In the passive warming study, the patient should be emerged into a full bath at approximately 42°C for 15 minutes, with goal to achieve a rise in core body temperature of greater than 1°C. When differentiating cholinergic urticaria with hypotension from exercise-induced anaphylaxis, patients with exercise-induced anaphylaxis will not react with passive heating.[99,126,128]

Treatment and Prevention

Because of the transient nature of acute urticaria, treatment may not be necessary. Most episodes of acute urticaria self-resolve within 2 to 3 weeks. Prolonged episodes have been associated with atopy.[129] If the lesions are prolonged or bothersome, an oral second-generation H1 antagonist is the first-line treatment.[90] Commonly prescribed second-generation H1 antagonists include cetirizine, levocetirizine, fexofenadine, loratidine, and desloratadine. Of these, cetirizine and levocetirizine seem to be the most clinically effective.[87,108,130] Older H1 antagonists, such as diphenhydramine and hydroxyzine, are also still commonly used in the acute management of urticaria, but have been associated with higher levels of sedation and cognitive impairment.[131] Although the addition of an H2 antagonist, leukotriene receptor antagonist, and/or oral corticosteroids may alleviate the duration and severity of symptoms, these medications are often not necessary in the management of acute urticaria.

After identification of triggers, urticaria owing to foods, medications, venom, latex, or contact with aeroallergens can be prevented with strict avoidance. When urticaria present in the setting of acute infection, the infection should be treated promptly.

The frequency, severity, and unpredictability of chronic urticaria have contributed to a decrease quality of life in affected individuals.[132] Multiple medications are often required for the management of chronic urticaria. As with acute urticaria, second-generation H1 antagonists are first-line treatment and may require multiple doses a day for chronic suppression of symptoms. Often patients are prescribed a second-generation H1 antagonist 1 to 2 times a day with a shorter acting, first-generation H1 antagonist, such as diphenhydramine or hydroxyzine, for breakthrough symptoms. Other patients may require a second-generation H1 antagonist 4 times a day.[87,133,134]

The combination of both H1 and H2 antagonists has had conflicting efficacy results compared with monotherapy with H1 antagonists.[87,135–137] Of the H2 antagonists available, ranitidine, famotidine, and cimetidine are the most commonly prescribed for chronic urticaria. Combination use of H1 antagonist with a leukotriene receptor antagonist, such as montelukast and zafirlukast, has also been studied with mixed results.[138–140] Leukotriene receptor antagonists have shown increased efficacy particularly in patients with positive autologous serum skin tests and those with aspirin intolerance.[141,142]

For refractory urticaria, several additional agents have been used with varied results. These include corticosteroids, doxepin, sulfasalazine, dapsone, hydroxychloroquine, colchicine, mycophenolate mofetil, cyclosporine, methotrexate, and omalizumab.

Corticosteroids are often effective at resolving the urticaria; however, recurrence during taper or after completion of a course has been described commonly.[138] Systemic side effects are also reported widely with oral corticosteroids. Because doxepin has activity at both the H1 and H2 receptors, it has been used in recalcitrant urticaria.[87] Although the addition of dapsone to medication regimens has not reduced urticaria activity scores, it has shown good efficacy in inducing complete remission.[143,144] Sulfasalazine has incidentally resolved urticaria, and hydroxychloroquine has shown significant improvement in quality of life, albeit not with a significant improvement in urticaria activity scores.[145–148] Cyclosporine has induced remission of disease in a majority of patients, but the patients must be closely monitored for development of side effects (eg, kidney dysfunction, liver dysfunction, hypertension). In multiple, recent, randomized, multicenter trials, omalizumab has been shown to reduce significantly clinical symptoms of chronic urticaria compared with placebo.[149–152]

Physical stimuli known to elicit urticaria should be avoided when possible. Most physical urticarias are treated with oral antihistamines, either preceding exposure to a known trigger or as maintenance therapy.[99] Omalizumab is also being explored in treatment of physical urticaria.[126]

SUMMARY

Anaphylaxis and urticaria are allergic reactions that commonly present to outpatient clinics and emergency departments. Diagnosis relies heavily on obtaining a thorough clinical history and physical examination. If an allergen is suspected as the cause of the reaction, the patient should be referred to an allergist–immunologist for further evaluation. When possible, triggers should be identified to ensure avoidance and prevent future reactions. Unfortunately, a significant portion of cases are idiopathic and subsequently unpredictable. Especially in the case of anaphylaxis, patient education is essential in reducing morbidity and mortality.

Future research should focus on better elucidating the pathogenesis of chronic urticaria and idiopathic anaphylaxis so that treatment can be better targeted at their cause.

REFERENCES

1. Lieberman P. Epidemiology of anaphylaxis. Curr Opin Allergy Clin Immunol 2008;8(4):316–20.
2. Lieberman P, Camargo CA Jr, Bohlke K, et al. Epidemiology of anaphylaxis: findings of the American College of Allergy, Asthma and Immunology Epidemiology of Anaphylaxis Working Group. Ann Allergy Asthma Immunol 2006;97(5): 596–602.
3. Gupta RS, Springston EE, Warrier MR, et al. The prevalence, severity, and distribution of childhood food allergy in the United States. Pediatrics 2011;128(1):e9–17.
4. Rona RJ, Keil T, Summers C, et al. The prevalence of food allergy: a meta-analysis. J Allergy Clin Immunol 2007;120(3):638–46.
5. Sampson HA, Mendelson L, Rosen JP. Fatal and near-fatal anaphylactic reactions to food in children and adolescents. N Engl J Med 1992;327(6):380–4.
6. Wood RA, Camargo CA Jr, Lieberman P, et al. Anaphylaxis in America: the prevalence and characteristics of anaphylaxis in the United States. J Allergy Clin Immunol 2014;133(2):461–7.
7. Clark S, Bock SA, Gaeta TJ, et al. Multicenter study of emergency department visits for food allergies. J Allergy Clin Immunol 2004;113(2):347–52.
8. Joint Task Force on Practice Parameters, American Academy of Allergy, Asthma and Immunology, American College of Allergy, Asthma and Immunology, et al. The diagnosis and management of anaphylaxis: an updated practice parameter. J Allergy Clin Immunol 2005;115(3 Suppl 2):S483–523.
9. Clark S, Long AA, Gaeta TJ, et al. Multicenter study of emergency department visits for insect sting allergies. J Allergy Clin Immunol 2005;116(3):643–9.
10. Decker WW, Campbell RL, Manivannan V, et al. The etiology and incidence of anaphylaxis in Rochester, Minnesota: a report from the Rochester Epidemiology Project. J Allergy Clin Immunol 2008;122(6):1161–5.
11. Sclar DA, Lieberman PL. Anaphylaxis: underdiagnosed, underreported, and undertreated. Am J Med 2014;127(Suppl 1):S1–5.
12. Gupta R, Sheikh A, Strachan D, et al. Increasing hospital admissions for systemic allergic disorders in England: analysis of national admissions data. BMJ 2003;327(7424):1142–3.
13. Moneret-Vautrin DA, Morisset M, Flabbee J, et al. Epidemiology of life-threatening and lethal anaphylaxis: a review. Allergy 2005;60(4):443–51.
14. Mulla ZD, Lin RY, Simon MR. Perspectives on anaphylaxis epidemiology in the United States with new data and analyses. Curr Allergy Asthma Rep 2011; 11(1):37–44.

15. Poulos LM, Waters AM, Correll PK, et al. Trends in hospitalizations for anaphylaxis, angioedema, and urticaria in Australia, 1993–1994 to 2004–2005. J Allergy Clin Immunol 2007;120(4):878–84.
16. Finkelman FD. Anaphylaxis: lessons from mouse models. J Allergy Clin Immunol 2007;120(3):506–15 [quiz: 516–7].
17. Kalesnikoff J, Galli SJ. Anaphylaxis: mechanisms of mast cell activation. Chem Immunol Allergy 2010;95:45–66.
18. Karasuyama H, Tsujimura Y, Obata K, et al. Role for basophils in systemic anaphylaxis. Chem Immunol Allergy 2010;95:85 97.
19. Khan BQ, Kemp SF. Pathophysiology of anaphylaxis. Curr Opin Allergy Clin Immunol 2011;11(4):319–25.
20. Ono E, Taniguchi M, Mita H, et al. Increased production of cysteinyl leukotrienes and prostaglandin D2 during human anaphylaxis. Clin Exp Allergy 2009; 39(1):72–80.
21. Lieberman P. Middleton's allergy: principles and practice. In: Adkinson NF, et al, editors. Anaphylaxis, chapter 59, vol. 2, Seventh edition. Philadelphia: Elsevier Inc; 2010. p. 1027–50.
22. Shibamoto T, Liu W, Cui S, et al. PAF, rather than histamine, participates in mouse anaphylactic hypotension. Pharmacology 2008;82(2):114–20.
23. Strait RT, Morris SC, Finkelman FD. IgG-blocking antibodies inhibit IgE-mediated anaphylaxis in vivo through both antigen interception and Fc gamma RIIb cross-linking. J Clin Invest 2006;116(3):833–41.
24. Ogawa Y, Grant JA. Mediators of anaphylaxis. Immunol Allergy Clin North Am 2007;27(2):249–60, vii.
25. Vadas P, Perelman B, Liss G. Platelet-activating factor, histamine, and tryptase levels in human anaphylaxis. J Allergy Clin Immunol 2013;131(1):144–9.
26. Sampson HA. Anaphylaxis and emergency treatment. Pediatrics 2003; 111(6 Pt 3):1601–8.
27. Webb LM, Lieberman P. Anaphylaxis: a review of 601 cases. Ann Allergy Asthma Immunol 2006;97(1):39–43.
28. Sicherer SH, Munoz-Furlong A, Sampson HA. Prevalence of seafood allergy in the United States determined by a random telephone survey. J Allergy Clin Immunol 2004;114(1):159–65.
29. Sicherer SH, Sampson HA. Peanut allergy: emerging concepts and approaches for an apparent epidemic. J Allergy Clin Immunol 2007;120(3):491–503 [quiz: 504–5].
30. Pumphrey RS, Gowland MH. Further fatal allergic reactions to food in the United Kingdom, 1999–2006. J Allergy Clin Immunol 2007;119(4):1018–9.
31. Sicherer SH, Sampson HA. Food allergy: epidemiology, pathogenesis, diagnosis, and treatment. J Allergy Clin Immunol 2013;133(2):291–307.
32. Commins SP, Platts-Mills TA. Delayed anaphylaxis to red meat in patients with IgE specific for galactose alpha-1,3-galactose (alpha-gal). Curr Allergy Asthma Rep 2013;13(1):72–7.
33. Hamsten C, Starkhammar M, Tran TA, et al. Identification of galactose-alpha-1,3-galactose in the gastrointestinal tract of the tick Ixodes ricinus; possible relationship with red meat allergy. Allergy 2013;68(4):549–52.
34. Brown AF, McKinnon D, Chu K. Emergency department anaphylaxis: a review of 142 patients in a single year. J Allergy Clin Immunol 2001;108(5):861–6.
35. Idsoe O, Guthe T, Willcox RR, et al. Nature and extent of penicillin side-reactions, with particular reference to fatalities from anaphylactic shock. Bull World Health Organ 1968;38(2):159–88.

36. Helbling A, Hurni T, Mueller UR, et al. Incidence of anaphylaxis with circulatory symptoms: a study over a 3-year period comprising 940,000 inhabitants of the Swiss Canton Bern. Clin Exp Allergy 2004;34(2):285–90.
37. Joint Task Force on Practice Parameters, American Academy of Allergy, Asthma and Immunology, American College of Allergy, Asthma and Immunology, et al. Drug allergy: an updated practice parameter. Ann Allergy Asthma Immunol 2010;105(4):259–73.
38. deShazo RD, Kemp SF. Allergic reactions to drugs and biologic agents. JAMA 1997;278(22):1895–906.
39. Hong DI, Bankova L, Cahill KN, et al. Allergy to monoclonal antibodies: cutting-edge desensitization methods for cutting-edge therapies. Expert Rev Clin Immunol 2012;8(1):43–52 [quiz: 53–4].
40. Oei HD, Tjiook SB, Chang KC. Anaphylaxis due to latex allergy. Allergy Proc 1992;13(3):121–2.
41. Ownby DR, Tomlanovich M, Sammons N, et al. Anaphylaxis associated with latex allergy during barium enema examinations. AJR Am J Roentgenol 1991; 156(5):903–8.
42. Kimata H. Latex allergy in infants younger than 1 year. Clin Exp Allergy 2004; 34(12):1910–5.
43. Golden DB. Insect sting anaphylaxis. Immunol Allergy Clin North Am 2007; 27(2):261–72, vii.
44. Golden DB, Moffitt J, Nicklas RA, et al. Stinging insect hypersensitivity: a practice parameter update 2011. J Allergy Clin Immunol 2011;127(4): 852–4.e1-23.
45. Lieberman PL. Idiopathic anaphylaxis. Allergy Asthma Proc 2014;35(1):17–23.
46. Ditto AM, Harris KE, Krasnick J, et al. Idiopathic anaphylaxis: a series of 335 cases. Ann Allergy Asthma Immunol 1996;77(4):285–91.
47. Farnam K, Chang C, Teuber S, et al. Nonallergic drug hypersensitivity reactions. Int Arch Allergy Immunol 2012;159(4):327–45.
48. Lang JH, Lasser EC, Kolb WP. Activation of serum complement by contrast media. Invest Radiol 1976;11(4):303–8.
49. Simon RA, Schatz M, Stevenson DD, et al. Radiographic contrast media infusions. Measurement of histamine, complement, and fibrin split products and correlation with clinical parameters. J Allergy Clin Immunol 1979;63(4): 281–8.
50. Szebeni J. Hypersensitivity reactions to radiocontrast media: the role of complement activation. Curr Allergy Asthma Rep 2004;4(1):25–30.
51. Bergamaschini L, Santangelo T, Faricciotti A, et al. Study of complement-mediated anaphylaxis in humans. The role of IgG subclasses (IgG1 and/or IgG4) in the complement-activating capacity of immune complexes. J Immunol 1996;156(3):1256–61.
52. Beaudouin E, Renaudin JM, Morisset M, et al. Food-dependent exercise-induced anaphylaxis–update and current data. Eur Ann Allergy Clin Immunol 2006;38(2):45–51.
53. Schwartz LB, Delgado L, Craig T, et al. Exercise-induced hypersensitivity syndromes in recreational and competitive athletes: a PRACTALL consensus report (what the general practitioner should know about sports and allergy). Allergy 2008;63(8):953–61.
54. Shadick NA, Liang MH, Partridge AJ, et al. The natural history of exercise-induced anaphylaxis: survey results from a 10-year follow-up study. J Allergy Clin Immunol 1999;104(1):123–7.

55. Sheffer AL, Tong AK, Murphy GF, et al. Exercise-induced anaphylaxis: a serious form of physical allergy associated with mast cell degranulation. J Allergy Clin Immunol 1985;75(4):479–84.

56. Tharp MD, Thirlby R, Sullivan TJ. Gastrin induces histamine release from human cutaneous mast cells. J Allergy Clin Immunol 1984;74(2):159–65.

57. Du Toit G. Food-dependent exercise-induced anaphylaxis in childhood. Pediatr Allergy Immunol 2007;18(5):455–63.

58. Oyefara BI, Bahna SL. Delayed food-dependent, exercise-induced anaphylaxis. Allergy Asthma Proc 2007;28(1):64–6.

59. Pourpak Z, Ghojezadeh L, Mansouri M, et al. Wheat anaphylaxis in children. Immunol Invest 2007;36(2):175–82.

60. Aihara M, Miyazawa M, Osuna H, et al. Food-dependent exercise-induced anaphylaxis: influence of concurrent aspirin administration on skin testing and provocation. Br J Dermatol 2002;146(3):466–72.

61. Harada S, Horikawa T, Ashida M, et al. Aspirin enhances the induction of type I allergic symptoms when combined with food and exercise in patients with food-dependent exercise-induced anaphylaxis. Br J Dermatol 2001;145(2):336–9.

62. Baldo BA, Pham NH. Histamine-releasing and allergenic properties of opioid analgesic drugs: resolving the two. Anaesth Intensive Care 2012;40(2):216–35.

63. Casale TB, Bowman S, Kaliner M. Induction of human cutaneous mast cell degranulation by opiates and endogenous opioid peptides: evidence for opiate and nonopiate receptor participation. J Allergy Clin Immunol 1984;73(6):775–81.

64. Metcalfe DD. Mast cells and mastocytosis. Blood 2008;112(4):946–56.

65. Valent P, Horny HP, Escribano L, et al. Diagnostic criteria and classification of mastocytosis: a consensus proposal. Leuk Res 2001;25(7):603–25.

66. Sperr WR, Jordan JH, Fiegl M, et al. Serum tryptase levels in patients with mastocytosis: correlation with mast cell burden and implication for defining the category of disease. Int Arch Allergy Immunol 2002;128(2):136–41.

67. Akin C. Molecular diagnosis of mast cell disorders: a paper from the 2005 William Beaumont Hospital Symposium on Molecular Pathology. J Mol Diagn 2006;8(4):412–9.

68. Campbell RL, Hagan JB, Manivannan V, et al. Evaluation of national institute of allergy and infectious diseases/food allergy and anaphylaxis network criteria for the diagnosis of anaphylaxis in emergency department patients. J Allergy Clin Immunol 2012;129(3):748–52.

69. Lieberman P, Nicklas RA, Oppenheimer J, et al. The diagnosis and management of anaphylaxis practice parameter: 2010 update. J Allergy Clin Immunol 2010;126(3):477–80.e1-42.

70. Simons FE, Ardusso LR, Bilo MB, et al. 2012 Update: World Allergy Organization Guidelines for the assessment and management of anaphylaxis. Curr Opin Allergy Clin Immunol 2012;12(4):389–99.

71. Lin RY, Schwartz LB, Curry A, et al. Histamine and tryptase levels in patients with acute allergic reactions: an emergency department-based study. J Allergy Clin Immunol 2000;106(1 Pt 1):65–71.

72. Boyce JA, Assa'ad A, Burks AW, et al. Guidelines for the diagnosis and management of food allergy in the United States: summary of the NIAID-sponsored expert panel report. J Allergy Clin Immunol 2010;126(6):1105–18.

73. Hill DJ, Hosking CS, Reyes-Benito LV. Reducing the need for food allergen challenges in young children: a comparison of in vitro with in vivo tests. Clin Exp Allergy 2001;31(7):1031–5.

74. Sporik R, Hill DJ, Hosking CS. Specificity of allergen skin testing in predicting positive open food challenges to milk, egg and peanut in children. Clin Exp Allergy 2000;30(11):1540–6.

75. Tole JW, Lieberman P. Biphasic anaphylaxis: review of incidence, clinical predictors, and observation recommendations. Immunol Allergy Clin North Am 2007; 27(2):309–26, viii.

76. Bock SA, Munoz-Furlong A, Sampson HA. Further fatalities caused by anaphylactic reactions to food, 2001–2006. J Allergy Clin Immunol 2007;119(4):1016–8.

77. Pumphrey RS. Lessons for management of anaphylaxis from a study of fatal reactions. Clin Exp Allergy 2000;30(8):1144–50.

78. Kemp SF, Lockey RF, Simons FE, et al. Epinephrine: the drug of choice for anaphylaxis. A statement of the World Allergy Organization. Allergy 2008; 63(8):1061–70.

79. Simons FE, Ardusso LR, Bilo MB, et al. World Allergy Organization anaphylaxis guidelines: summary. J Allergy Clin Immunol 2011;127(3):587–93.e1-22.

80. Simons FE, Gu X, Simons KJ. Epinephrine absorption in adults: intramuscular versus subcutaneous injection. J Allergy Clin Immunol 2001;108(5):871–3.

81. Simons FE, Roberts JR, Gu X, et al. Epinephrine absorption in children with a history of anaphylaxis. J Allergy Clin Immunol 1998;101(1 Pt 1):33–7.

82. Soar J, Pumphrey R, Cant A, et al. Emergency treatment of anaphylactic reactions–guidelines for healthcare providers. Resuscitation 2008;77(2):157–69.

83. Lin RY, Curry A, Pesola GR, et al. Improved outcomes in patients with acute allergic syndromes who are treated with combined H1 and H2 antagonists. Ann Emerg Med 2000;36(5):462–8.

84. Choo KJ, Simons FE, Sheikh A. Glucocorticoids for the treatment of anaphylaxis. Cochrane Database Syst Rev 2012;(4):CD007596.

85. Greenberger PA, Rotskoff BD, Lifschultz B. Fatal anaphylaxis: postmortem findings and associated comorbid diseases. Ann Allergy Asthma Immunol 2007; 98(3):252–7.

86. Joint Task Force on Practice Parameters. The diagnosis and management of urticaria: a practice parameter part I: acute urticaria/angioedema part II: chronic urticaria/angioedema. Joint Task Force on Practice Parameters. Ann Allergy Asthma Immunol 2000;85(6 Pt 2):521–44.

87. Kaplan A. Middleton's allergy: principles and practice. In: Adkinson NF, et al, editors. Urticaria and angioedema, chapter 61, vol. 2, Seventh edition. Philadelphia: Elsevier Inc; 2010. p. 1063–82.

88. Sabroe RA. Acute urticaria. Immunol Allergy Clin North Am 2014;34(1):11–21.

89. Sheldon JM, Mathews KP, Lovell RG. The vexing urticaria problem: present concepts of etiology and management. J Allergy 1954;25(6):525–60.

90. Bernstein JA, Lang DM, Khan DA, Joint Task Force on Practice Parameters, et al. The diagnosis and management of acute and chronic urticaria: 2014 update. J Allergy Clin Immunol 2014;133:1270–7.

91. Huang SW. Acute urticaria in children. Pediatr Neonatol 2009;50(3):85–7.

92. Humphreys F, Hunter JA. The characteristics of urticaria in 390 patients. Br J Dermatol 1998;138(4):635–8.

93. Nettis E, Pannofino A, D'Aprile C, et al. Clinical and aetiological aspects in urticaria and angio-oedema. Br J Dermatol 2003;148(3):501–6.

94. Nizami RM, Baboo MT. Office management of patients with urticaria: an analysis of 215 patients. Ann Allergy 1974;33(2):78–85.

95. Sehgal VN, Rege VL. An interrogative study of 158 urticaria patients. Ann Allergy 1973;31(6):279–83.

96. Gaig P, Olona M, Munoz Lejarazu D, et al. Epidemiology of urticaria in Spain. J Investig Allergol Clin Immunol 2004;14(3):214–20.
97. Greaves MW. Chronic idiopathic urticaria. Curr Opin Allergy Clin Immunol 2003; 3(5):363–8.
98. Juhlin L. Recurrent urticaria: clinical investigation of 330 patients. Br J Dermatol 1981;104(4):369–81.
99. Dice JP. Physical urticaria. Immunol Allergy Clin North Am 2004;24(2):225–46, vi.
100. Poon E, Seed PT, Greaves MW, et al. The extent and nature of disability in different urticarial conditions. Br J Dermatol 1999;140(4):667–71.
101. Kulthanan K, Jiamton S, Thumpimukvatana N, et al. Chronic idiopathic urticaria: prevalence and clinical course. J Dermatol 2007;34(5):294–301.
102. Hennino A, Berard F, Guillot I, et al. Pathophysiology of urticaria. Clin Rev Allergy Immunol 2006;30(1):3–11.
103. Brodell LA, Beck LA, Saini SS. Pathophysiology of chronic urticaria. Ann Allergy Asthma Immunol 2008;100(4):291–7 [quiz: 297–9, 322].
104. Horn MP, Pachlopnik JM, Vogel M, et al. Conditional autoimmunity mediated by human natural anti-Fc(epsilon)RIalpha autoantibodies? FASEB J 2001;15(12): 2268–74.
105. Saini SS. Chronic spontaneous urticaria: etiology and pathogenesis. Immunol Allergy Clin North Am 2014;34(1):33–52.
106. Mortureux P, Leaute-Labreze C, Legrain-Lifermann V, et al. Acute urticaria in infancy and early childhood: a prospective study. Arch Dermatol 1998;134(3): 319–23.
107. Wu CC, Kuo HC, Yu HR, et al. Association of acute urticaria with *Mycoplasma pneumoniae* infection in hospitalized children. Ann Allergy Asthma Immunol 2009;103(2):134–9.
108. Zuberbier T, Asero R, Bindslev-Jensen C, et al. EAACI/GA(2)LEN/EDF/WAO guideline: definition, classification and diagnosis of urticaria. Allergy 2009; 64(10):1417–26.
109. Kobayashi H, Aiba S, Yamagishi T, et al. Cholinergic urticaria, a new pathogenic concept: hypohidrosis due to interference with the delivery of sweat to the skin surface. Dermatology 2002;204(3):173–8.
110. Nakamizo S, Kurosawa M, Sawada Y, et al. A case of cholinergic urticaria associated with acquired generalized hypohidrosis and reduced acetylcholine receptors: cause and effect? Clin Exp Dermatol 2011;36(5):559–60.
111. Shelley WB, Shelley ED, Ho AK. Cholinergic urticaria: acetylcholine-receptor-dependent immediate-type hypersensitivity reaction to copper. Lancet 1983; 1(8329):843–6.
112. Sanchez-Borges M, Capriles-Hulett A, Caballero-Fonseca F. NSAID-induced urticaria and angioedema: a reappraisal of its clinical management. Am J Clin Dermatol 2002;3(9):599–607.
113. Losol P, Yoo HS, Park HS. Molecular genetic mechanisms of chronic urticaria. Allergy Asthma Immunol Res 2014;6(1):13–21.
114. Aoki T, Kojima M, Horiko T. Acute urticaria: history and natural course of 50 cases. J Dermatol 1994;21(2):73–7.
115. Kulthanan K, Chiawsirikajorn Y, Jiamton S. Acute urticaria: etiologies, clinical course and quality of life. Asian Pac J Allergy Immunol 2008;26(1):1–9.
116. Ricci G, Giannetti A, Belotti T, et al. Allergy is not the main trigger of urticaria in children referred to the emergency room. J Eur Acad Dermatol Venereol 2010; 24(11):1347–8.
117. Stibich AS, Schwartz RA. Papular urticaria. Cutis 2001;68(2):89–91.

118. Pite H, Wedi B, Borrego LM, et al. Management of childhood urticaria: current knowledge and practical recommendations. Acta Derm Venereol 2013;93(5): 500–8.

119. Sackesen C, Sekerel BE, Orhan F, et al. The etiology of different forms of urticaria in childhood. Pediatr Dermatol 2004;21(2):102–8.

120. Cowdrey SC, Reynolds JS. Acute urticaria in infectious mononucleosis. Ann Allergy 1969;27(4):182–7.

121. Koehn GG, Thorne EG. Urticaria and viral hepatitis. Arch Dermatol 1972; 106(3):422.

122. Di Campli C, Gasbarrini A, Nucera E, et al. Beneficial effects of Helicobacter pylori eradication on idiopathic chronic urticaria. Dig Dis Sci 1998;43(6):1226–9.

123. Jirapongsananuruk O, Pongpreuksa S, Sangacharoenkit P, et al. Identification of the etiologies of chronic urticaria in children: a prospective study of 94 patients. Pediatr Allergy Immunol 2010;21(3):508–14.

124. Wedi B, Raap U, Wieczorek D, et al. Urticaria and infections. Allergy Asthma Clin Immunol 2009;5(1):10.

125. Shakouri A, Compalati E, Lang DM, et al. Effectiveness of Helicobacter pylori eradication in chronic urticaria: evidence-based analysis using the grading of recommendations assessment, development, and evaluation system. Curr Opin Allergy Clin Immunol 2010;10(4):362–9.

126. Abajian M, Schoepke N, Altrichter S, et al. Physical urticarias and cholinergic urticaria. Immunol Allergy Clin North Am 2014;34(1):73–88.

127. Peroni A, Colato C, Schena D, et al. Urticarial lesions: if not urticaria, what else? The differential diagnosis of urticaria: part I. Cutaneous diseases. J Am Acad Dermatol 2010;62(4):541–55 [quiz: 555–6].

128. Magerl M, Borzova E, Gimenez-Arnau A, et al. The definition and diagnostic testing of physical and cholinergic urticarias–EAACI/GA2LEN/EDF/UNEV consensus panel recommendations. Allergy 2009;64(12):1715–21.

129. Lin YR, Liu TH, Wu TK, et al. Predictive factors of the duration of a first-attack acute urticaria in children. Am J Emerg Med 2011;29(8):883–9.

130. Sanchez-Borges M, Asero R, Ansotegui IJ, et al. Diagnosis and treatment of urticaria and angioedema: a worldwide perspective. World Allergy Organ J 2012; 5(11):125–47.

131. McDonald K, Trick L, Boyle J. Sedation and antihistamines: an update. Review of inter-drug differences using proportional impairment ratios. Hum Psychopharmacol 2008;23(7):555–70.

132. O'Donnell BF, Lawlor F, Simpson J, et al. The impact of chronic urticaria on the quality of life. Br J Dermatol 1997;136(2):197–201.

133. Staevska M, Popov TA, Kralimarkova T, et al. The effectiveness of levocetirizine and desloratadine in up to 4 times conventional doses in difficult-to-treat urticaria. J Allergy Clin Immunol 2010;125(3):676–82.

134. Asero R, Tedeschi A, Cugno M. Treatment of chronic urticaria. Immunol Allergy Clin North Am 2014;34(1):105–16.

135. Burland WL, Duncan WA, Hesselbo T, et al. Pharmacological evaluation of cimetidine, a new histamine H2-receptor antagonist, in healthy man. Br J Clin Pharmacol 1975;2(6):481–6.

136. Monroe EW, Cohen SH, Kalbfleisch J, et al. Combined H1 and H2 antihistamine therapy in chronic urticaria. Arch Dermatol 1981;117(7):404–7.

137. Paul E, Bodeker RH. Treatment of chronic urticaria with terfenadine and ranitidine. A randomized double-blind study in 45 patients. Eur J Clin Pharmacol 1986;31(3):277–80.

138. Asero R, Tedeschi A, Cugno M. Treatment of refractory chronic urticaria: current and future therapeutic options. Am J Clin Dermatol 2013;14(6):481–8.
139. Di Lorenzo G, Pacor ML, Mansueto P, et al. Randomized placebo-controlled trial comparing desloratadine and montelukast in monotherapy and desloratadine plus montelukast in combined therapy for chronic idiopathic urticaria. J Allergy Clin Immunol 2004;114(3):619–25.
140. Nettis E, Colanardi MC, Soccio AL, et al. Desloratadine in combination with montelukast suppresses the dermographometer challenge test papule, and is effective in the treatment of delayed pressure urticaria: a randomized, double-blind, placebo-controlled study. Br J Dermatol 2006;155(6):1279–82.
141. Bagenstose SE, Levin L, Bernstein JA. The addition of zafirlukast to cetirizine improves the treatment of chronic urticaria in patients with positive autologous serum skin test results. J Allergy Clin Immunol 2004;113(1):134–40.
142. Pacor ML, Di Lorenzo G, Corrocher R. Efficacy of leukotriene receptor antagonist in chronic urticaria. A double-blind, placebo-controlled comparison of treatment with montelukast and cetirizine in patients with chronic urticaria with intolerance to food additive and/or acetylsalicylic acid. Clin Exp Allergy 2001; 31(10):1607–14.
143. Cassano N, D'Argento V, Filotico R, et al. Low-dose dapsone in chronic idiopathic urticaria: preliminary results of an open study. Acta Derm Venereol 2005;85(3):254–5.
144. Engin B, Ozdemir M. Prospective randomized non-blinded clinical trial on the use of dapsone plus antihistamine vs. antihistamine in patients with chronic idiopathic urticaria. J Eur Acad Dermatol Venereol 2008;22(4):481–6.
145. Hartmann K, Hani N, Hinrichs R, et al. Successful sulfasalazine treatment of severe chronic idiopathic urticaria associated with pressure urticaria. Acta Derm Venereol 2001;81(1):71.
146. McGirt LY, Vasagar K, Gober LM, et al. Successful treatment of recalcitrant chronic idiopathic urticaria with sulfasalazine. Arch Dermatol 2006;142(10): 1337–42.
147. Reeves GE, Boyle MJ, Bonfield J, et al. Impact of hydroxychloroquine therapy on chronic urticaria: chronic autoimmune urticaria study and evaluation. Intern Med J 2004;34(4):182–6.
148. Orden RA, Timble H, Saini SS. Efficacy and safety of sulfasalazine in patients with chronic idiopathic urticaria. Ann Allergy Asthma Immunol 2014;112(1): 64–70.
149. Maurer M, Rosen K, Hsieh HJ, et al. Omalizumab for the treatment of chronic idiopathic or spontaneous urticaria. N Engl J Med 2013;368(10):924–35.
150. Baskan EB, Tunali S, Turker T, et al. Comparison of short- and long-term cyclosporine A therapy in chronic idiopathic urticaria. J Dermatolog Treat 2004;15(3): 164–8.
151. Khan DA. Alternative agents in refractory chronic urticaria: evidence and considerations on their selection and use. J Allergy Clin Immunol Pract 2013; 1(5):433–40.e1.
152. Saini S, Rosen KE, Hsieh HJ, et al. A randomized, placebo-controlled, dose-ranging study of single-dose omalizumab in patients with H1-antihistamine-refractory chronic idiopathic urticaria. J Allergy Clin Immunol 2011;128(3): 567–73.e1.

Drug and Vaccine Allergy

John M. Kelso, MD

KEYWORDS

- Allergy • Beta-lactam • Penicillin • Egg allergy • Influenza vaccination

KEY POINTS

- Children labeled as allergic to penicillin should undergo penicillin skin testing and oral challenge to identify the vast majority who are not currently penicillin-allergic.
- Children with a distant history of a mild reaction to penicillin can safely be administered oral cephalosporins.
- Reactions to carbapenems among children with penicillin allergy are rare, and such medications can be administered cautiously under observation.
- Leaving egg-allergic patients unvaccinated against influenza leaves them at risk for morbidity and mortality from influenza.
- Studies involving thousands of egg-allergic subjects, including hundreds with histories of severe reactions to the ingestion of eggs, have shown a low rate of minor reactions that is not different from nonegg-allergic controls.
- Current guidelines from the American Academy of Pediatrics (AAP) and Centers for Disease Control and Prevention (CDC) recommend that egg-allergic patients receive annual influenza vaccine and be observed for 30 minutes afterward; however, given the safety data, even this precaution may be unnecessary.

INTRODUCTION

It is important to identify children who are allergic to drugs and vaccines, because administration of these substances to such children can lead to serious, even life-threatening systemic allergic reactions (anaphylaxis). Recent updates of practice parameters on adverse reactions to drugs[1] and vaccines[2] provide excellent resources on these topics.

However, it is also important not to overdiagnose such allergy (ie, label children as allergic when they are not), because this deprives them of the most appropriate treatment. This article specifically reviews allergic reactions to beta-lactam antibiotics and the administration of influenza vaccine to egg-allergic recipients. These are areas where recent evidence has allowed the administration of these treatments to children from whom they had previously been withheld.

Division of Allergy, Asthma, and Immunology, Scripps Clinic, 3811 Valley Centre Drive, San Diego, CA 92130, USA
E-mail address: kelso.john@scrippshealth.org

Immunol Allergy Clin N Am 35 (2015) 221–230
http://dx.doi.org/10.1016/j.iac.2014.09.013   immunology.theclinics.com

BETA-LACTAM ANTIBIOTICS

Penicillin and it is derivatives are regarded as the most common cause of drug allergy,[1] due to propensity to cause such reactions, but also because of frequent use. However, the incidence of penicillin allergy appears to be falling over time, perhaps related to the less frequent use of penicillin by the potentially more sensitizing parenteral route in the outpatient setting.[3,4] Approximately 6% of children are reported to be allergic to penicillin.[5] However, only approximately 4% to 9% of such children have positive immediate type (immunoglobulin E [IgE]) skin tests to penicillin reagents.[6-9] The remainder were either never allergic to penicillin or the allergy was lost with the passage of time.[10] Those who were never allergic may have been mislabeled, because they suffered a nonimmunologic side effect from the medication such as emesis, or because they suffered an adverse event that was coincidental to, but not caused by the penicillin administration. Thus, most children labeled as penicillin-allergic are not, and are inappropriately denied treatment with this class of antibiotics. The use of alternative antibiotics may be associated with suboptimal treatment and higher costs and may promote antibiotic resistance.[11] Thus, a strong argument can be made for testing such patients in advance of need in order to identify the vast majority who are not currently allergic to penicillin.[1,10]

It had previously been advocated that penicillin skin testing be performed in patients with suspected penicillin allergy only at the time of infection and only when there were no acceptable alternatives.[12] The rationale for this recommendation was based in part on a concern that skin testing and challenge with penicillin could resensitize previously allergic children who had lost sensitivity over time, placing them at risk for allergic reactions when administered penicillin in the future. However, such resensitization is rare with orally administered penicillins,[6,9] although it may be somewhat higher after parenterally administered penicillin.[13]

Penicillin is a small molecule and must act as a hapten with a protein carrier to have a large enough size and high enough valency to elicit an IgE-mediated response. Penicillin is metabolized to so-called major and minor determinants. The majority of the drug is metabolized to the penicilloyl (major) determinant, while the remainder is metabolized to penilloate and penicilloate (minor) determinants. Unmetabolized benzylpenicillin, known as penicillin G, is also typically regarded as a minor determinant. Penicillin G has always been available as a skin test reagent simply as a dilution of the drug used for treatment. The penicilloyl (major) determinant is available commercially as benzylpenicilloyl polylysine, where multiple penicilloyl determinants (haptens) are linked to an amino acid polymer (carrier). Penilloate and penicilloate (minor) determinants have never been available commercially in the United States, although many allergists with access to laboratory facilities have generated these reagents from penicillin G through acid and alkaline hydrolysis, respectively.[14] The rationale for including penilloate and penicilloate minor determinants for skin testing patients with suspected penicillin allergy is that some patients with such histories will have positive skin test results only to these reagents.[6,15] Some centers perform penicillin skin testing with the readily available benzylpenicilloyl polylysine and penicillin G, and if negative perform an oral amoxicillin challenge under observation to identify those patients who are clinically allergic to penicillin despite negative skin test with these 2 reagents, some of whom would presumably have had positive skin tests to penilloate, penicilloate, or amoxicillin.[16] However, when 496 patients with suspected penicillin allergy but negative benzylpenicilloyl polylysine and penicillin G skin tests underwent amoxicillin challenge, only 4 (0.8%) were positive, all developing only hives within 1 hour. The authors calculated that 3375 patients would have to be tested with a panel also including penilloate, penicilloate, and amoxicillin to avoid 1 additional positive oral challenge with amoxicillin.[16] Thus, until such time as a minor determinant mixture is commercially available, skin testing with benzylpenicilloyl polylysine and penicillin G, and if negative, observed oral amoxicillin challenge, is a reasonable approach to the evaluation of penicillin allergy.

A common clinical scenario is for a child to develop up a rash, often urticarial, several days into a course of penicillin. Thus, the nature of this adverse event (urticaria) is consistent with an IgE-mediated mechanism, but the timing (delayed) is not, given that the typical IgE-mediated reaction should occur within minutes to hours of the first dose in a previously sensitized child. Children also often develop maculopapular rashes in this setting, which can be difficult to distinguish from urticarial reactions without a careful history and physical examination. Nonetheless, given the potential danger of a more serious reaction with subsequent exposure if the child does have an IgE-mediated penicillin allergy, such children are typically labeled as penicillin-allergic and do not receive the drug again in the future. A study published in 2011 examined the likelihood of penicillin allergy in this clinical situation.[17] Eighty-eight children who had developed urticarial (53%) or maculopapular (47%) rashes an average of 4.9 days into the course of treatment with a beta-lactam antibiotic underwent intradermal penicillin skin tests and an oral challenge test (OCT) with the culprit antibiotic testing 2 months later. The skin test results were positive in 11 of the 88 patients (12.5%), yet 7 of these patients did not develop a rash on OCT. Six of the 88 patients (6.8%) developed a rash on OCT, 4 urticarial and 2 maculopapular. Three of the 4 patients who developed urticarial reactions on OCT had positive skin tests, as did 1 of the 2 patients who developed a maculopapular rash. Thus, most children who develop a delayed-onset rash during the course of treatment with a beta-lactam antibiotic are not allergic to the antibiotic and will not develop a rash on subsequent exposure. Penicillin skin testing and oral challenge performed 1 or 2 months after the event will confirm the absence of allergy in most children so that they need not be inappropriately labeled as penicillin-allergic.

Penicillins and cephalosporins are both beta-lactam class antibiotics, and thus there is at least the theoretic potential that a child who is allergic to penicillin would also react to cephalosporins due to immunologic cross-reactivity (ie, that IgE antibodies directed against a particular penicillin epitope would also bind a similar cephalosporin epitope). However, most penicillin-allergic children tolerate cephalosporins.[18] The potential for cross-reactivity appears largely related to the similarity of side chains on various penicillins and cephalosporins.[18] There are several other factors that may increase the risk of a reaction to a cephalosporin in a penicillin-allergic child. The severity of a past anaphylactic reaction may predict the severity of a future reaction; penicillin allergy tends to wane over time, and anaphylactic reactions are more common with parenteral (as opposed to oral) administration. Thus, in a child with a recent history of a severe reaction to penicillin, caution is warranted with the administration of a parenteral cephalosporin, particularly one with a side chain similar to the penicillin that caused the initial reaction. On the other hand, a child with a distant history of a mild reaction to penicillin will almost certainly tolerate administration of an oral cephalosporin, particularly one with a side chain dissimilar to the penicillin that caused the initial reaction.

Carbapenems and monobactams are beta-lactam antibiotic classes with chemical structures that are dissimilar to other beta-lactam antibiotics, and the rate of cross-reactivity between these antibiotics and penicillin is low. One-hundred-eight children with histories of immediate-type allergic reactions to penicillin and positive penicillin skin tests were skin tested with the carbapenem meropenem.[19] Only 1 child had a positive meropenem skin test and was not challenged; however the remaining 107 children had negative meropenem skin tests and tolerated a meropenem challenge. Similarly, 124 children with histories of immediate-type allergic reactions to penicillin and positive penicillin skin tests were skin tested with the carbapenem imipenem.[20] Only 1 child had a positive imipenem skin test and was not challenged. Interestingly, this was the same child who had a positive skin test to meropenem in a study described previously. However, the remaining 123 children had negative imipenem skin tests and tolerated an imipenem challenge. Thus, in a child with a history of penicillin allergy who is to receive a carbapenem, skin testing with penicillin reagents and the carbapenem proposed for administration may be considered; however, given the low rate of cross-reactivity, cautious administration of the carbapenem under observation may be an acceptable alternative. Patients who are allergic to penicillin have not shown skin test reactivity or clinical reactions to the monobactam aztreonam.[21]

ADMINISTRATION OF INFLUENZA VACCINE TO EGG-ALLERGIC CHILDREN

Most influenza vaccines are literally grown in chicken eggs.[22,23] Although the virus is subsequently purified, some residual egg protein remains in the final product. For decades, it had been assumed that administration of influenza vaccines containing this residual egg protein to egg-allergic recipients would result in systemic allergic reactions. For this reason, egg allergy had been considered a contraindication to the receipt of influenza vaccine. This approach may be regarded as conservative or prudent, because it avoids this risk of an allergic reaction. However, it neglects the risk of remaining unimmunized. Each year in the United States, over 20,000 children are hospitalized with influenza, and over 100 children die from the disease.[24,25] Thus, not vaccinating egg-allergic children with influenza vaccine avoids the theoretic risk of an allergic reaction, but leaves the children at risk of hospitalization or death from influenza.

Many studies have been conducted to assess the risk of administration of egg-based influenza vaccines to egg allergic recipients.[26–53] Most such recipients are children, as egg allergy is quite common among children, but almost always outgrown. The inclusion criteria for these studies have included both a recent history of reaction to the ingestion of egg, where the nature and timing of this reaction are consistent with an IgE-mediated event, as well as demonstration of IgE antibody either by immediate-type allergy skin testing or serum-specific IgE antibody to egg. Some studies excluded patients with histories of anaphylactic as opposed to less severe allergic reactions to egg; however, most studies specifically included those with anaphylactic egg allergy. Many studies included skin testing with the influenza vaccine as part of the study protocol. Although some studies withheld the vaccine from egg-allergic patients with positive vaccine skin tests, in the majority of studies, the vaccine was administered even to those with positive vaccine skin tests. Some studies took the precautionary step of administering 10% of the vaccine dose followed by a 30-minute observation, after which, if no reaction occurred, the remaining 90% of the vaccine dose was given. Other studies administered the vaccine as a single (100%) age-appropriate dose in the usual manner. Some studies have also included control groups of nonegg-allergic children who were also carefully observed for adverse reactions after immunization.

Collectively, these studies evaluated 4315 patients with egg allergy, including 656 with severe reactions to the ingestion of egg. Including booster doses, 4872 doses of influenza vaccine were administered to these patients. No anaphylactic reactions were reported. Occasional patients developed hives or mild wheezing; however, the rate of these reactions was similar in control patients without egg allergy. These rare reactions were no more common in patients who were skin test positive to the vaccine than in those who were skin test negative. The vaccine was tolerated equally well whether given in divided doses or as a single dose.

The actual amount of egg protein in the various influenza vaccines has also been measured by the manufacturers and in independent laboratories. Although other egg proteins may be present in the vaccine, the particular egg protein measured in the vaccines is ovalbumin, with the concentration typically expressed as micrograms of ovalbumin per milliliter or per 0.5 mL vaccine dose. According to the manufacturers, all currently available influenza vaccines contain less than 1 μg of ovalbumin per 0.5 mL dose.[23] Analysis in independent laboratories has often revealed levels of ovalbumin much lower than the amounts claimed by the manufacturers.[54–56]

It is likely that the reason that egg-allergic patients can receive the egg-containing influenza vaccine without reaction is that the amount of egg protein present in the vaccine is simply not high enough to induce a reaction. Although there are no dose–response studies on the injection of egg protein as occurs with vaccination, attempts have been made to establish the lowest dose of egg protein that could elicit a reaction in egg-allergic patients by ingestion.[57,58] The lowest amount of egg protein ever reported to provoke an allergic reaction is 130 μg.[57] A calculated dose of egg protein that "would be predicted to elicit no reaction in 99% of the allergic population [and]…would likely provoke mostly mild allergic reactions in the remainder of the patients" is 30 μg.[58] Thus, although not subject to digestion, the at most 1 μg of egg protein present in the influenza vaccine is likely below the threshold required to elicit an allergic reaction.

These considerations have led to major changes in official guidance regarding the administration of influenza vaccines to egg allergic recipients. Beginning in 2011, both the CDC's Advisory Committee On Immunization Practices (ACIP)[59] and the AAP's Committee on Infectious Diseases[60] began recommending that egg-allergic patients should receive annual influenza vaccines, with the latter stating "Although both trivalent influenza vaccine (TIV) (now called IIV, inactivated influenza vaccine) and LAIV (live attenuated influenza vaccine) are produced in eggs, recent data have shown that influenza vaccine administered in a single, age-appropriate dose is well tolerated by nearly all recipients who have egg allergy. More conservative approaches, such as skin testing or a 2-step graded challenge, are no longer recommended." In subsequent influenza seasons, since this change in recommendation, there has been no disproportionate reporting of allergic reactions after influenza vaccine.[23]

Recently 2 new influenza vaccines have been introduced that are not grown in eggs. One is made from virus grown in cell culture,[61] and the other consists of recombinant hemagglutinin proteins produced in an insect cell line.[62] There is no mention of egg allergy in the package inserts for either of these 2 vaccines. The cell culture-based vaccine is approved for patients 18 years of age and older. The recombinant vaccine is approved for patients 18 to 49 years of age. Thus, these vaccines are acceptable alternatives for egg-allergic adults; however, this constitutes a tiny fraction of the population of egg-allergic patients, most of whom are children. It may be tempting to use one of these to vaccines off label (ie, outside the approved age range) for children with egg allergy; however, this is not appropriate. The safety and effectiveness of these vaccines have not been demonstrated in younger patients, and antibody responses to the recombinant vaccine in children ages 6 months to 3 years were less than those generated to a standard influenza vaccine. Further, the safety of egg-based vaccines has been demonstrated in egg-allergic children.

Recommendations from the CDC and AAP for the 2013 to 2014 influenza season[22,23] are summarized in **Fig. 1**. This algorithm points out that patients who can consume egg directly without reaction are not egg-allergic and require no special precautions for influenza vaccination. Most patients who have had allergic reactions to the ingestion of egg have had hives as their only symptom. Such patients can receive influenza vaccine in a primary care setting with a 30-minute observation period afterward. It is recommended that patients who have had more severe reactions to the ingestion of egg, or who are sensitized but who have never knowingly ingested egg and thus whose reaction severity cannot be known, be referred to an allergist. The 2012 update of the adverse reactions to vaccines practice parameter for allergists recommends that influenza vaccine be administered (as a single, age-appropriate dose without prior vaccine skin testing) to patients with egg allergy of any severity (including anaphylaxis) with a 30-minute observation period afterward.[2] However, given the

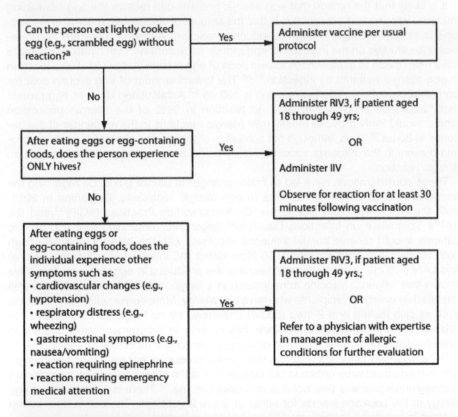

Abbreviations: IIV = inactivated influenza vaccine; RIV3 = recombinant influenza vaccine, trivalent
[a] Persons with egg allergy might tolerate egg in baked products (e.g. bread or cake). Tolerance to egg-containing foods does not exclude the possibility of egg allergy. For persons who have no known history of exposure to egg but who are suspected of being egg-allergic on the basis of previously performed allergy testing, consultation with a physician with expertise in the management of allergic conditions should be obtained prior to vaccination. Alternatively, RIV3 may be administered if the recipient is aged 18 through 49 years.

Fig. 1. Recommendations regarding influenza vaccination of persons who report allergy to eggs. IIV, inactivated influenza vaccine; RIV3, recombinant influenza vaccine, trivalent. (*From* Advisory Committee on Immunization Practices, United States, 2013–2014 influenza season.)

overwhelming safety data on the administration of egg-based influenza vaccines to egg-allergic recipients, a statement endorsed by the Joint Task Force on Practice Parameters has recommended that all patients with egg allergy receive annual influenza vaccination without any special precautions.[63] Although all studies published to date have examined the safety of inactivated influenza vaccines (IIV) in egg-allergic recipients, the LAIV for intranasal administration contains less than 0.24 μg of ovalbumin per 0.2 mL dose[23] and would also not be expected to cause reactions in egg-allergic subjects.

FUTURE CONSIDERATIONS/SUMMARY

Given the general principle that patients who are allergic to a particular allergen should avoid exposure to the allergen, it seemed reasonable for children with a prior history of reactions to penicillin not to receive subsequent courses of beta-lactam antibiotics and for egg-allergic children not to receive influenza vaccines containing egg protein. However, this conservative approach is not without risks of its own. Denying patients treatment with beta-lactam antibiotics when they are able to tolerate them leads to their treatment with antibiotics that may be less effective and more expensive and have greater side effects. Denying egg-allergic patients influenza vaccines when they are able to tolerate them leaves them at risk of the morbidity and mortality associated with the disease itself. Thus, children with a history of penicillin allergy should undergo penicillin skin testing and oral challenge to identify those who never were or are no longer allergic, allowing them to be treated with beta-lactam antibiotics, and children with egg allergy of any severity should receive annual influenza vaccination. In the future, efforts could be directed toward applying the same approach to other drugs and vaccines. For example, sulfa allergy is also commonly reported. If reliable skin test reagents could be developed for sulfonamide antibiotics, testing and challenge might reveal that most of these patients are also not allergic to this antibiotic. Similarly, for patients reporting egg allergy, yellow fever vaccine skin testing and graded dose and are currently recommended; however, carefully conducted studies such as those performed with influenza vaccine might determine that these precautions are unnecessary. Allergists routinely provide an important service in determining what patients are allergic to and need to avoid, but can also provide an equally important service in determining what patients are not allergic to and need not avoid.

REFERENCES

1. Joint Task Force on Practice Parameters, American Academy of Allergy, Asthma and Immunology, American College of Allergy, Asthma and Immunology, Joint Council of Allergy, Asthma and Immunology.. Drug allergy: an updated practice parameter. Ann Allergy Asthma Immunol 2010;105:259–73.
2. Kelso JM, Greenhawt MJ, Li JT, et al. Adverse reactions to vaccines practice parameter 2012 update. J Allergy Clin Immunol 2012;130:25–43.
3. Jost BC, Wedner HJ, Bloomberg GR. Elective penicillin skin testing in a pediatric outpatient setting. Ann Allergy Asthma Immunol 2006;97:807–12.
4. Macy E, Schatz M, Lin C, et al. The falling rate of positive penicillin skin tests from 1995 to 2007. Perm J 2009;13:12–8.
5. Kraemer MJ, Caprye-Boos H, Berman HS. Increased use of medical services and antibiotics by children who claim a prior penicillin sensitivity. West J Med 1987;146:697–700.

6. Mendelson LM, Ressler C, Rosen JP, et al. Routine elective penicillin allergy skin testing in children and adolescents: study of sensitization. J Allergy Clin Immunol 1984;73:76–81.
7. Langley JM, Halperin SA, Bortolussi R. History of penicillin allergy and referral for skin testing: evaluation of a pediatric penicillin allergy testing program. Clin Invest Med 2002;25:181–4.
8. Macy E, Poon KY. Self-reported antibiotic allergy incidence and prevalence: age and sex effects. Am J Med 2009;122(778):e1–7.
9. Hershkovich J, Broides A, Kirjner L, et al. Beta lactam allergy and resensitization in children with suspected beta lactam allergy. Clin Exp Allergy 2009;39:726–30.
10. Solensky R. The time for penicillin skin testing is here. J Allergy Clin Immunol Pract 2013;1:264–5.
11. Macy E, Contreras R. Health care use and serious infection prevalence associated with penicillin "allergy" in hospitalized patients: a cohort study. J Allergy Clin Immunol 2014;133:790–6.
12. Disease management of drug hypersensitivity: a practice parameter. Ann Allergy Asthma Immunol 1999;83:665–700.
13. Parker PJ, Parrinello JT, Condemi JJ, et al. Penicillin resensitization among hospitalized patients. J Allergy Clin Immunol 1991;88:213–7.
14. Macy E, Richter PK, Falkoff R, et al. Skin testing with penicilloate and penilloate prepared by an improved method: amoxicillin oral challenge in patients with negative skin test responses to penicillin reagents. J Allergy Clin Immunol 1997;100:586–91.
15. Pichichero ME, Pichichero DM. Diagnosis of penicillin, amoxicillin, and cephalosporin allergy: reliability of examination assessed by skin testing and oral challenge. J Pediatr 1998;132:137–43.
16. Macy E, Ngor EW. Safely diagnosing clinically significant penicillin allergy using only penicilloyl-poly-lysine, penicillin, and oral amoxicillin. J Allergy Clin Immunol Pract 2013;1:258–63.
17. Caubet JC, Kaiser L, Lemaitre B, et al. The role of penicillin in benign skin rashes in childhood: a prospective study based on drug rechallenge. J Allergy Clin Immunol 2011;127:218–22.
18. Pichichero ME. A review of evidence supporting the American Academy of Pediatrics recommendation for prescribing cephalosporin antibiotics for penicillin-allergic patients. Pediatrics 2005;115:1048–57.
19. Atanaskovic-Markovic M, Gaeta F, Medjo B, et al. Tolerability of meropenem in children with IgE-mediated hypersensitivity to penicillins. Allergy 2008;63:237–40.
20. Atanaskovic-Markovic M, Gaeta F, Gavrovic-Jankulovic M, et al. Tolerability of imipenem in children with IgE-mediated hypersensitivity to penicillins. J Allergy Clin Immunol 2009;124:167–9.
21. Patriarca G, Schiavino D, Lombardo C, et al. Tolerability of aztreonam in patients with IgE-mediated hypersensitivity to beta-lactams. Int J Immunopathol Pharmacol 2008;21:375–9.
22. Committee on Infectious Diseases. Recommendations for prevention and control of influenza in children, 2013-2014. Pediatrics 2013;132:e1089–104.
23. Centers for Disease Control and Prevention (CDC). Prevention and control of seasonal influenza with vaccines. Recommendations of the Advisory Committee on Immunization Practices–United States, 2013-2014. MMWR Morb Mortal Wkly Rep 2013;62:1–43.
24. Thompson WW, Shay DK, Weintraub E, et al. Influenza-associated hospitalizations in the United States. JAMA 2004;292:1333–40.

25. Centers for Disease Control and Prevention (CDC). Estimates of deaths associated with seasonal influenza—United States, 1976-2007. MMWR Morb Mortal Wkly Rep 2010;59:1057–62.
26. Bierman CW, Shapiro GG, Pierson WE, et al. Safety of influenza vaccination in allergic children. J Infect Dis 1977;136:S652–5.
27. James JM, Zeiger RS, Lester MR, et al. Safe administration of influenza vaccine to patients with egg allergy. J Pediatr 1998;133:624–8.
28. Zeiger RS. Current issues with influenza vaccination in egg allergy. J Allergy Clin Immunol 2002;110:834–40.
29. Dorsey MJ, Song L, Geha T, et al. Influenza vaccine in 55 patients with egg allergy. J Allergy Clin Immunol 2005;115:S250.
30. Hotte SL, Lejtenyi C, Primeau M. A 6-year experience with influenza vaccination in egg allergic patients. J Allergy Clin Immunol 2008;121:S239.
31. Esposito S, Gasparini C, Martelli A, et al. Safe administration of an inactivated virosomal adjuvanted influenza vaccine in asthmatic children with egg allergy. Vaccine 2008;26:4664–8.
32. Park AY, Pien GC, Stinson R, et al. Administration of influenza vaccine to patients with egg allergy. J Allergy Clin Immunol 2008;121:S240.
33. Saltzman RW, Park AY, Pien GC, et al. Administration of influenza vaccine to pediatric patients with egg allergy. J Allergy Clin Immunol 2009;123:S175.
34. Thanik ES, Cox AL, Sampson HA. Administration of a low egg-containing influenza vaccine [Fluarix®] in an egg-allergic pediatric population. J Allergy Clin Immunol 2010;125:AB25.
35. Chung EY, Huang L, Schneider L. Safety of influenza vaccine administration in egg-allergic patients. Pediatrics 2010;125:e1024–30.
36. Gagnon R, Primeau MN, Des Roches A, et al. Safe vaccination of patients with egg allergy with an adjuvanted pandemic H1N1 vaccine. J Allergy Clin Immunol 2010;126:317–23.
37. Greenhawt MJ, Chernin AS, Howe L, et al. The safety of the H1N1 influenza A vaccine in egg allergic individuals. Ann Allergy Asthma Immunol 2010;105:387–93.
38. Leo S, Dean J, Chan E. Safety of H1N1 and seasonal influenza vaccines in egg allergic patients in British Columbia. Allergy Asthma Clin Immunol 2010;6:P4.
39. Pien GC, LeBenger KS, Carotenuto DR, et al. Coordination of multidisciplinary resources for vaccination of egg-allergic individuals during an H1N1 (novel) influenza pandemic. Allergy Asthma Proc 2010;31:507–10.
40. Siret-Alatrista A, Bouali F, Demoly M, et al. The 2009-2010 H1N1 vaccination campaign for patients with egg allergy in a region of France. Allergy 2011;66:298–9.
41. Boden SR, LaBelle VS, Sedlak DA, et al. Safe administration of flu vaccine in egg allergic patients. J Allergy Clin Immunol 2011;127:AB114.
42. Paschall VL, Siles RI, Bhatti H, et al. Do egg-specific IgE levels predict reactions to seasonal influenza or H1N1 vaccination? J Allergy Clin Immunol 2011;127:AB182.
43. Owens G, Macginnitie A. Higher-ovalbumin-content influenza vaccines are well tolerated in children with egg allergy. J Allergy Clin Immunol 2011;127:264–5.
44. Howe LE, Conlon AS, Greenhawt MJ, et al. Safe administration of seasonal influenza vaccine to children with egg allergy of all severities. Ann Allergy Asthma Immunol 2011;106:446–7.
45. Webb L, Petersen M, Boden S, et al. Single-dose influenza vaccination of patients with egg allergy in a multicenter study. J Allergy Clin Immunol 2011;128:218–9.

46. Pitt T, Kalicinsky C, Warrington R, et al. Assessment of epicutaneous testing of a monovalent influenza A (H1N1) 2009 vaccine in egg allergic patients. Allergy Asthma Clin Immunol 2011;7:3.
47. Schuler JE, King WJ, Dayneka NL, et al. Administration of the adjuvanted pH1N1 vaccine in egg-allergic children at high risk for influenza A/H1N1 disease. Can J Public Health 2011;102:196–9.
48. Forsdahl BA. Reactions of Norwegian children with severe egg allergy to an egg-containing influenza A (H1N1) vaccine: a retrospective audit. BMJ Open 2012;2: e000186.
49. Fung I, Spergel JM. Administration of influenza vaccine to pediatric patients with egg-induced anaphylaxis. J Allergy Clin Immunol 2012;129:1157–9.
50. Khan FS, Virant FS, Furukawa CT, et al. Influenza vaccine administration in egg allergic children. J Allergy Clin Immunol 2012;129:AB70.
51. Upton J, Hummel D, Kasprzak A, et al. No systemic reactions to influenza vaccination in egg-sensitized tertiary-care pediatric patients. Allergy Asthma Clin Immunol 2012;8:2.
52. Des Roches A, Paradis L, Gagnon R, et al. Egg-allergic patients can be safely vaccinated against influenza. J Allergy Clin Immunol 2012;130:1213–6.e1.
53. Greenhawt MJ, Spergel JM, Rank MA, et al. Safe administration of the seasonal trivalent influenza vaccine to children with severe egg allergy. Ann Allergy Asthma Immunol 2012;109:426–30.
54. McKinney KK, Webb L, Petersen M, et al. Ovalbumin content of 2010-2011 influenza vaccines. J Allergy Clin Immunol 2011;127:1629–32.
55. Waibel KH, Gomez R. Ovalbumin content in 2009 to 2010 seasonal and H1N1 monovalent influenza vaccines. J Allergy Clin Immunol 2010;125:749–51, 751.e1.
56. Li JT, Rank MA, Squillace DL, et al. Ovalbumin content of influenza vaccines. J Allergy Clin Immunol 2010;125:1412–3.
57. Taylor SL, Hefle SL, Bindslev-Jensen C, et al. Factors affecting the determination of threshold doses for allergenic foods: how much is too much? J Allergy Clin Immunol 2002;109:24–30.
58. Allen KJ, Remington BC, Baumert JL, et al. Allergen reference doses for precautionary labeling (VITAL 2.0): clinical implications. J Allergy Clin Immunol 2014; 133:156–64.
59. Centers for Disease Control and Prevention (CDC). Prevention and control of influenza with vaccines: recommendations of the advisory committee on immunization practices (ACIP), 2011. MMWR Morb Mortal Wkly Rep 2011;60:1128–32.
60. American Academy of Pediatrics Committee on Infectious Diseases. Recommendations for prevention and control of influenza in children, 2011-2012. Pediatrics 2011;128:813–25.
61. FLUCELVAX (Novartis, Cambridge MA) [Package Insert]. 2013.
62. FLUBLOK (Protein Sciences, Meriden CT) [Package Insert]. 2013.
63. Kelso JM, Greenhawt MJ, Li JT. Update on influenza vaccination of egg allergic patients. Ann Allergy Asthma Immunol 2013;111:301–2.

Moving?

Make sure your subscription moves with you!

To notify us of your new address, find your **Clinics Account Number** (located on your mailing label above your name), and contact customer service at:

Email: journalscustomerservice-usa@elsevier.com

800-654-2452 (subscribers in the U.S. & Canada)
314-447-8871 (subscribers outside of the U.S. & Canada)

Fax number: 314-447-8029

Elsevier Health Sciences Division
Subscription Customer Service
3251 Riverport Lane
Maryland Heights, MO 63043

*To ensure uninterrupted delivery of your subscription, please notify us at least 4 weeks in advance of move.

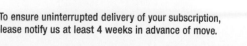

Printed and bound by CPI Group (UK) Ltd, Croydon, CR0 4YY

03/10/2024

01040490-0004